THAI STEP-BY-STEP MASSAGE

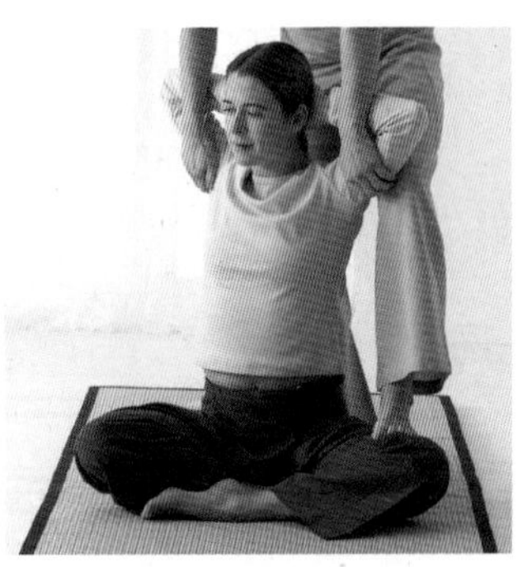

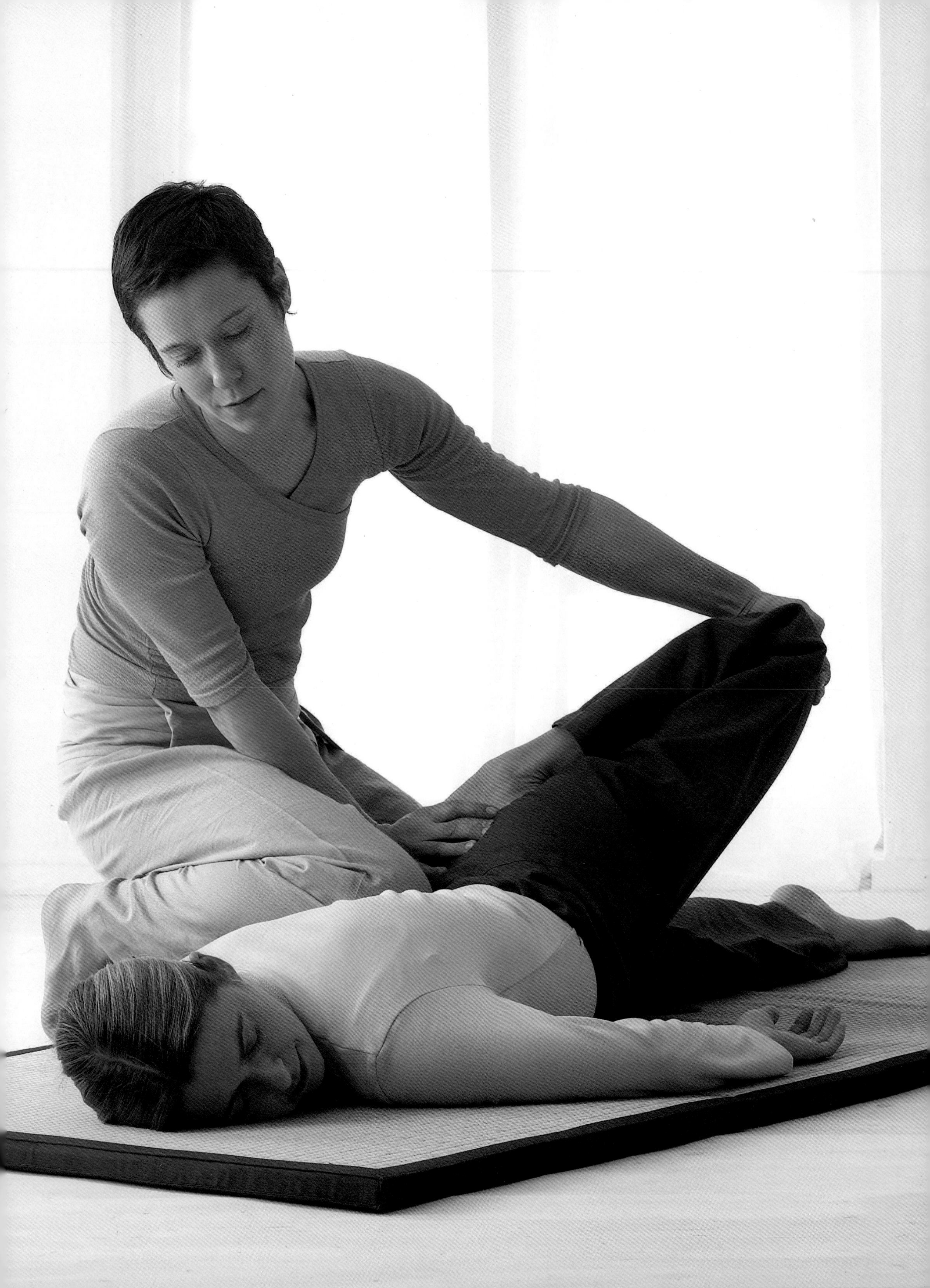

THAI STEP-BY-STEP MASSAGE

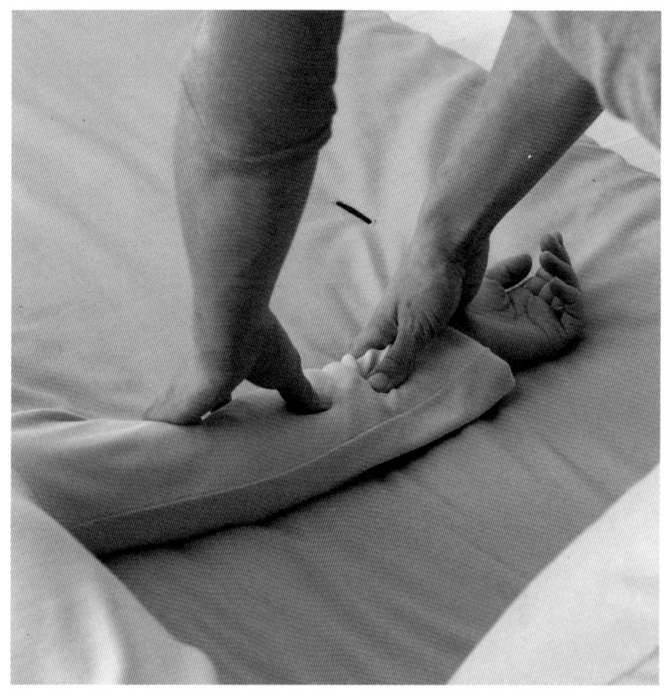

The perfect introduction to using massage, yoga and acupressure to balance the body's natural energies, with easy-to-follow techniques shown in 400 photographs

NICKY SMITH

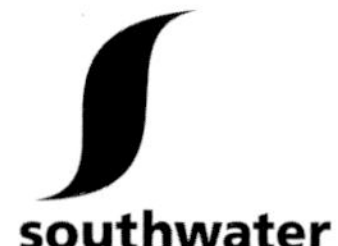

southwater

This edition is published by Southwater,
an imprint of Anness Publishing Ltd

info@anness.com
www.southwaterbooks.com
www.annesspublishing.com

A CIP catalogue record for this book is available from the British Library.

Publisher Joanna Lorenz
Editorial Director Helen Sudell
Project Editor Ann Kay
Copy Editor Beverley Jollands
Editorial Reader Penelope Goodare
Designer Lisa Tai
Photography Paul Bricknell
Illustrator Sam Elmhurst
Production Controller Ben Worley

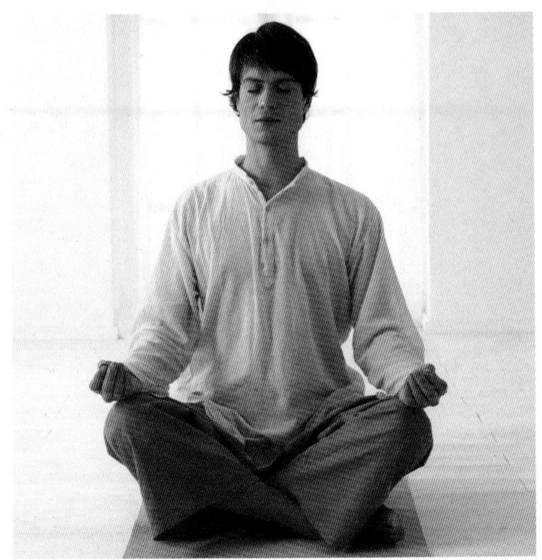

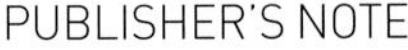

PUBLISHER'S NOTE

The author and publishers have made every effort to ensure that all instructions contained within this book are accurate and safe, and cannot accept liability for any resulting injury, damage or loss to persons or property, however it may arise. If you do have any special needs or problems, consult your doctor or a physiotherapist. This book cannot replace medical consultation and should be used in conjunction with professional advice. You should not attempt Thai massage without training from a properly qualified practitioner.

Contents

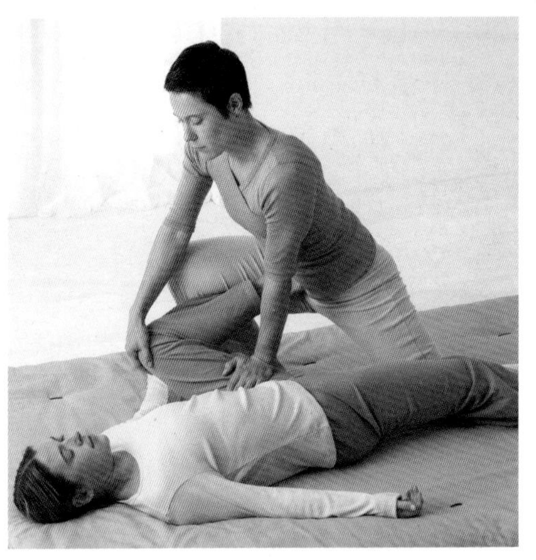

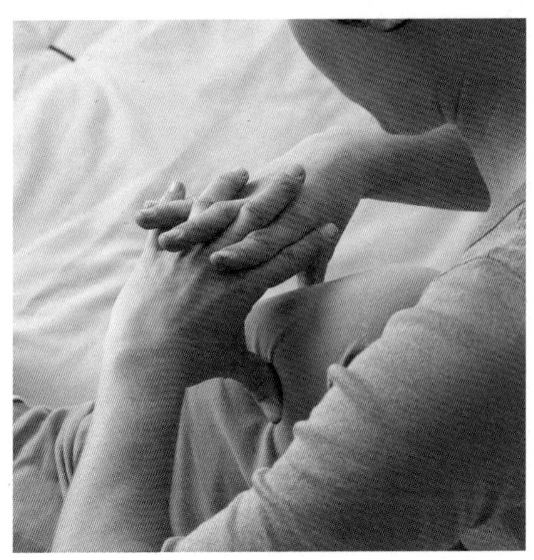

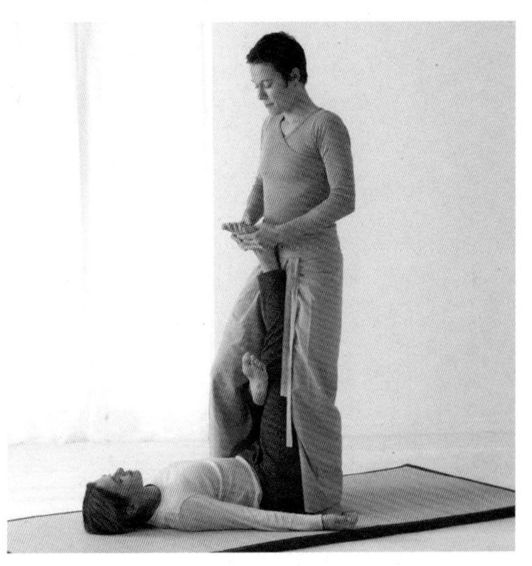

Foreword

Nicky Smith has put her heart into creating an authentic and thorough introduction to this fascinating form of energy balancing, which was barely known outside Thailand just a few short years ago. As well as producing a book that is both authoritative and accessible, she has also stayed true to the spirit of tradition, and offers us a refreshingly unique and personal perspective that makes this so much more than simply an instructional manual.

Nicky Smith has been studying with me for several years, with great enthusiasm. She is now one of my senior authorized teachers and she has a profound understanding of the healing power of her work, an understanding that she shares here with the readers of this book. I am sure that the approach she has taken will prove to be a real inspiration for anyone wanting to learn more about a tradition that has only become popular worldwide very recently.

Traditional Thai massage, or Thai yoga massage as it is often called, is a unique and powerful massage therapy. It combines acupressure, energy balancing, stretching and applied yoga exercises. As well as improving flexibility, relaxation and energy levels, a Thai massage can relieve headaches, asthma, constipation and frozen shoulder, improve flexibility for those who enjoy sports, help recovery after a heart attack or stroke, and provide exercise for the disabled – to mention only a few possibilities.

Thai massage therapists are in demand for working with everyone from performance athletes to stressed office workers and anyone seeking to find greater calm and

Asokananda

Asokananda is our principal teacher and we are deeply inspired and grateful for his work. Originally from Germany, he founded The Sunshine Network, a sangha of connected friends from around the world who teach and practise Thai Massage. He dedicated his life to spreading the gift of Thai massage to the rest of the world and was the first person to write about Thai massage in English in "The Art of Traditional Thai Massage" in 1990. He primarily taught from his School in a Lahu hill tribe village near Chiang Mai in Northern Thailand. He was our teacher and our friend and with each massage we give and every student we teach, we remain thankful for his teaching and the legacy he left.

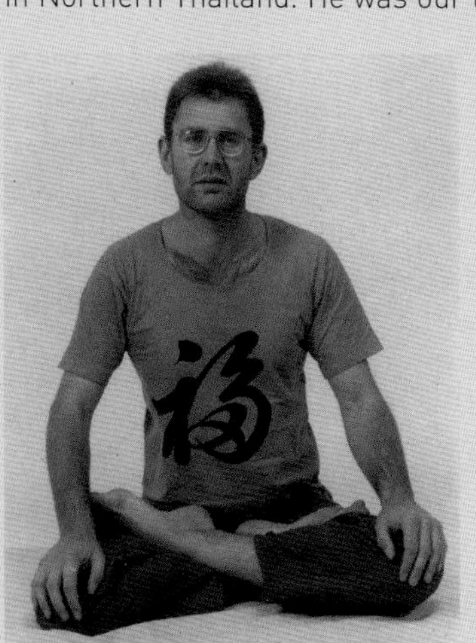

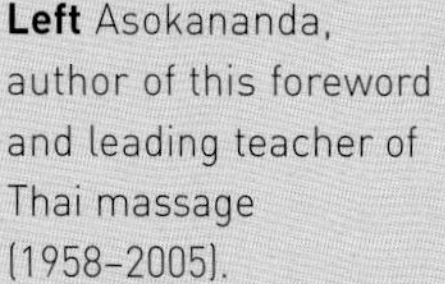

Left Asokananda, author of this foreword and leading teacher of Thai massage (1958–2005).

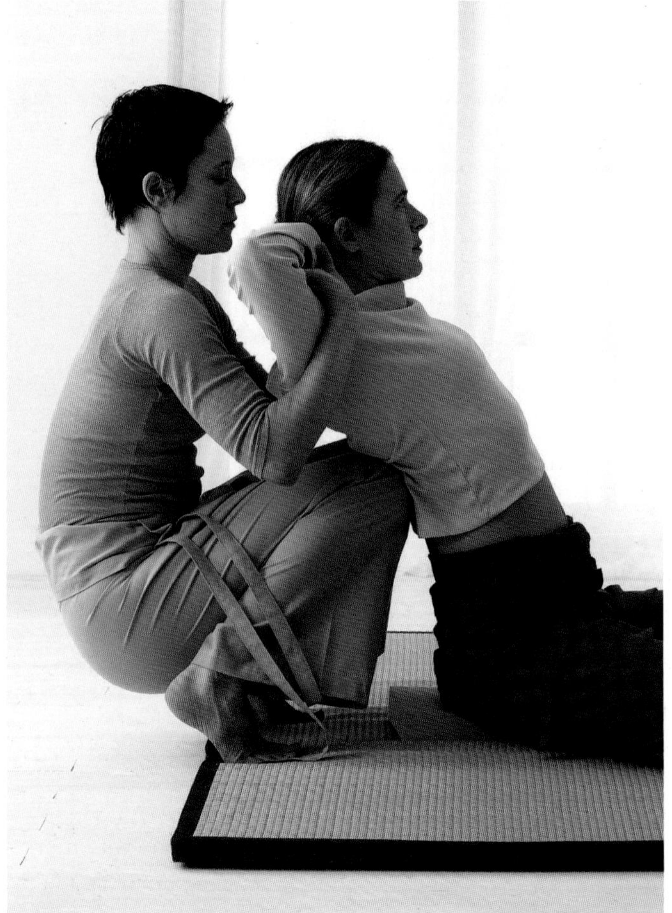

Below Givers of Thai massage need to learn to work with both sensitivity and grace, to enable their partners to open up their bodies freely and completely.

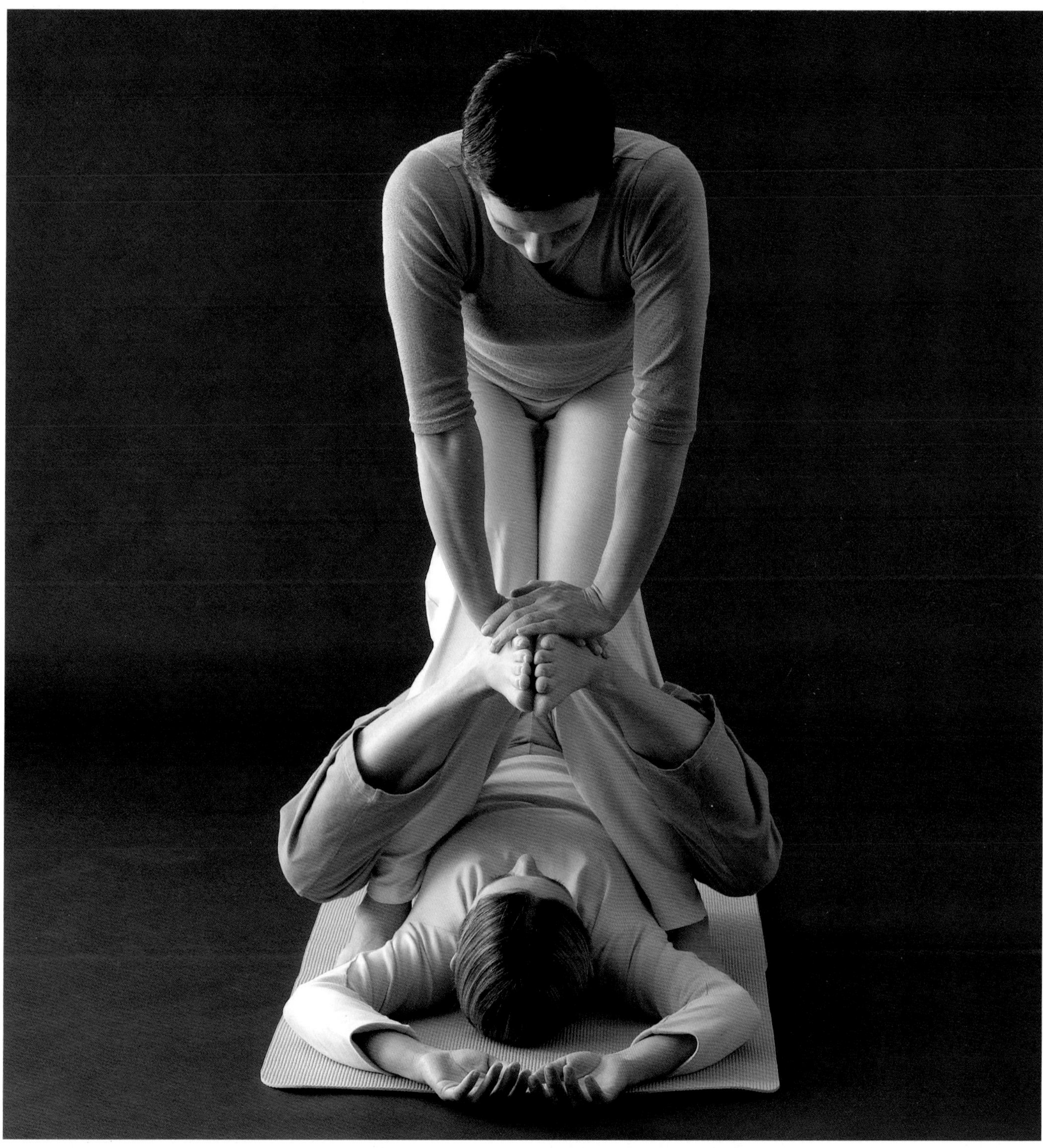

Above It is extremely important that the giver and receiver of a Thai massage treatment maintain good communication throughout, especially during the deeper stretches.

improve their energy levels. In offering relief for such a wide range of current health issues, this art is as useful and valid for our age as it has been for thousands of years. I am convinced that the current increase in popularity of Thai yoga massage will continue in the years to come with more and more people experiencing the balancing benefits of a whole body Thai massage.

THE PERFECT GROUNDING

With growing popularity will come an increasing need for quality training, and Nicky's book is the perfect guide. It offers a detailed outline of everything you need to get started and to find your way into the heart and spirit of the art. She follows the traditional structure, doesn't alter principles in order to "Westernize", and finds a language that is easy for anyone to follow. The instructions are both thorough and clear. Thai massage has found a dedicated advocate in Nicky Smith and her book is a testimony to her love for this fascinating branch of Ayurvedic bodywork.

Introduction

Traditional Thai massage, also known today in the West as Thai yoga massage, is a powerful form of energy rebalancing and physical massage. A fusion of Buddhist spiritual practice and Indian Ayurvedic bodywork, it combines hatha yoga techniques and the spiritual commitment of working with "loving kindness". This approach of working intuitively and without judgement supports our body's natural inclination to heal itself.

Thai massage has been practised widely across what is now known as Thailand for several hundred years, exchanged among family members as a healing art. Only relatively recently has it become known in the West, where people are now discovering its ability to rebalance body and mind on many different levels, harmonizing the physical, the energetic and the emotional bodies to give the recipient a truly holistic treatment.

This book is intended as an introduction to the joy and art of traditional Thai massage. It gives practical guidance on everything from preparing to give a massage with yoga and meditation, through a step-by-step breakdown of specific techniques for a full-body massage, to taking care of yourself and your partner after a massage. It has been written as a guide to help get you started, but the essence, the quality and the art of the massage will come from you, from your dedication to practise with an open heart and with sensitivity towards your partner. Once you have become familiar with the physical exercises in each sequence you can begin to shift your focus, massaging less from your head and more from your heart, surrendering yourself, more and more, to simply being present in the moment.

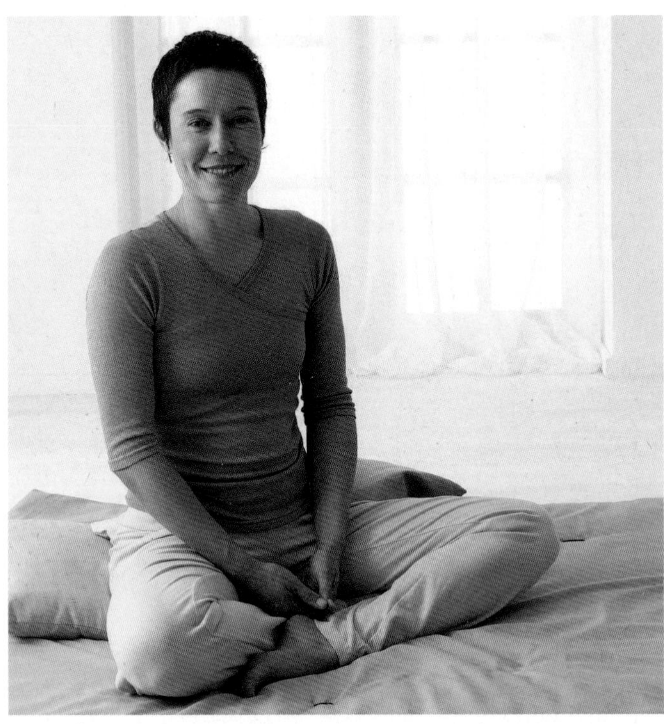

Above Thai massage has been a gift in my life and writing this book has given me the opportunity to pass on this gift to others.

DISCOVERING THAI MASSAGE

My introduction to Thai massage came many years ago, when I received a treatment from a friend. I was highly impressed by the completeness of the massage, and it touched me in a way that I had not previously experienced with other forms of bodywork.

My first opportunity to find out more about this fascinating form of massage came totally out of the blue, with a last-minute trip to Thailand. I went to study with Asokananda, a German man who was living in a small tribal community in the north of Thailand and teaching northern-style Thai massage. I had repeatedly come across Asokananda in several other contexts in my life, and was intrigued by these recurring personal connections and by my new discovery of the delights of Thai massage. So, when the opportunity to learn more presented itself, I took it without hesitation.

I already had an interest in bodywork through physical theatre, performance art and Western massage. But learning Thai massage started me on a deeper journey with myself, introducing me to meditation and a committed yoga practice, and setting me on a path of self-enquiry. My initial two-week trip extended into many months of study, exploring the world of Thai massage. Over the years I served a kind of apprenticeship, living in a Lahu hill tribe village and in Chiang Mai for several months at a time.

I feel personally that Thai massage connects me with my body. Its physical and dynamic nature opens my eyes to hidden parts of myself. Through both the giving and receiving I learn more about my own and other people's bodies. Its underlying spiritual principle of working with loving kindness also affords me the opportunity to accept myself more fully and with greater compassion. The hands on approach of Thai Massage allows the work to be absorbed bodily rather than mentally, encouraging a sense of feeling and 'listening' through the hands and it offers a wonderful breadth of techniques to suit all body types and abilities.

I feel blessed to have been able to incorporate the richness of Thai massage practice into my life, integrating its elements not only into my massage practice as a therapist and teacher but also into many aspects of my everyday life.

HOW TO USE THIS BOOK

The first chapter, *What is Thai Massage?*, provides useful background and history, while the following chapter, *Preparing Body and Mind*, leads you through a variety of mental and physical practices that will lay the foundations for giving a good Thai massage. The third chapter, *A Complete Body Routine*, makes up a large section of this book. It takes you step by step through how to give a full-body massage, illustrating a balance of Thai massage techniques for you to practise and share with your friends or family. The routine is broken down into sequences for each part of the body, showing how to open up your partner's (the recipient's) body gradually, resulting in a well-balanced treatment. It is worth mentioning here that the techniques and the sequence shown in this chapter represent only one way of working within this incredibly broad and varied tradition. The next chapter, *After a Massage*, gives useful and effective grounding and relaxation techniques – what you do afterwards is just as vital as good preparation if you are going to look after yourself properly.

The book is not intended as a substitute for hands-on teaching. If you are serious about wanting to learn, I hope it will inspire you to explore further under the guidance of an experienced teacher. If you are already a student of Thai massage, I hope it provides a stimulating addition to your practice. There are many excellent teachers worldwide and it is not necessary to go to Thailand to learn traditional Thai massage. What is important is that your teacher's approach should resonate with you. Try out different teachers by attending workshops and receiving massage.

Below The teacher-student relationship is a crucial one. Take your time trying out different teachers, and trust that your intuition will lead you to the right teacher when you are ready.

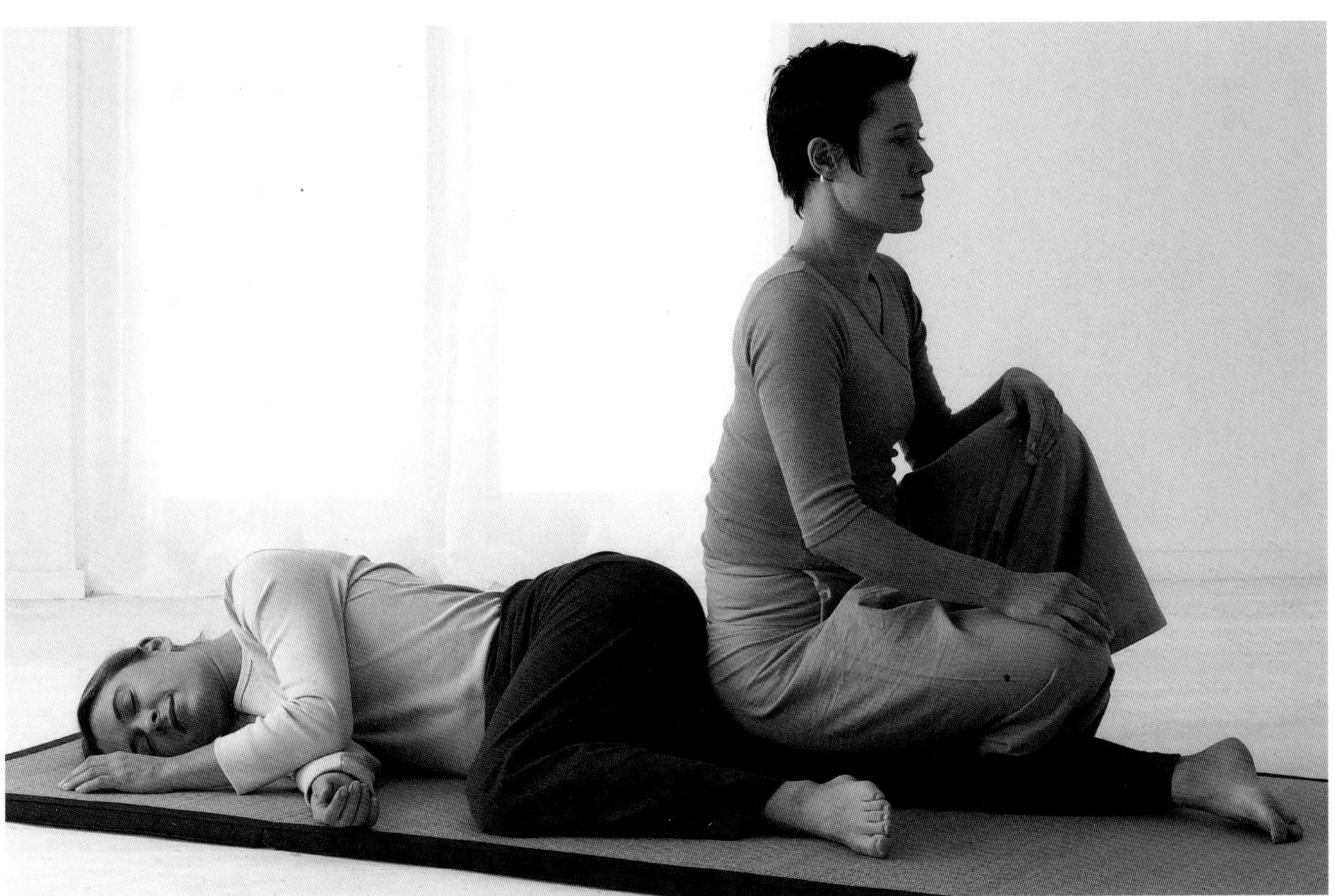

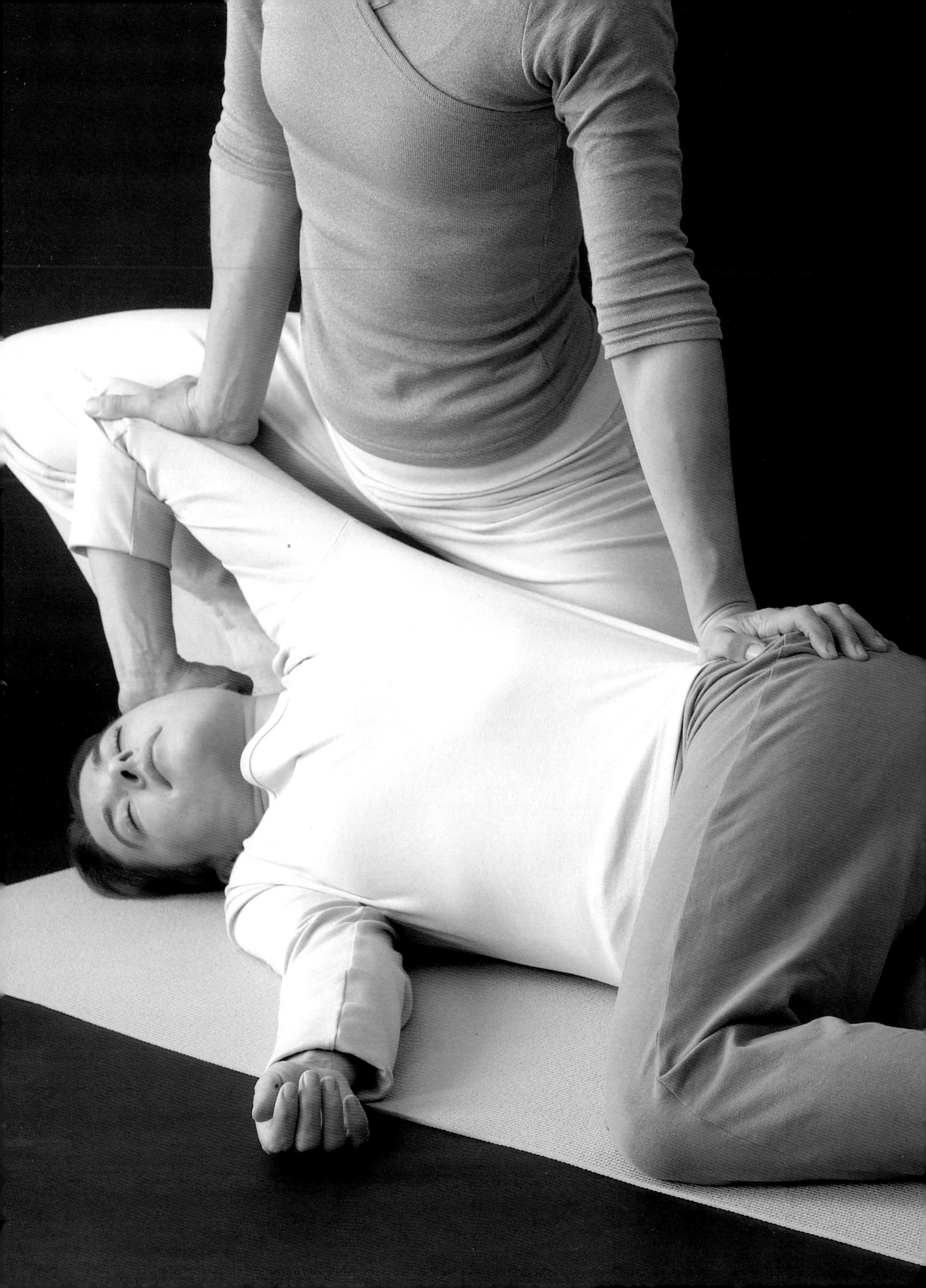

What is Thai Massage?

Traditional Thai Massage, Thai Yoga Massage or Thai Massage are all different labels to describe a highly physical, hands-on branch of traditional Thai medicine. Other branches include the use of herbs or steam baths.

Learning a little about the history behind this form of bodywork, and about some of the underlying theories and practices, will start the process of understanding this extraordinarily simple, yet profoundly effective, healing art form.

The History of Thai Massage

Traditional Thai massage has its roots in India, in the Indian yoga tradition and in Buddhism. The practices that grew into Thai massage travelled to what we now call Thailand from India over 2,000 years ago. They were brought by Indian Buddhist monks and Ayurvedic practitioners who had been invited to northern Thailand by the Mon rulers of that region. Thai massage has been a part of traditional Thai medicine ever since.

In massage schools and practices right across modern-day Thailand, it is a man called Jivaka Kumar Bhaccha who is revered and honoured as the father of traditional Thai medicine. His name appears in ancient Buddhist scriptures as he was a physician to the Buddha himself, and to the spiritual community, around 2,500 years ago. Consequently, Jivaka Kumar Bhaccha became closely associated with what is now known as traditional Thai massage. In Thailand today, practitioners still offer up a prayer to him in thanks before they give each massage.

Detailed knowledge about the ways in which the practice of Thai massage developed over the centuries is limited, as most of the historical texts dealing with its theoretical background were destroyed by a Burmese invasion of the old capital, Ayuthia, in 1767. However, some remnants of these texts did survive – and they form the basis for carvings that can be seen today on the walls of the Phra Chetuphon Temple (known as Wat Pho) in Bangkok.

PAST AND PRESENT PRACTICES

In most parts of Thailand, the practice and developing knowledge of Thai medicine and Thai massage was and still is passed directly from teacher to student, leading to a

Below These Buddha statues, from around the 1200s, are found at the ancient city of Satchanalai, in northern Thailand.

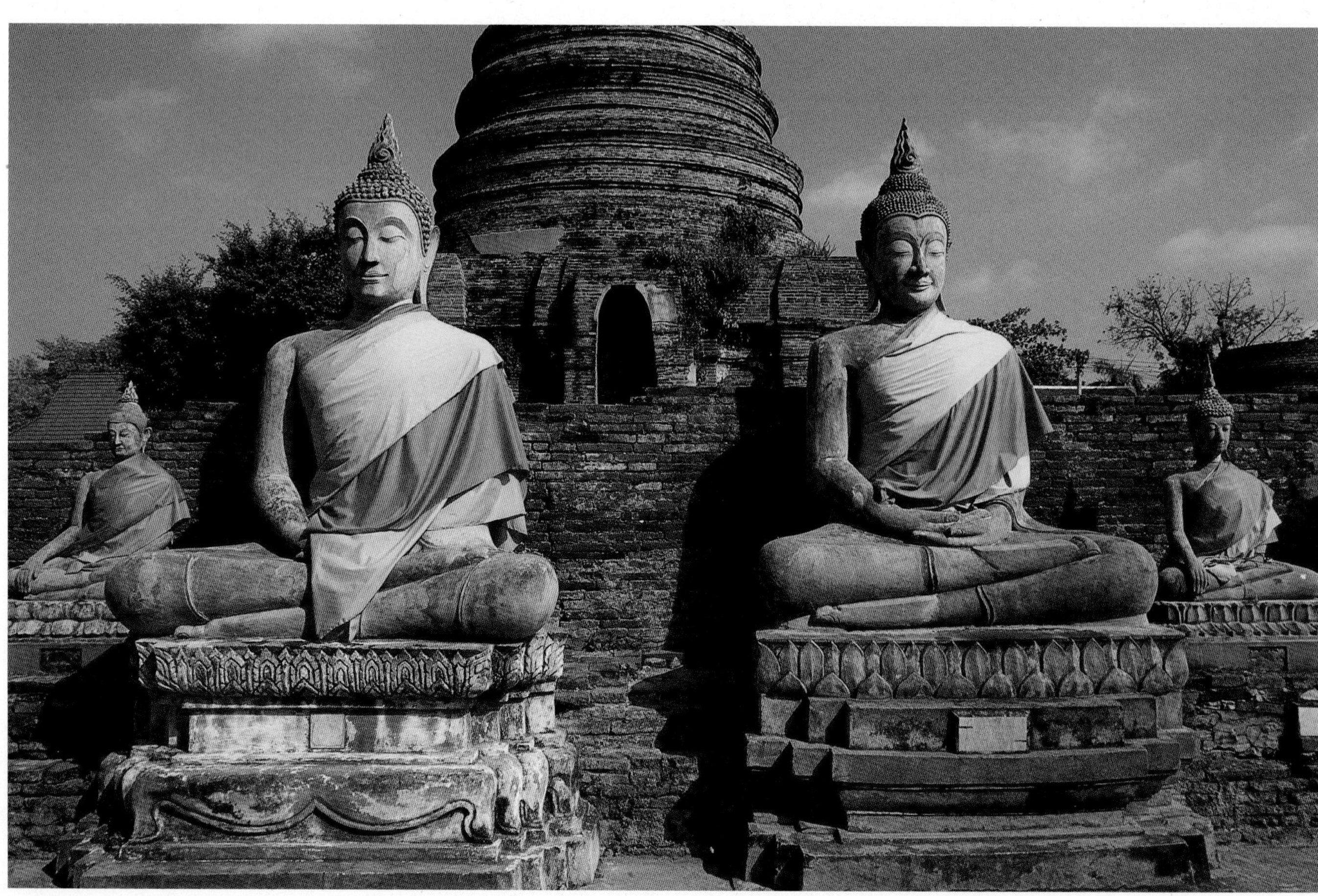

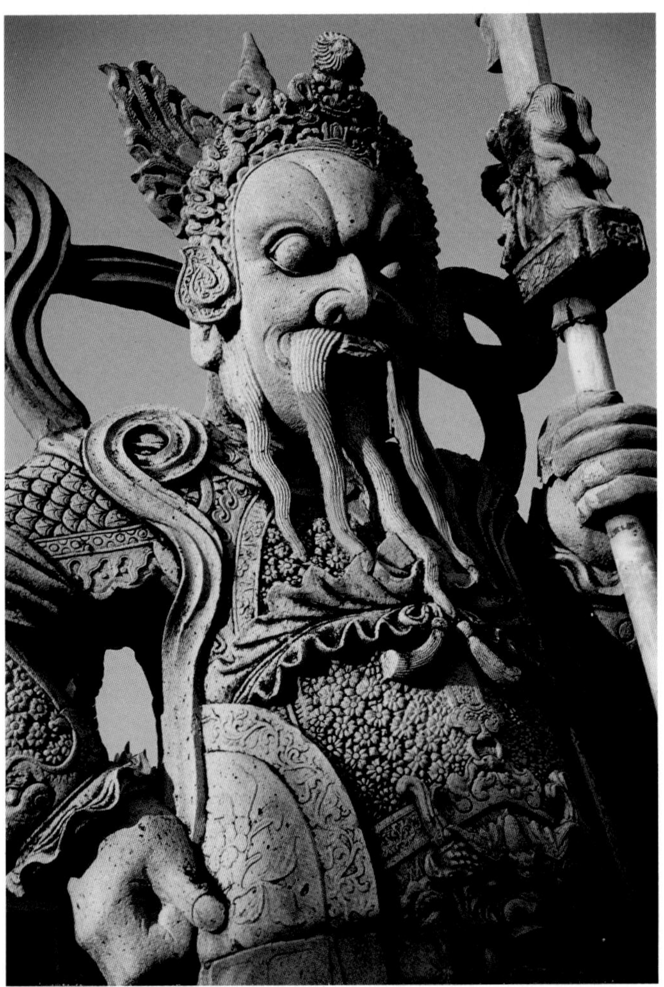

Northern-style Thai massage

There are two quite distinct styles of traditional massage that are practised in Thailand today: northern style and southern style. Both approaches adhere to similar principles, but their emphasis is slightly different. The methods described throughout this book broadly follow the tradition of northern-style Thai massage. This developed among the farming communities that lived in the hills of northern Thailand, and so the massage methods physically reflect their way of life by placing a particular emphasis on leg work and on dynamic stretches.

Left This sixteenth-century stone figure is a guardian statue at the temple of Wat Pho in Bangkok. Inside this temple lie carvings that tell us something of the early history of this healing art.

Below Today, traditional Thai massage is offered all over the country. Receiving this kind of massage in Thailand is a profoundly invigorating experience. The practitioners' relaxed manner and matter-of-fact approach to bodywork comes across very strongly.

wonderfully broad and eclectic approach to this ancient art. Traditionally, Thai massage was practised within temple compounds – not by monks, but by ordinary people who happily offered their healing arts to the community.

In modern-day Thailand, temples continue to function as the centre of the community, as a place where people come together and enjoy all kinds of social gatherings. Among Thai people, massage is still seen as a form of hands-on healing and therapeutic touch that is an everyday part of a normal and healthy life.

HEALTHY RESURGENCE

For many years, as Thailand began to open up to increased tourism, the only understanding that many Westerners had of "Thai massage" was in the context of the tourism and sex industries. However, over the last 15–20 years this rather sordid image has been shed and traditional Thai massage has enjoyed a serious resurgence within the country's mainstream culture. This revival was helped by Westerners, who were intrigued by Thai massage's unique combination of spiritual practice and physical therapy. As is the case with therapies in any country, there are still poorly trained masseurs who aim their services at the tourist trade, but if you avoid these you can now enjoy an excellent standard of traditional massage throughout Thailand.

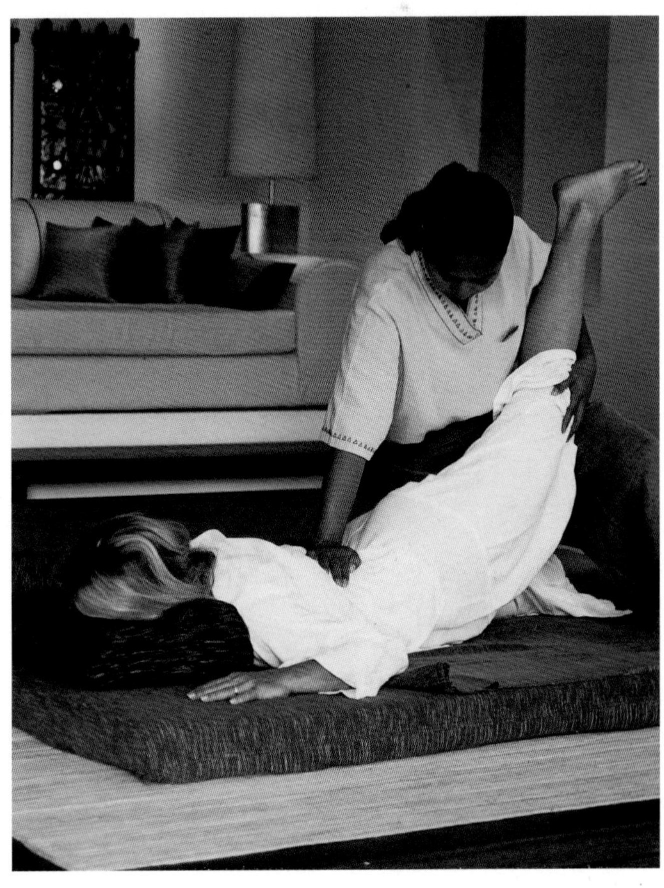

The Practice of Thai Massage

According to the Eastern philosophy underlying Thai massage, the body is made up of an interconnecting web of energy lines through which *prana*, or life energy, flows. This is the force that supports and maintains all the vital functions of the body. It permeates all life and sustains all living things. It is in the air that we breathe and the food that we eat. When this energy flows freely we enjoy good mental, physical and spiritual health.

If the energy lines become blocked and the flow of prana is interrupted, it causes disruption and imbalance throughout the system. So in Thai massage, practitioners stimulate the energy lines by using pressure and passive stretches to maintain a free flow of energy through the whole body.

THE ENERGY SYSTEM

Like yoga, Thai massage is based on the concept of a human being consisting of more than just their physical body. According to the Indian yoga tradition, we are made up of five different bodies, or *koshas*. These are the physical body (*anamaya kosha*), the prana or energy body (*pranamaya kosha*), the memory body (*manamaya kosha*), the subconscious body (*vijnanamaya kosha*) and the all-encompassing cosmic body (*anandamaya kosha*), within which all the koshas are interconnected. This concept can be useful to embrace as a metaphor with which to appreciate the many layers of physical, mental and emotional experience within us.

It is the pranamaya kosha, the energy body, that we work with primarily in Thai massage and yoga. In the pranamaya kosha, yoga philosophy perceives many thousands of *nadis*, or energy lines. Thai massage has selected ten of these lines, called *sen*, which are all worked on during a treatment to rebalance the energy flow within the whole body.

THE NADIS AND CHAKRAS OF YOGA

Thai massage has strong links with yoga, not least in the yogic energy lines called nadis and the yogic energy centres known as chakras.

The links between the sen and the nadis are evident in the names of the three main nadis: *sushumna nadi* in yoga corresponds directly with *sen sumana*, and *ida nadi* and *pingala nadi* with *sen ittha* and *pingkhala*. Sushumna nadi runs through the spine; the other two run from each nostril down either side of the spine.

Chakras are energy centres located along the spine and up to the brow. Eastern treatments such as yoga and Thai massage aim to activate these, or their equivalents, in various ways.

Pingala nadi stands for the sun's awakening power

Sushumna nadi is the most important of the nadis

Ida nadi stands for the relaxing energy of the moon

The crown chakra (*sahasrara*) is related to spiritual understanding

The brow chakra (*ajna*), also known as the third eye, is related to intuition

The throat chakra (*vishuddha*) is related to communication

The heart chakra (*anahata*) is the centre of compassion and all-embracing love

The solar plexus chakra (*manipura*) is the energetic centre for all bodily activities

The sacral chakra (*swadisthana*) is the centre of unconsciousness and of sexual desire

The base chakra (*muladhara*) relates to our fundamental survival needs

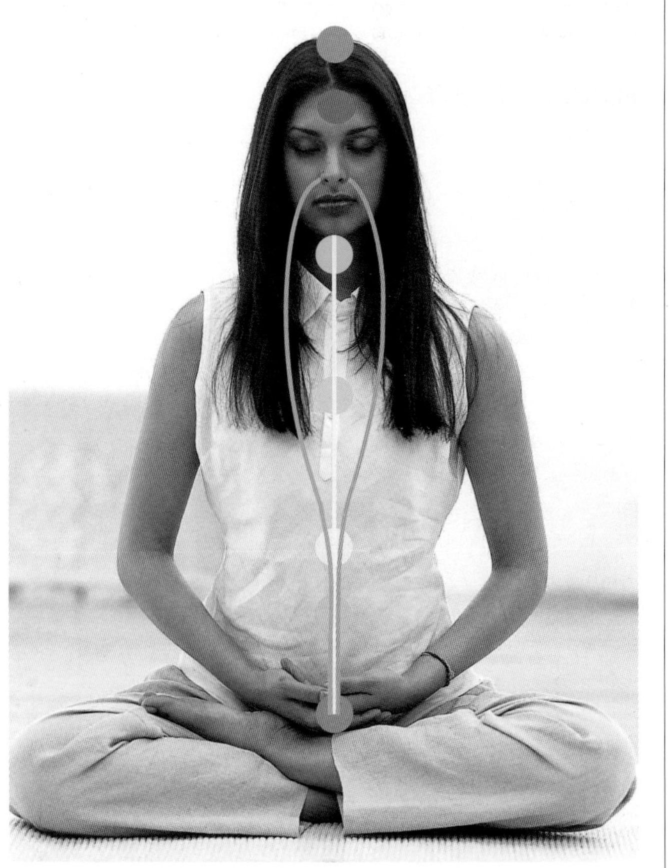

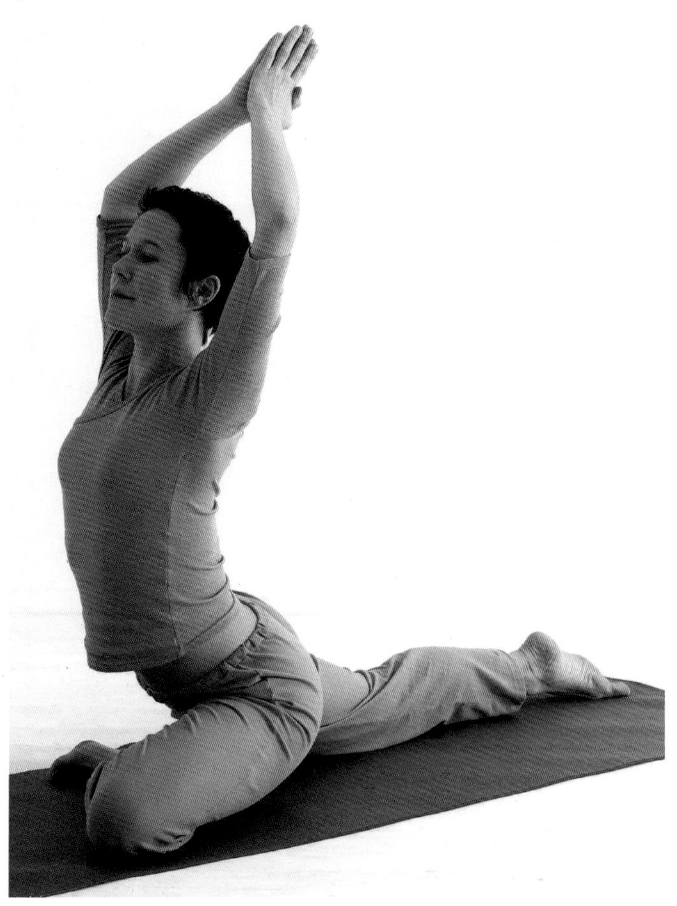

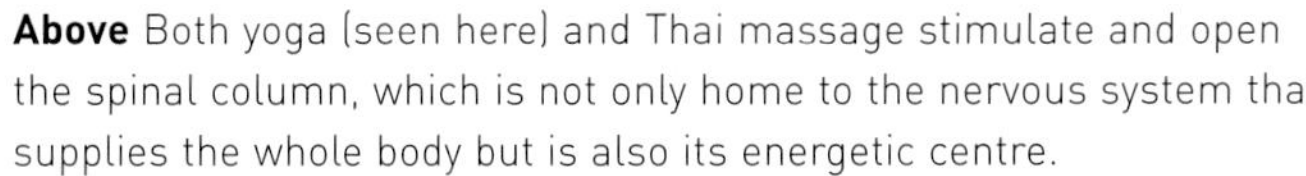

Above Both yoga (seen here) and Thai massage stimulate and open the spinal column, which is not only home to the nervous system that supplies the whole body but is also its energetic centre.

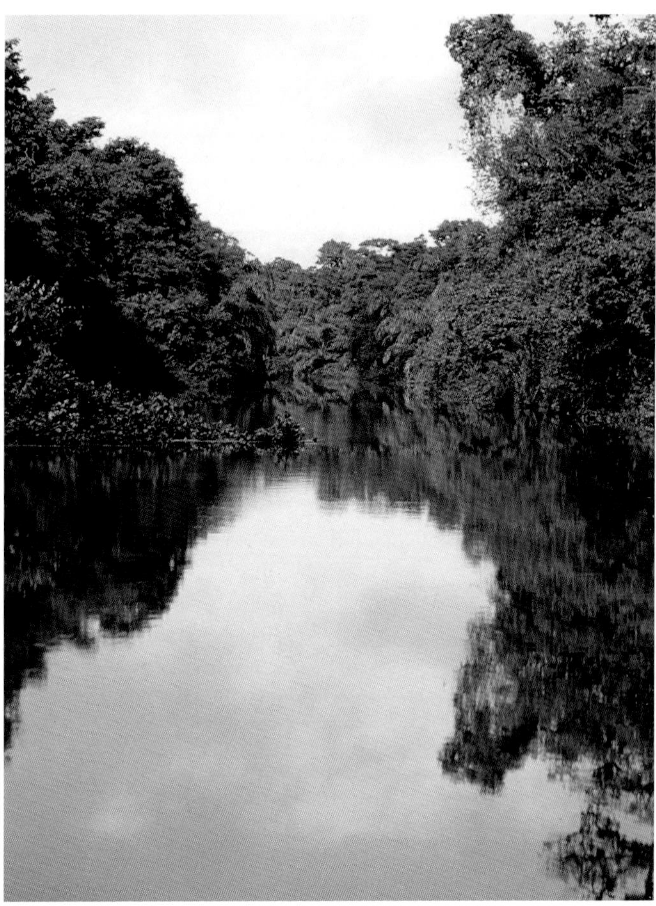

Above The body's energy flows just like water. If its pathways are kept clear, the energy can run freely, and this helps to maintain optimum physical and mental health.

THAI MASSAGE AND YOGA

Other healing practices, such as Chinese medicine and Japanese shiatsu, also view the body as a map of energy lines, which are known as meridians. There are many crossover points and areas of common ground among the Eastern systems, but Thai massage is more closely linked to the Indian yoga tradition. We can see quite strongly the links between yoga and Thai massage as it is practised today. It is often referred to as Thai yoga massage, highlighting the use of applied and passive hatha yoga stretches that give the massage its dynamic flow.

People often ask why Thai massage involves such a physically dynamic workout if it is a form of energy rebalancing. One way of looking at this is to understand that we manifest energy physically in the form of bones, muscle, skin and so on. So, the physical body can be seen as a point of access through which we are able to contact the more subtle aspects of the self. When we open the body with passive yoga stretches we feel it physically but, as in a yoga practice, the intention is ultimately to stimulate the energy flow within the body. This principle is important to remember – it is a reminder that Thai massage is not based upon the anatomical system that is understood in the West, but has its own logic and methodology.

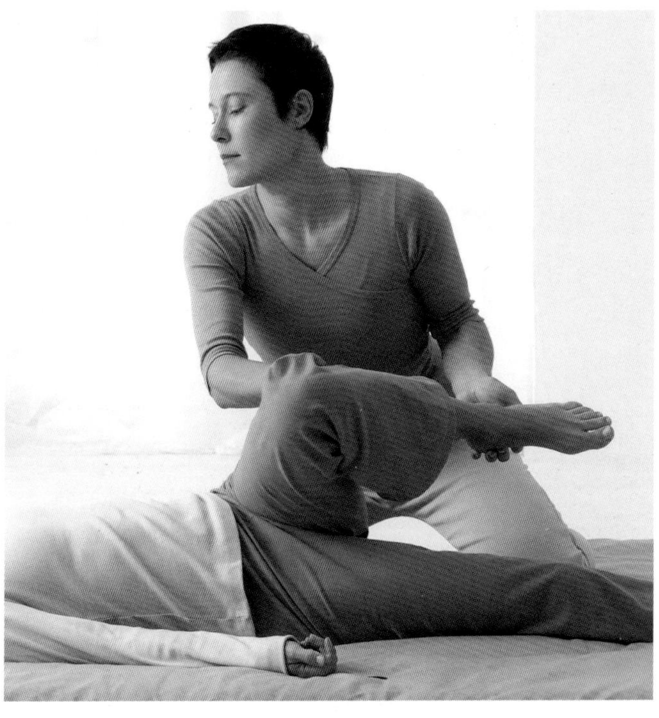

Above Energy is easily trapped in the joints; the constant, repeated movements of the body in Thai massage help to release deeply held tension in under-worked joints such as the hips.

The Sen

The practice of traditional Thai massage works on the sen, or energy lines, to keep the body in healthy balance. The sen, like the nadis of the yoga tradition, form a kind of map of the body that illustrates the subtle concept of the movement of energy within us. The sen lines sit neither inside nor on the body; they cannot be seen but only felt – as a subtle difference in the quality of the body.

When you are working the energy lines on your partner you may at times sense a kind of denseness, a feeling of something different from your own hands, a tingling or heat, a fullness or an emptiness. These kinds of sensation are extremely difficult to put into words, but you will know when you feel them. In order to give a good massage you don't have to understand such feelings; you should simply be open to experiencing them with your hands, and allow yourself to be guided by them.

The ten sen are always worked as an interconnecting unit. They do have their own individual strengths but as a general rule you would not select one line to work separately. Instead, you work all the energy lines throughout the body to create a feeling of balance. In the beginning it is not necessary to remember the functioning and exact therapeutic role of each line in order to give sensitive and relaxing massage. It can be useful to familiarize yourself with maps of the sen, but don't become so preoccupied with them that you forget to enjoy the scenery.

THE SEN AND THEIR FUNCTIONS

The diagrams featured on the following few pages indicate where the sen flow through the body. Though all ten lines are normally worked during Thai massage, each has a different therapeutic value and more experienced practitioners may place an emphasis on particular lines to achieve certain results.

Sen sumana

This line runs through the centre of the body. It supports the source of life – the breathing mechanism – affecting conditions such as asthma, bronchitis, coughs and colds.

Sen ittha and sen pingkhala

These are two aspects of the same line – the main treatment lines for problems with the internal organs. Sen ittha runs through the left side of the body; sen pingkhala runs through the right side. They are used therapeutically for abdominal pains, intestinal and digestive problems and diseases, diseases of the urinary tract and back pain.

Sen kalathari

This line criss-crosses the whole body, and its potency comes from this crossover effect. As it runs from left to right and from right to left, it joins the feminine and masculine elements within the body.

Sen kalathari supports or encourages emotional release, depending on how deeply and repeatedly it is worked. Stress is often related to the emotions, so it is good for tension headaches, sciatica and high blood pressure.

Sen sahatsarangsi and sen thawari

These two lines are simply different aspects of the same line. Sen sahatsarangsi runs down the left-hand side of the body and sen thawari down the right-hand side of the body. Working both these lines is especially effective for the treatment of knee pain.

Sen lawusang and sen ulangka

These are also two different aspects of the same line. Sen lawusang runs down the left side of the head and chest, and sen ulangka down the right side. Their main therapeutic use is for deafness and ear infections.

Sen nanthakrawat and sen khitchana

Both of these lines are part of sen sumana. Sen nanthakrawat splits into two: one aspect runs from the navel down through the urethra, while the other aspect runs from the navel down to the anus. Sen khitchana runs from the navel down through the vagina or penis.

In practical terms, both of these lines are accessed by working the abdomen from the navel down to the pubic bone. Their main areas of treatment are urinary problems, menstruation problems, infertility and impotence.

Right This artwork shows, in detail, the paths of the sen across the front of the body. Study this and the artworks over the next couple of pages to build up a picture of how these energy lines travel around the body, and where they interconnect and diverge. Notice also the places where certain pressure points lie on particular sen lines.

THE FRONT OF THE BODY

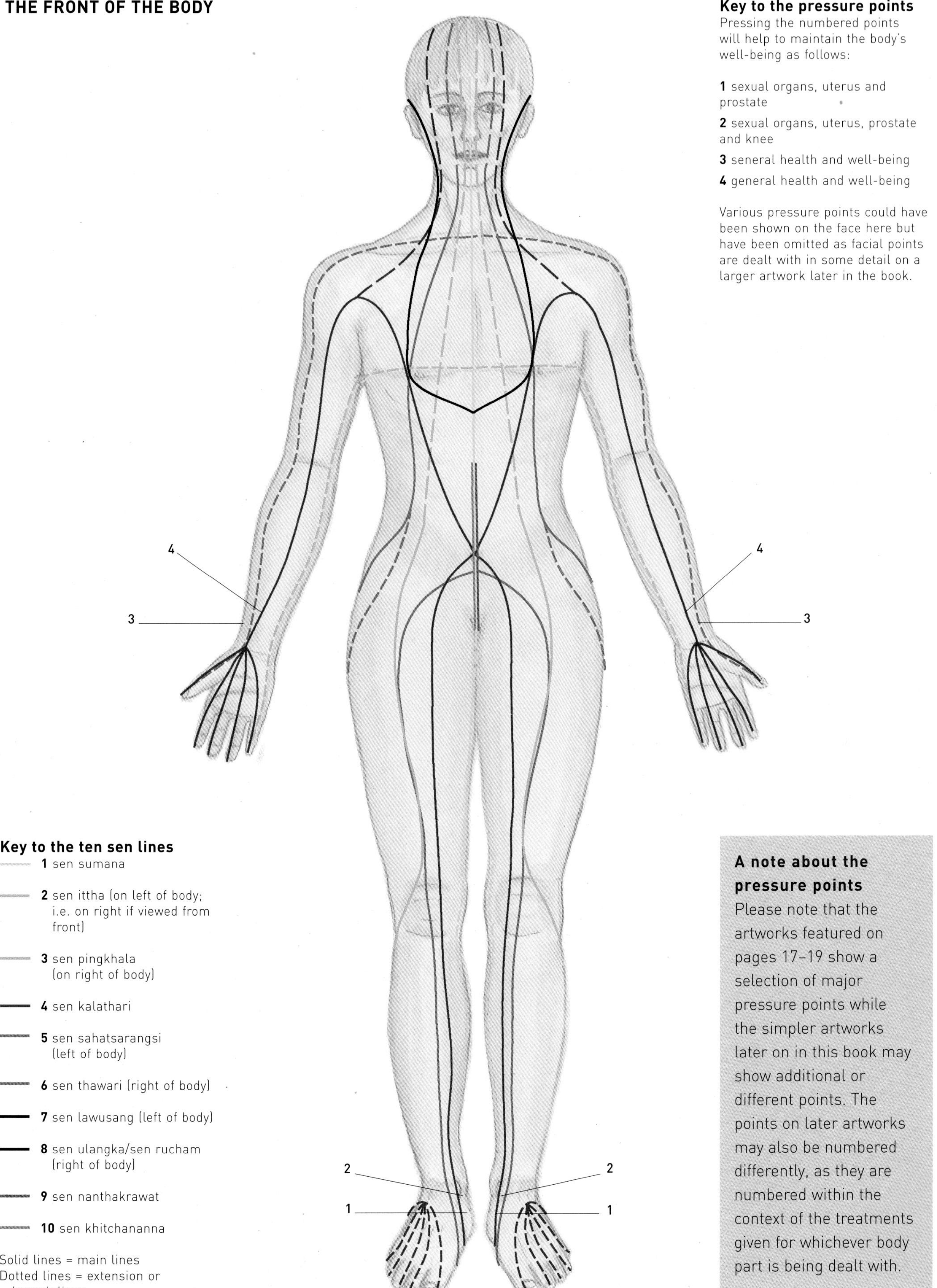

Key to the pressure points
Pressing the numbered points will help to maintain the body's well-being as follows:

1 sexual organs, uterus and prostate

2 sexual organs, uterus, prostate and knee

3 seneral health and well-being

4 general health and well-being

Various pressure points could have been shown on the face here but have been omitted as facial points are dealt with in some detail on a larger artwork later in the book.

Key to the ten sen lines

- **1** sen sumana
- **2** sen ittha (on left of body; i.e. on right if viewed from front)
- **3** sen pingkhala (on right of body)
- **4** sen kalathari
- **5** sen sahatsarangsi (left of body)
- **6** sen thawari (right of body)
- **7** sen lawusang (left of body)
- **8** sen ulangka/sen rucham (right of body)
- **9** sen nanthakrawat
- **10** sen khitchananna

Solid lines = main lines
Dotted lines = extension or branch lines

A note about the pressure points
Please note that the artworks featured on pages 17–19 show a selection of major pressure points while the simpler artworks later on in this book may show additional or different points. The points on later artworks may also be numbered differently, as they are numbered within the context of the treatments given for whichever body part is being dealt with.

Right This artwork shows the paths of the sen across the back of the body.

For explanatory colour key, see previous artwork

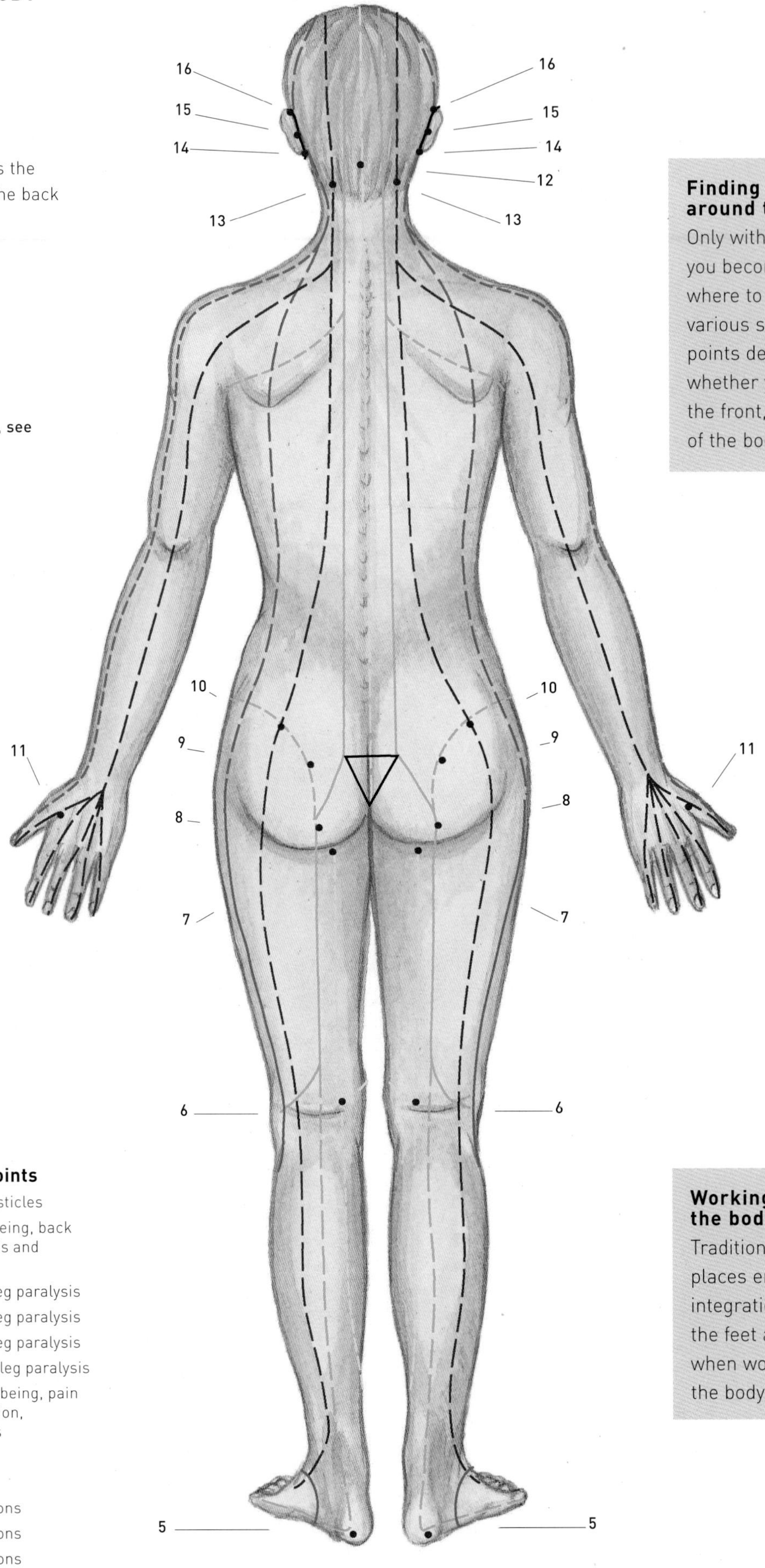

16 15 14 13 16 15 14 12 13 10 10 9 9 11 11 8 8 7 7 6 6 5 5

Finding your way around the body

Only with practice can you become familiar with where to locate the various sen and pressure points depending on whether you are working the front, back or side of the body.

Key to the pressure points

5 sexual organs, ovaries, testicles
6 general health and well-being, back pain, knee pain, leg paralysis and bloated stomach
7 lower back, sciatica and leg paralysis
8 lower back, sciatica and leg paralysis
9 lower back, sciatica and leg paralysis
10 lower back, sciatica and leg paralysis
11 general health and well-being, pain in general, lungs, constipation, tonsillitis, coughs and colds
12 headache and dizziness
13 headache
14 deafness and ear infections
15 deafness and ear infections
16 deafness and ear infections

Working the back of the body

Traditional Thai massage places emphasis on the integration of the legs, the feet and the back when working the back of the body.

THE SIDE OF THE BODY

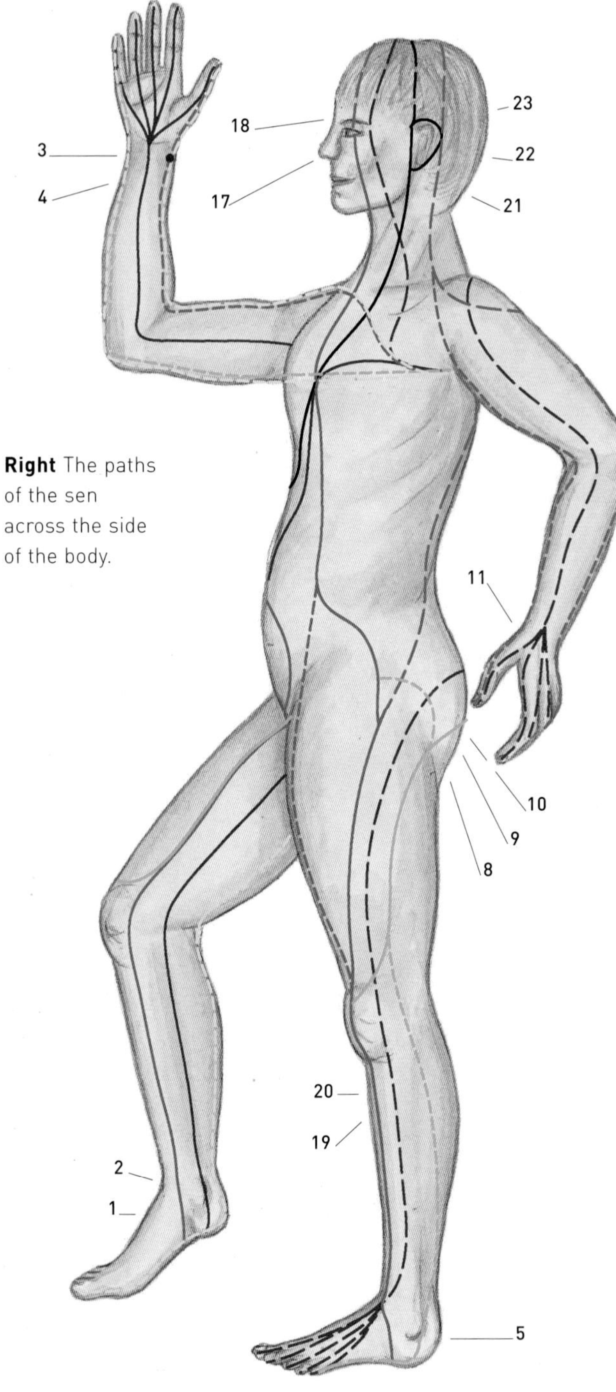

Right The paths of the sen across the side of the body.

Key to the pressure points

1 sexual organs, uterus and prostate
2 sexual organs, uterus, prostate and knee
3 general health and well-being
4 general health and well-being
5 sexual organs, ovaries and testicles
8–10 lower back, sciatica and leg paralysis
11 general health and well-being, pain in general, lungs, constipation, tonsillitis, coughs and colds
17 migraine
18 headache
19 general health and well-being, numbness, lower back and leg pain
20 general health and well-being, knee pain and bloated stomach
21–23 deafness and ear infections

THE TOP OF THE HEAD

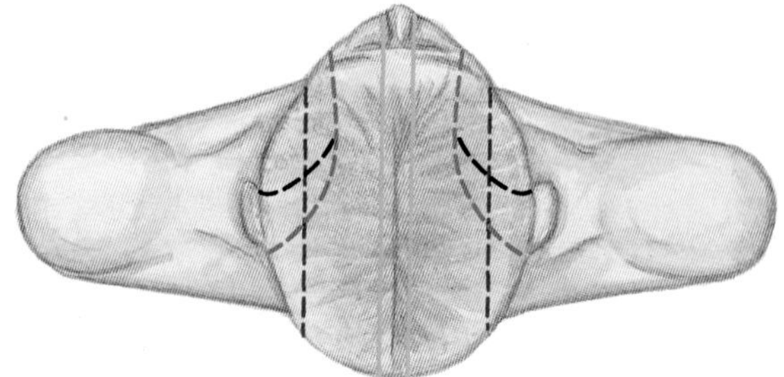

Above The paths of the sen across the top of the head.

THE SOLES OF THE FEET

Key to the pressure points

24 insomnia, foot pain, heart and mental disturbance
25 shock, sunstroke and hypertension

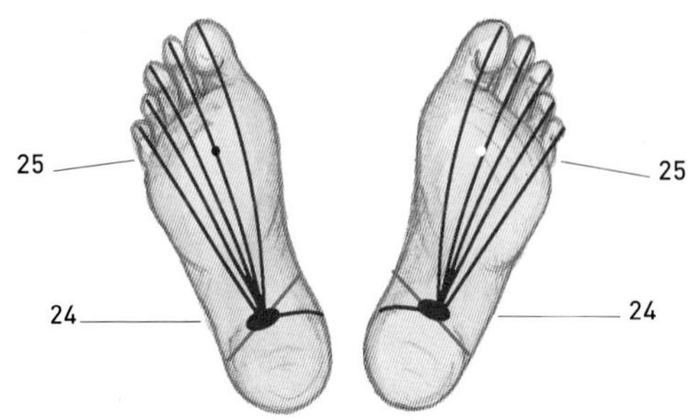

Above The paths of the sen across the soles of the feet.

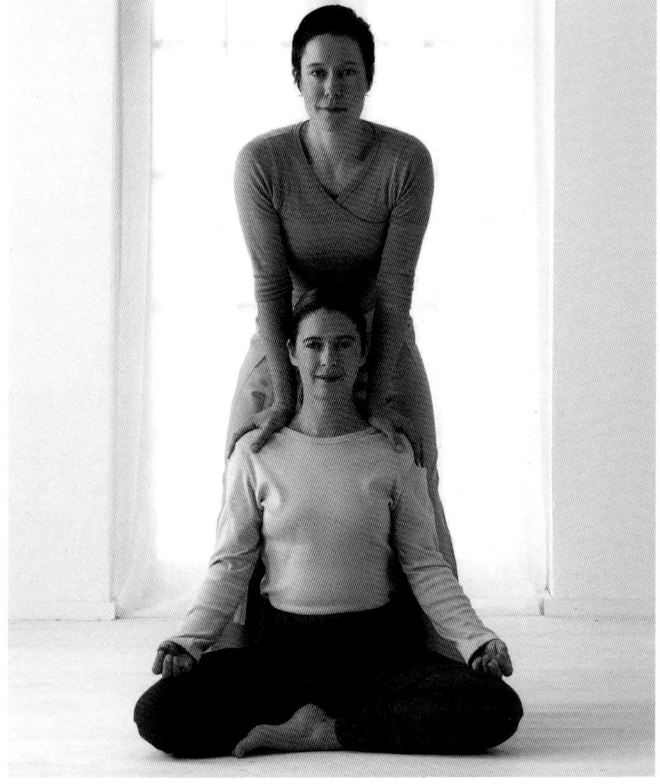

Above It is possible to work the energy lines in Thai massage from a variety of very different positions.

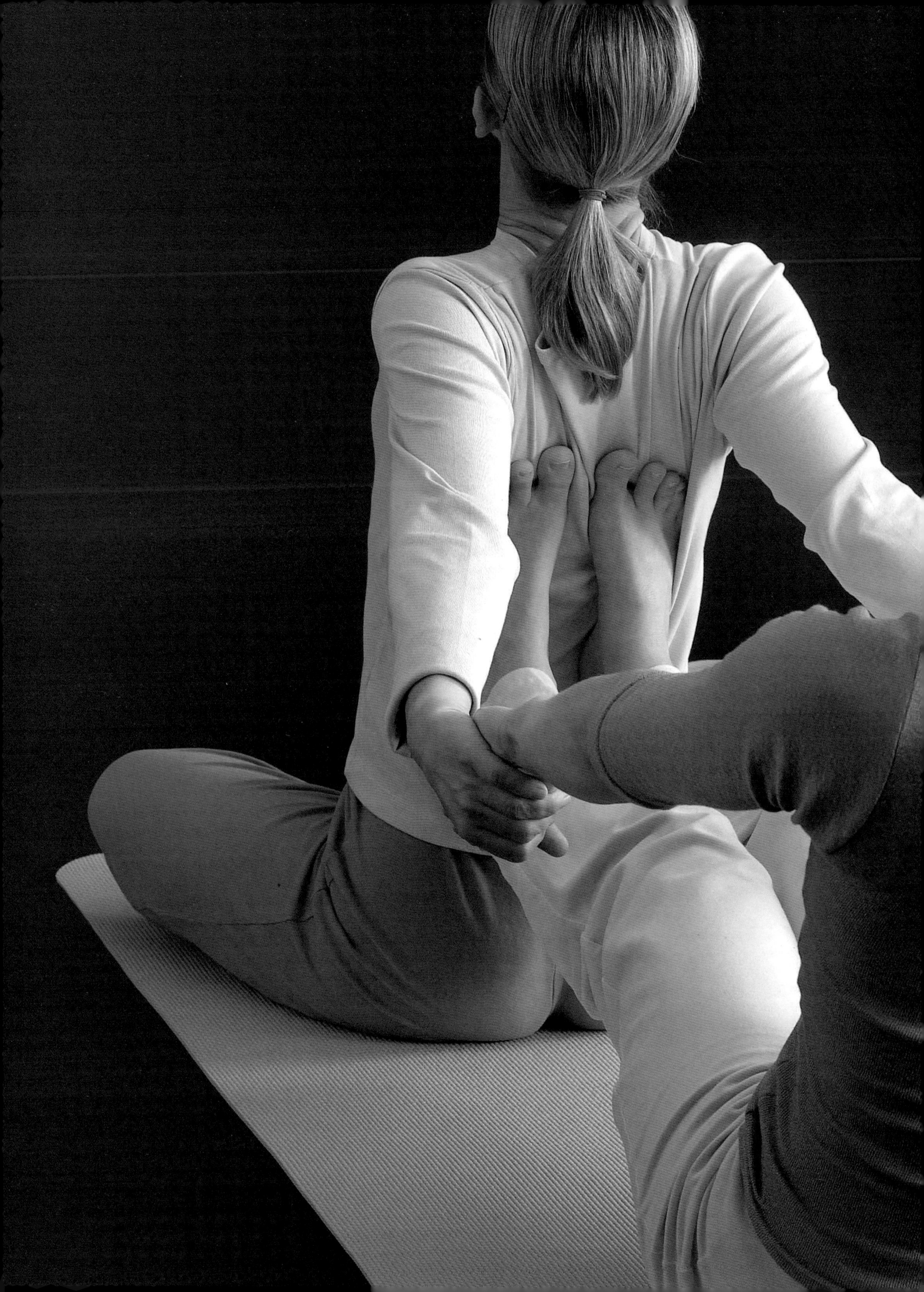

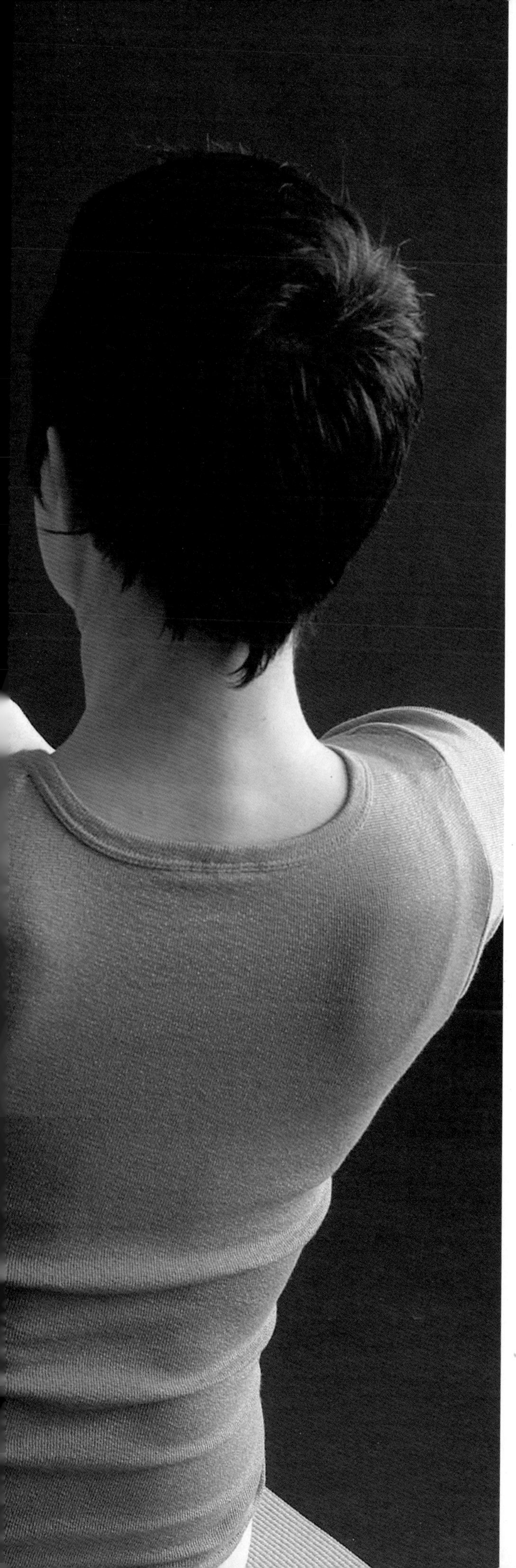

Preparing Body and Mind

In Thai massage the way you work is as important as what you do. As the giver, you need to ensure that the lines of energy are flowing freely in your own body so that you can be an example to your partner, the receiver. It is therefore vital to prepare yourself before giving a massage. Exercise will make your body supple and flexible so that you can move smoothly through the routine, and a regular meditation practice will help quieten your thoughts, allowing you to approach the massage session in a state of mindfulness and with an open heart. The spiritual roots of Thai massage can be acknowledged by creating a sacred space in which to work.

Preparing Your Body

Thai massage is a physical experience for both the giver and the receiver. It is therefore important to open and prepare your body thoroughly so that you feel physically at ease when giving a massage. Once you begin to feel more comfortable in your own body, the massage you give will be a much more relaxing and enjoyable experience for both you and your partner. The simple but effective exercises shown below have been specially devised to open up the joints of the feet, hands and spine – all vital areas for the giver.

The Feet

Since Thai massage is given on the floor, you need to develop flexibility in your feet in order to feel comfortable in your working postures. Try to do these exercises daily.

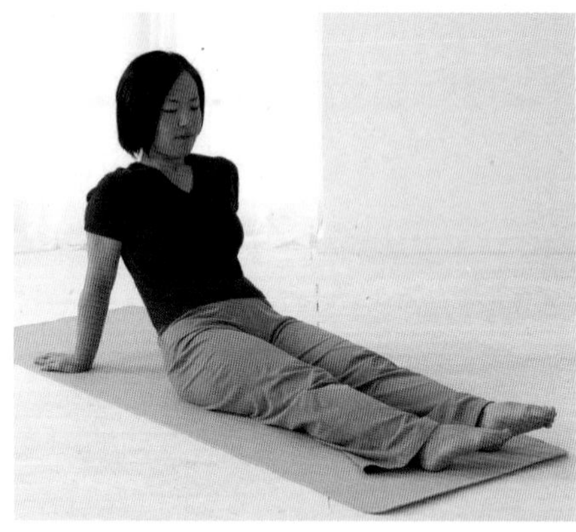

1 Circling the feet This opens and strengthens the ankle and hip joints. Sit as shown. With your feet at least hip-width apart, circle both feet slowly clockwise, and then anticlockwise.

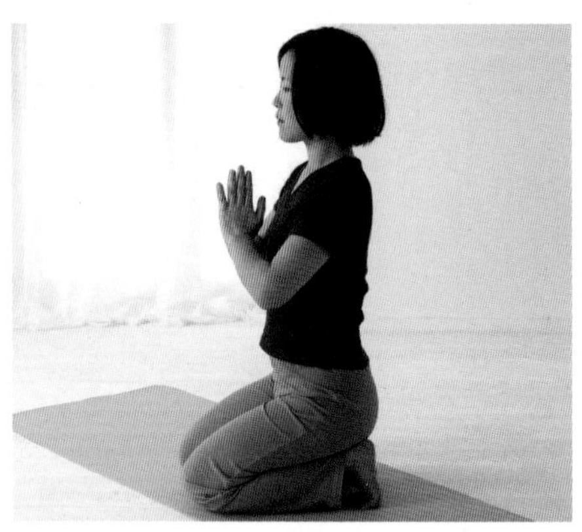

2 Waking up the insteps Kneel down with the knees and feet together. Inhale and kneel up, tucking your toes under. Exhale and sink slowly back on to your heels. Repeat at least three times.

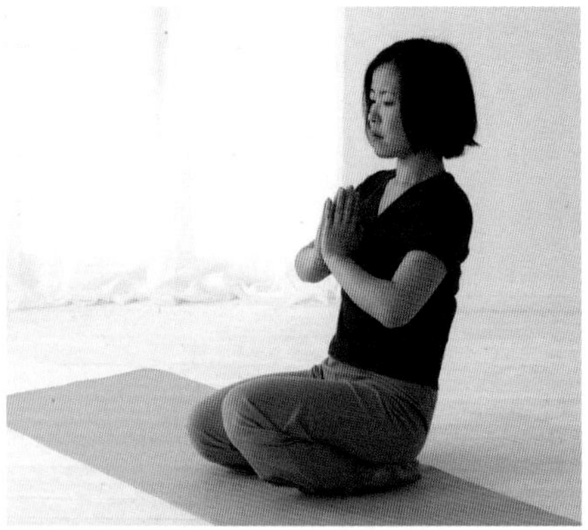

3 Knee lifts This opens the front of the ankles. Kneel down as shown. Lift one knee gently and return it to the floor. Work alternate knees, three times each. If you find this easy, lift both together.

The Hands

You will mostly be using your hands to apply pressure to the energy lines. Use these exercises to release any tension in your hands before or after giving a massage.

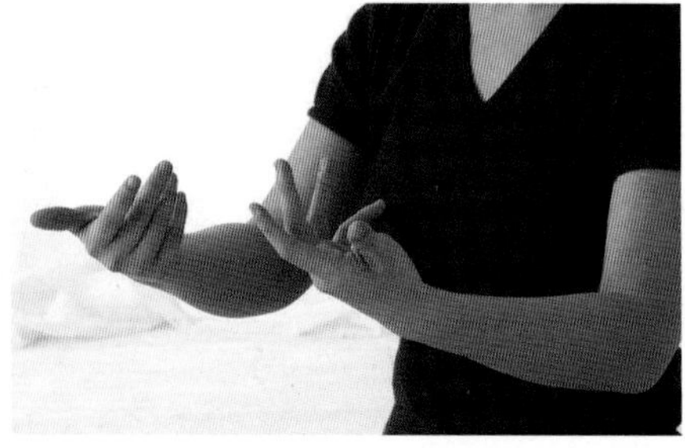

1 Wrist circles Check that your shoulders are relaxed and move your hands through full circles, both clockwise and anticlockwise, to loosen and strengthen the wrists.

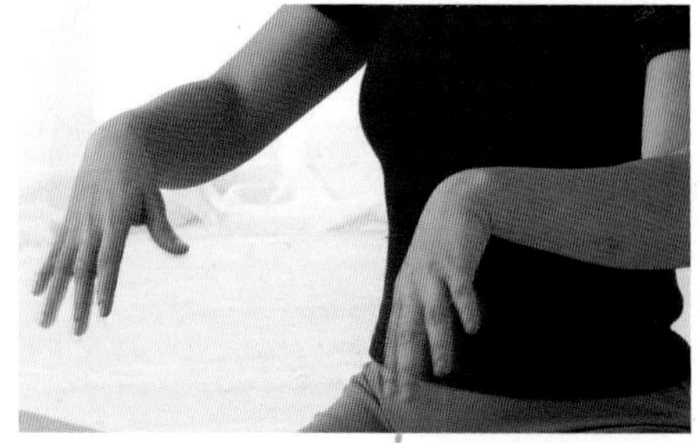

2 Shaking the wrists This is a very effective and quick way to release excess tension and energy in the joints of the fingers and the wrists.

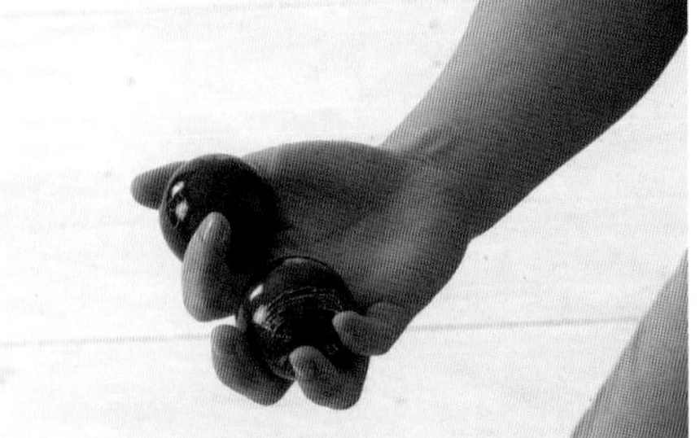

3 Strengthening the fingers Help to strengthen the hands and make your finger joints more flexible by rolling a pair of hard balls (ping pong balls are an option) around in your hands.

The Spine

When giving massage, aim to work with a sense of ease and freedom throughout your spine. This keeps you grounded in your own body and aware of your posture. These exercises help to free up the spine, from the pelvis all the way up to the base of the skull.

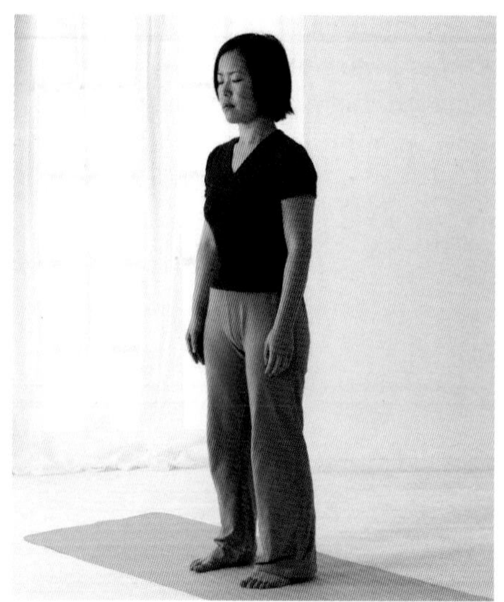

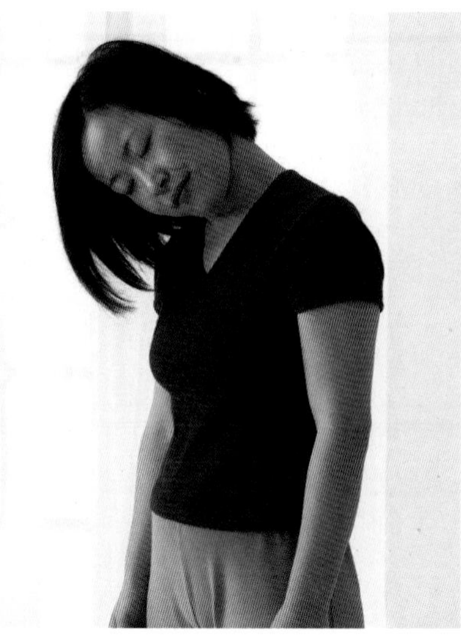

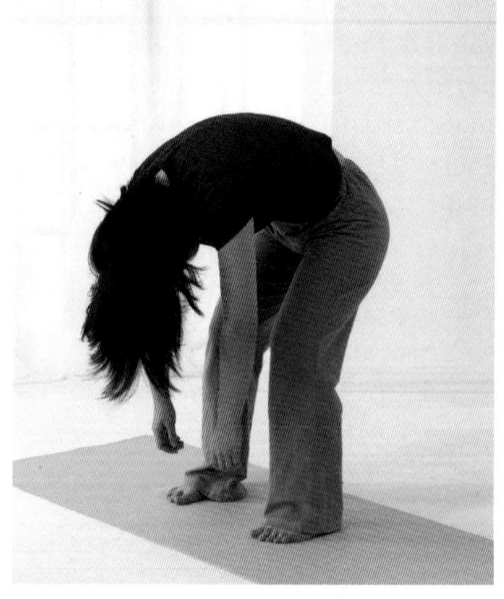

1 Standing Place your feet parallel and hip-width apart. Make sure that your weight is spread evenly throughout each foot – shift the weight until you feel yourself come to rest in the centre. Keep your knees straight but not locked. Let your tailbone drop towards the floor, and the back of your neck become very long. Stand like this for a short while, letting your breath flow freely and easily in and out of your nostrils.

2 Loosening the neck Drop your right ear towards your right shoulder, and let the weight of your head roll forward, keeping your shoulders relaxed back. Continue this soft, slow, rolling movement until the left ear is sinking towards the left shoulder. Repeat this semicircling three times. Do not roll your head back in a complete circle, as this would compromise the delicate spinal vertebrae.

3 Forward fold This provides a release between the spinal vertebrae. Stand with your feet hip-width apart, or slightly wider, with your knees a little bent to give the hips more freedom of movement. Let your forehead drop and feel each vertebra open, from the base of the neck down to the base of the spine. Fold from your hips, not your back. Exhale as you release forward, breathe smoothly and deeply as you fold fully. Roll slowly back to standing.

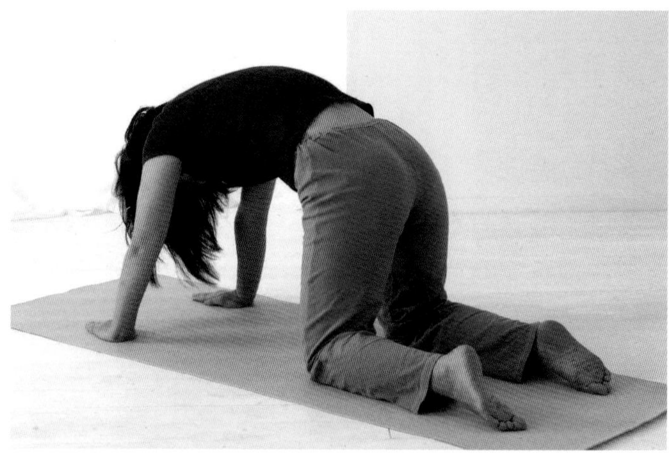

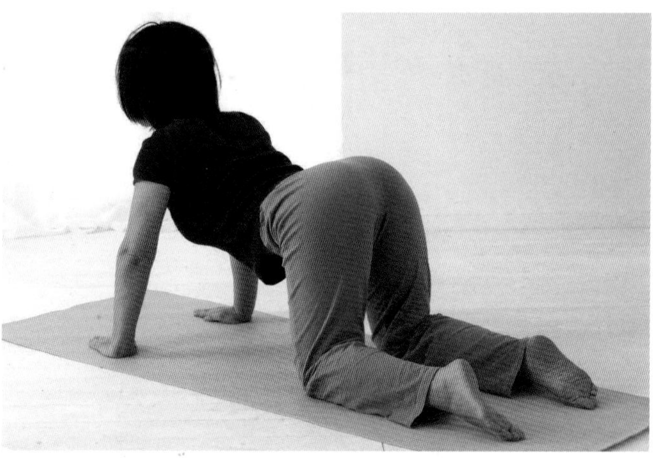

4 Cat tilt The cat and dog tilts bring greater flexibility to the entire spine. As you start to inhale, feel as if you are being drawn up between the shoulder blades, rounding your upper back. Tuck your tailbone under and let your chin move down towards your chest. Look between your legs. Feel your ribcage broaden.

5 Dog tilt As you begin to exhale, feel the whole of your spinal column lengthen. Lengthen your tailbone away from the crown of your head and open through the front of your body, looking up gently. Repeat this wavelike movement slowly and smoothly once or twice, letting your breath guide you.

Preparing Your Mind

A good Thai massage is more than just a series of physical stretches and manipulations. Practising your massage in a meditative frame of mind enhances its potential for deeper healing. It is the influence of Buddhist spiritual practice that gives Thai massage its unique spiritual depth. By familiarizing yourself with some of these practices you can start to embody specific mental states so that they become a natural part of your massage work. The practices described below, of observation meditation, *metta* meditation and chanting, help to settle the activity of the mind and open the heart. It is these qualities of stillness and open-heartedness that we can aspire to bring to our practice of Thai massage. There are many different approaches to meditation. It doesn't matter which you choose as each individual needs to find a way that suits them.

Meditation of Mindfulness

This exercise introduces you to the practice of vipassana, or observation meditation. This practice can be expanded to include an open observation of all sensations in the body – hearing, smell, thought or touch. But begin here simply, by just observing your breath.

Right Sit comfortably and notice how your breath feels as it passes in and out through your nostrils, then notice how your abdomen feels as it rises and falls with the inhalation and exhalation. If your attention wanders, gently remind it to come back to your breathing. You can begin by sitting for five minutes and then gradually extend your practice for up to an hour.

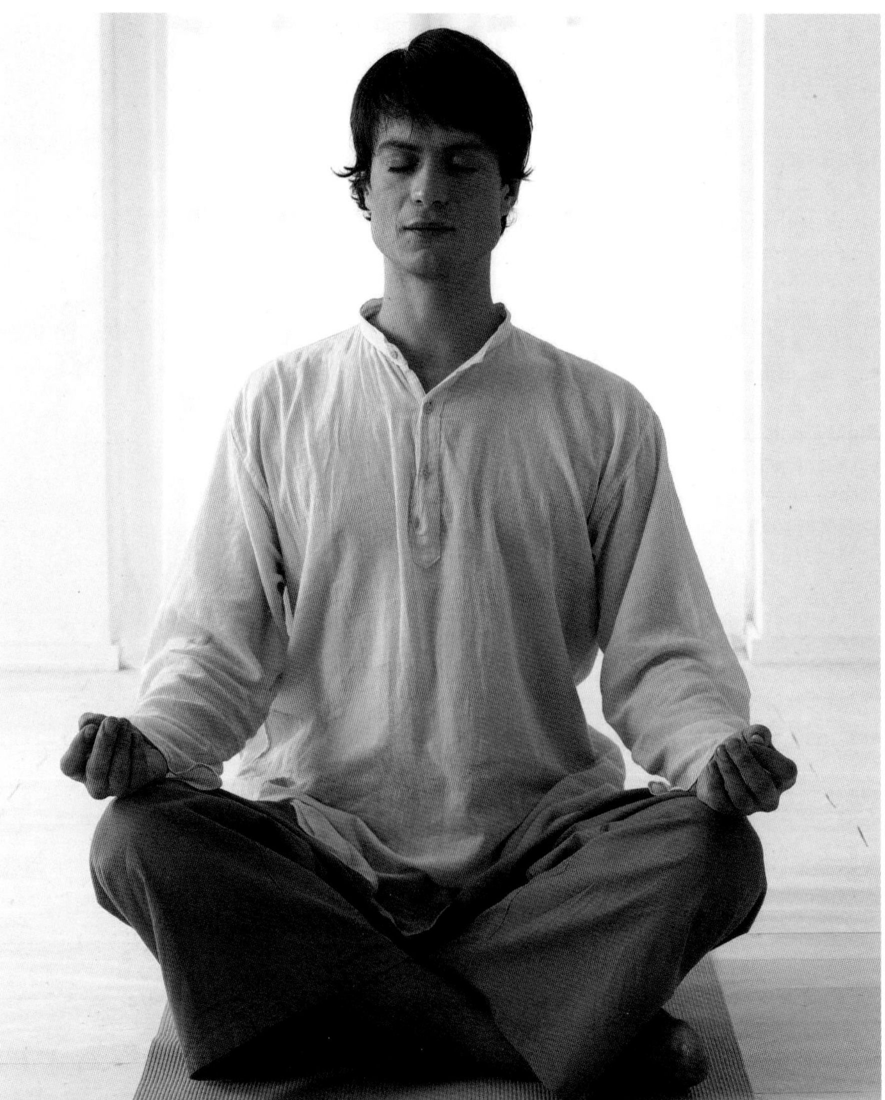

Below Spiritual practice is an inherent part of daily life in Thailand.

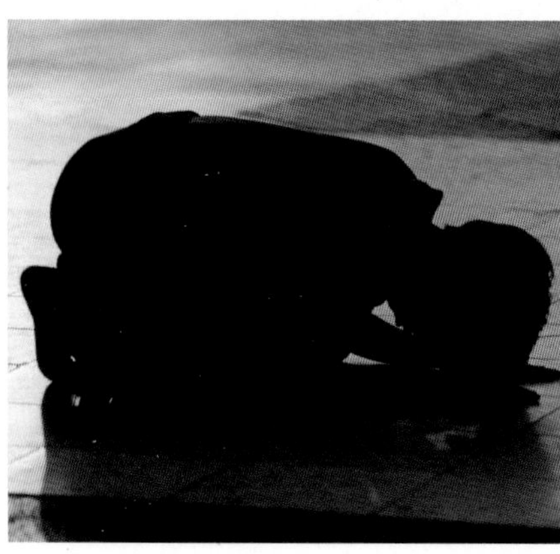

Metta Meditation

Metta is the word, from the ancient Indian Pali language, that means "loving kindness". Cultivating a compassionate and non-judgemental attitude is the foundation of Buddhist spiritual practice and is an important aspect of the spiritual practice of Thai massage.

When we choose to do this meditation of loving kindness it is important that we begin with ourselves. For only by fully accepting who we are, without any judgement, can we begin to extend this feeling out towards others. You can use the simple mantra below as a starting point.

May all beings be happy
May all beings be at peace
May all beings be well

Find a quiet, comfortable place to sit and allow yourself 5–15 minutes. Begin by focusing on yourself; on what you like and what you don't like or find difficult about yourself. You can repeat the mantra above with yourself in mind, focusing on the sensations around your heart centre. Imagine yourself in the role of your closest friend. If they were standing in front of you now, what would they wish for you? What would they say to you in order that you might feel more loving towards yourself? Receive this gift from your friend with an open heart. Once familiar with this practice, we can develop goodwill not just to relatives, friends and colleagues, but to everything around us and eventually the whole of creation.

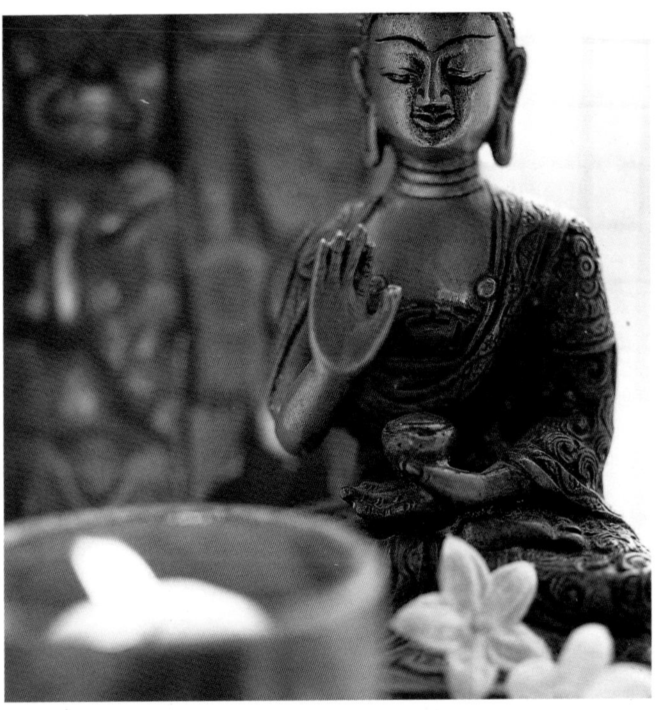

Above The Buddha is the embodiment of loving kindness. The development of loving kindness always begins with ourselves.

Om Mani Padme Hum

Widely used in Tibetan Buddhist practice today, this mantra originated in India and the Sanskrit language. Expressing this mantra evokes the qualities of the Buddha of Compassion.

Om is the sound vibration that is all existence.
Mani is the jewel, a diamond that uses the clarity and precision of wisdom to cut through ignorance.
Padme is the lotus, the symbol of beauty, purity and compassion, that rises and blooms out of the muddy depths of the clouded waters of ignorance.
Hum is the open heart that unifies all with kindness and love.

This lovely mantra or prayer can be very roughly translated as:

"May the jewel of the lotus flower send out a light of love and compassion to unite all existence as one."

It is a beautiful mantra to sing either out loud or in your head just before or even during a massage treatment. It opens up the heart centre and helps to focus your attention on working from your heart more than from your head.

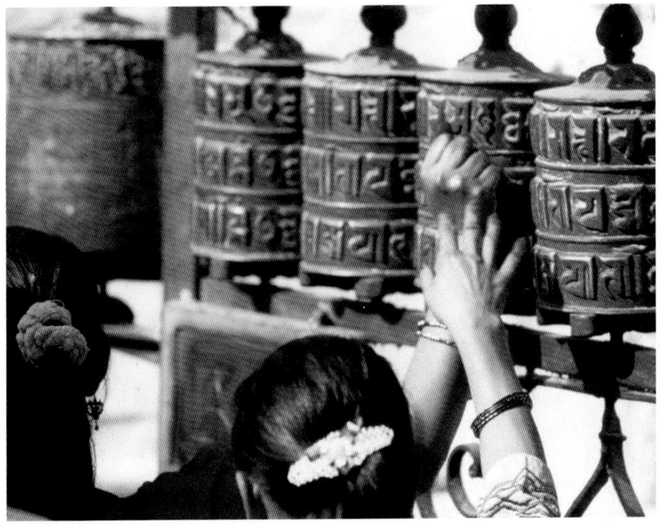

Above Prayer wheels inscribed with the *Om Mani Padme Hum* mantra are commonly used in Tibet and Nepal to ensure that the energy of the mantra is expressed continually throughout the day.

Nurturing Touch

For many people, nurturing touch is, sadly, very far from being an integral part of our everyday lives. Learning to give and to receive massage can be a wonderful way to reintroduce this important aspect of communication and to bring its benefits into your life. In order to give a good massage, you really do need to know what it feels like to receive a good massage. Receiving is always just as important as giving.

Through your sense of touch you feel your body and come to understand it better. Movement is also a way of getting to know the body, and people explore and express the feeling in their bodies in many different ways, such as through dance, yoga, swimming or sport.

Thai massage is movement and nurturing touch combined: as giver and receiver, you and your partner are in constant motion, dancing together. The dynamic quality of the passive yoga stretches makes them beneficial to the stiffest of bodies and helps to wake up those parts that may have been asleep for years.

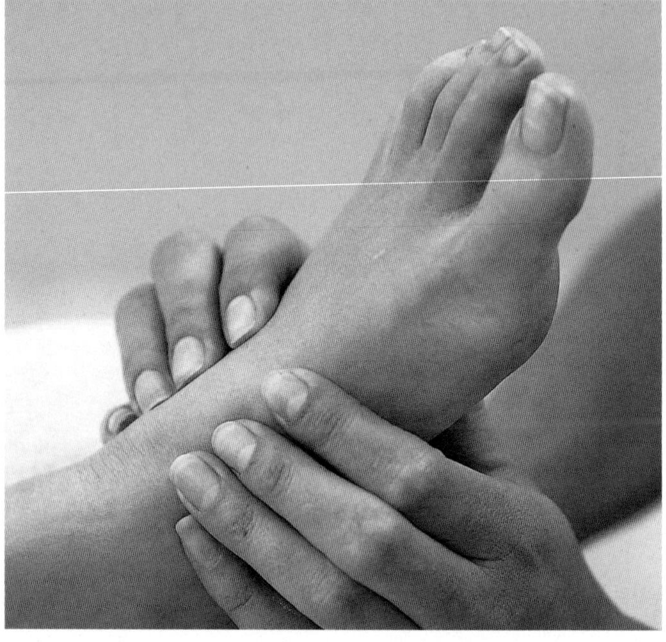

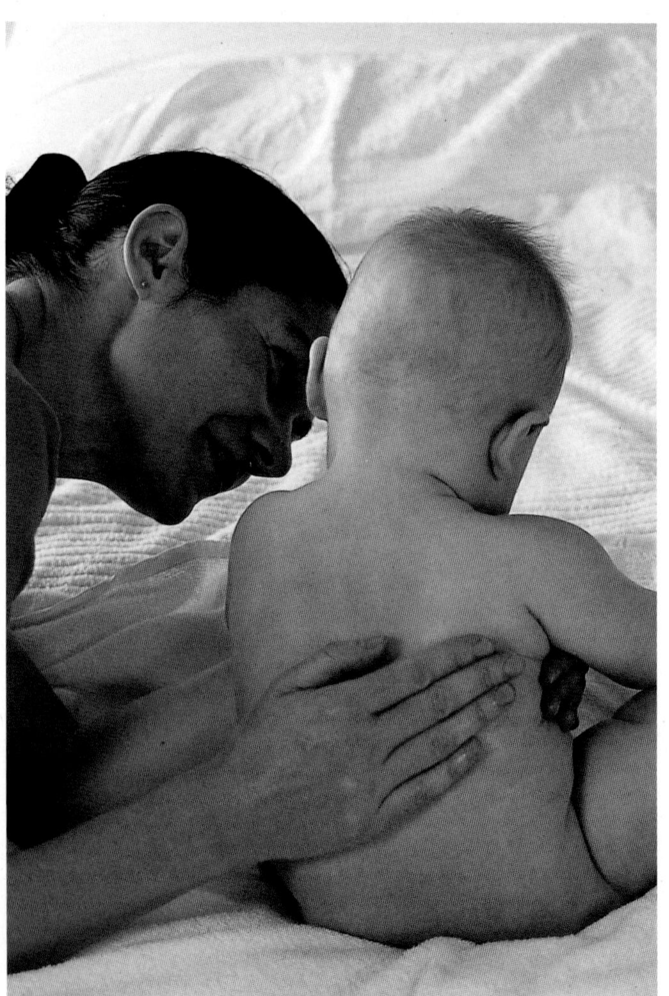

LEARNING THROUGH GIVING AND RECEIVING

Part of the learning process is to know what it feels like to surrender to the flow of the treatment. If you only ever give massage, and never receive it, you can become very unbalanced. A good practitioner is able to receive as well as they can give. It may sound obvious but it is surprising how many massage therapists don't take the time to receive massage and so never fully realize what helps them to relax. If you are a keen student it is recommended that you receive as much massage as you can from different people so that you can familiarize yourself with the feelings of release and letting go that come from a good massage. Your experience will, in turn, help you to facilitate greater relaxation for your massage partner.

Remember that Thai massage should be something that the giver and receiver share, like a conversation between two people. If you learn how to listen more acutely with your hands, it follows that you will develop far greater sensitivity and a more naturally intuitive approach to your massage.

Above The feet are a good place to start giving nurturing touch – most people enjoy a relaxing foot massage.

Left Touch is a natural way for a mother to talk to her child. It is the first form of communication that we learn as babies.

Sticky Hands

This exercise is a playful way to develop your sense of touch. One person leads the other by suggesting a movement with their hand. Try to tune into where your partner wants to go and to move with them, keeping your eyes closed and working by touch alone.

1 (right) Stand facing each other. Place the palm of one hand very gently against your partner's. Your touch should be light but firm, your elbows bent and your shoulders totally relaxed. Close your eyes and feel the connection between the surfaces of your palms. Make sure you are standing with your feet apart and your knees slightly soft, in a stable stance, so that you can be ready to move comfortably and easily in any direction.

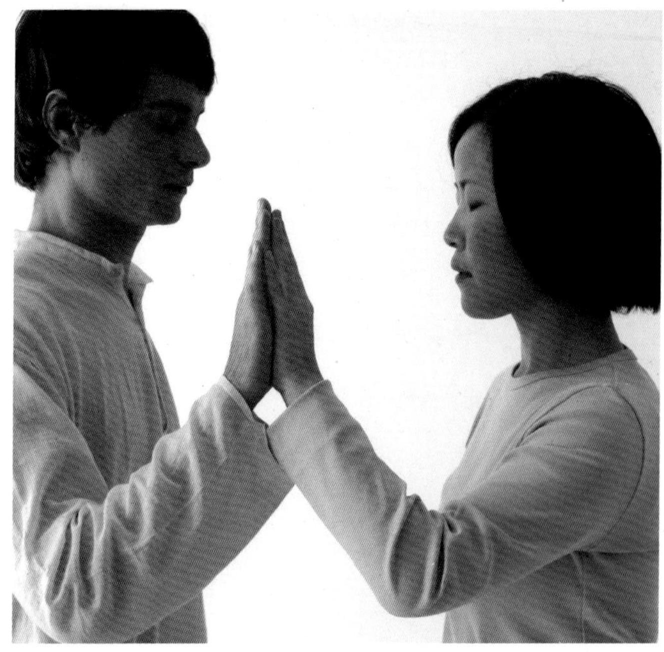

2 (below) Decide which of you is going to take the lead first. Now start to move around, keeping your palms together as you move in order to maintain that close connection with each other. Your movements can be either small or expansive, but you should always try to keep them as smooth as possible.

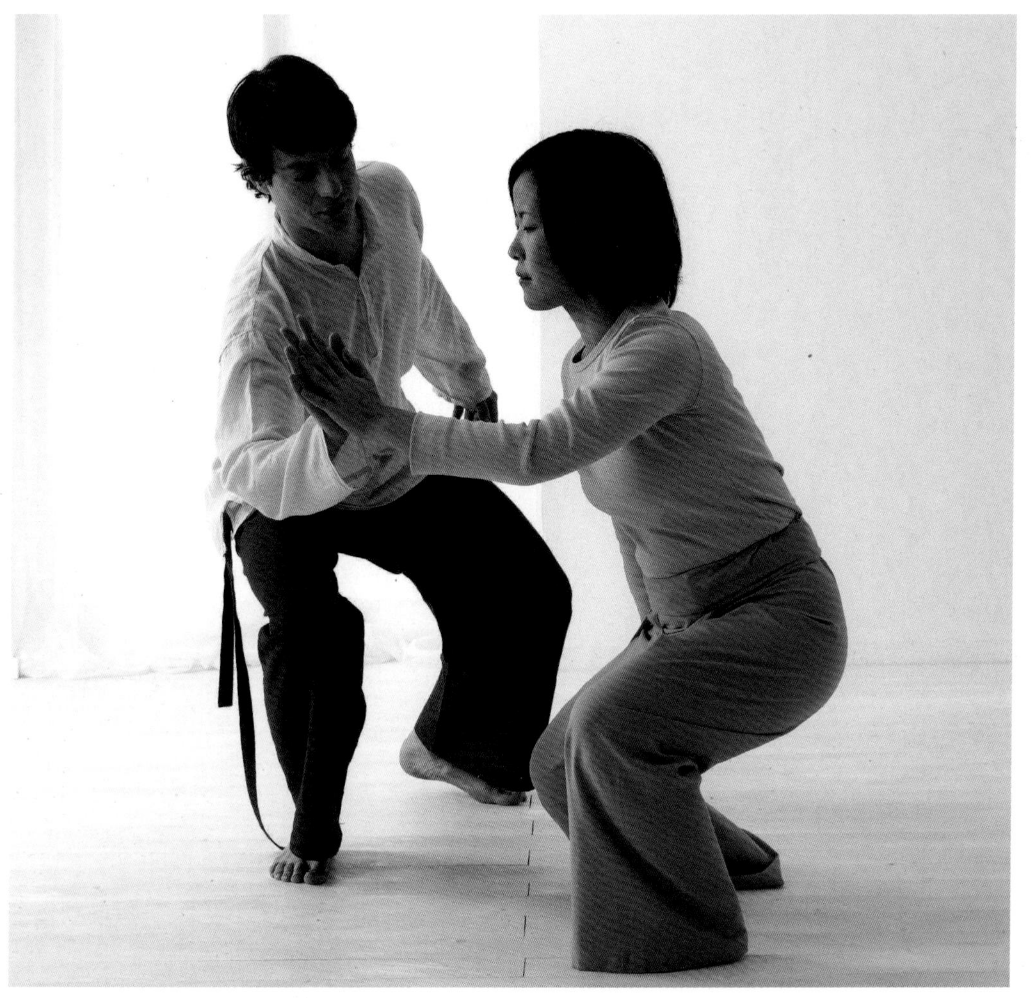

Ways of moving

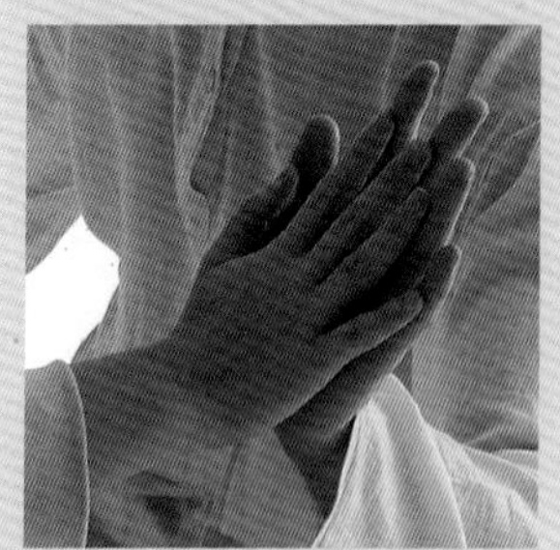

Always keep your palms together, but softly – do not force it. Also, remember that when you are moving around in this exercise you are not trying to outwit your partner but rather seeing how much you can move together in synchronicity.

Preparing the Space

Setting up the room for Thai massage can be like a ritual, defining the space as somewhere special where you put aside everyday distractions. This preparation encourages a shift in your mindset by creating a place where thoughts quieten, the body slows down and deeper healing can take place.

Apart from the practical necessity of providing a space where your partner will be able to relax, it is important to create the right atmosphere in the room where you are giving the massage. Set up the space exactly as you would like it to be if you were receiving the massage yourself. Make sure that it is quiet and warm, switch off the phone and choose a time when you can ensure that there will be no interruptions.

Burning a candle is recommended while you give massage. Not only does it provide a lovely soft light for working, but as fire is purifying you can use it as a means of clearing the energy in the room. The burning of incense or oils also has a cleansing and purifying effect on the space and creates a very welcoming and pleasant ambience, as long as the scent is not overpowering.

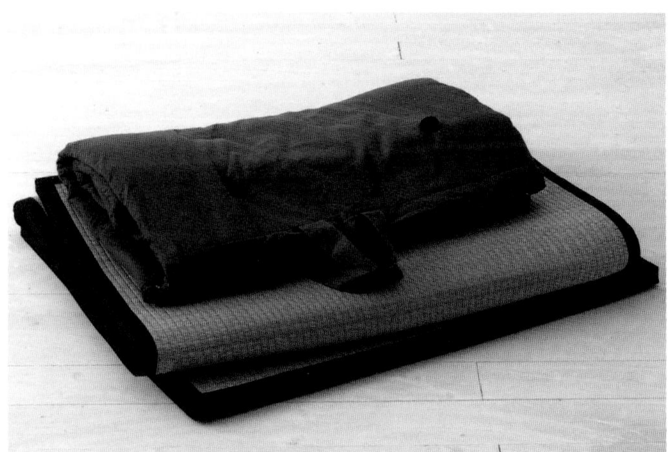

Right A bed roll, a thick exercise mat, a foam mattress, or even a folded duvet or thick blanket are good alternatives to a proper futon, but any working surface must be padded, firm and non-slip.

Below The ideal equipment includes a futon, cushions and bolsters, foam blocks and a blanket, but you can easily improvise.

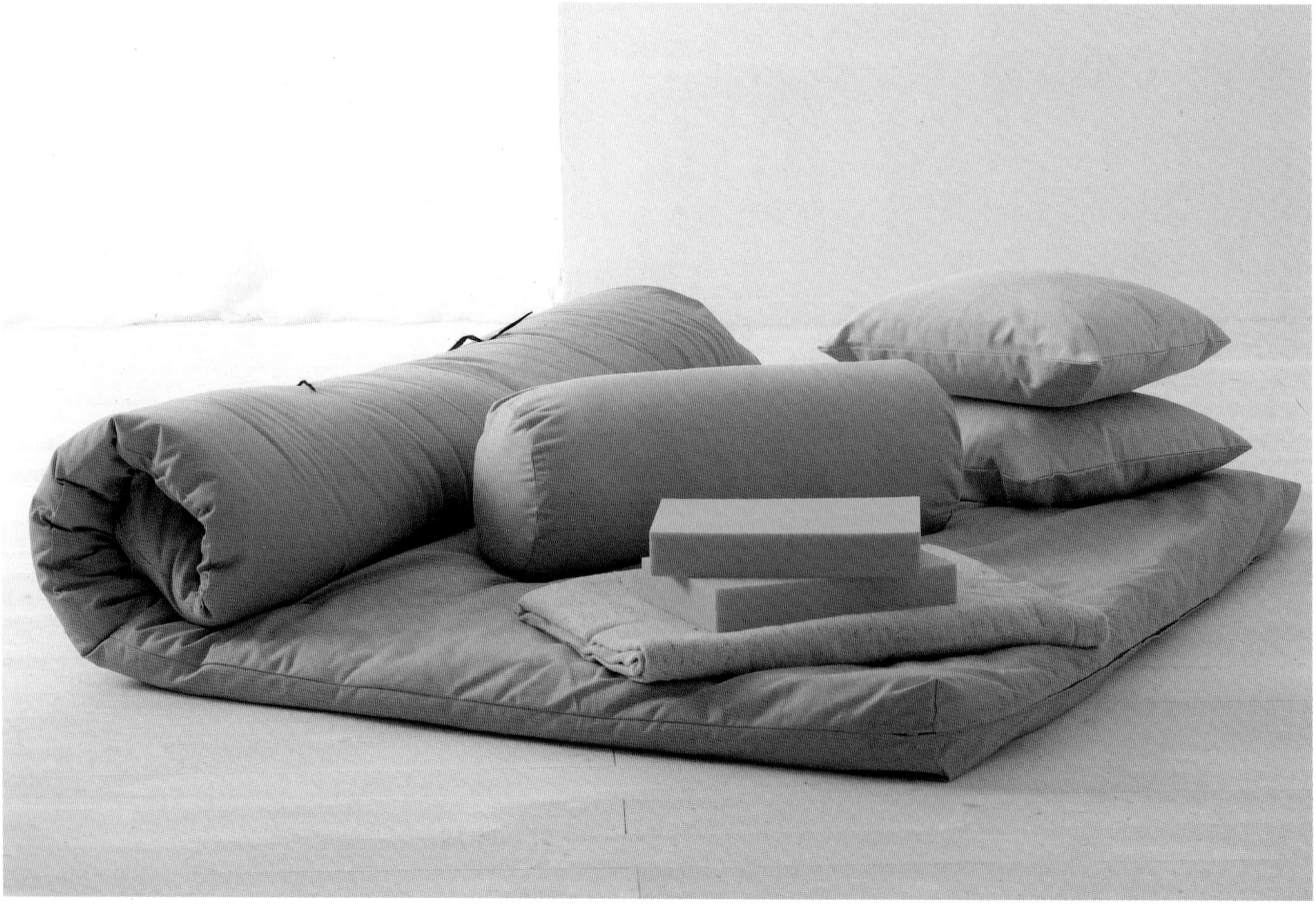

WHAT YOU NEED
Before you start your massage, ensure that you have everything that you will need close at hand. You may already have some of the following items, but if you don't you can always adapt similar everyday items that you own to use for your massage practice.

- **Futon or firm mat** This should preferably be wide enough so that you can kneel on it comfortably at either side of your partner.
- **Cushions or pillows** A couple of firm cushions will provide support for your partner's body.
- **Bolster** This will give additional support under the knees or the fronts of the ankles. Alternatively, you can use a rolled-up blanket.
- **Blanket cover** You may need to cover your partner at some point during the massage – their body temperature will drop as they become more relaxed.
- **Yoga blocks** A couple of foam blocks can be very helpful. They can be used as support either for your own posture or for your partner's, especially in the various seated positions.

WHAT TO WEAR
As Thai massage is a physical form of bodywork, you need to make sure that you are able to move very freely and easily, unrestricted by your clothing, while you are giving the massage treatment. You don't need any special clothing, but avoid anything with zips or buckles that could catch on your partner.

Your partner, the receiver, should also wear something unrestricting. Ideal garments are a t-shirt with sleeves and trousers rather than shorts. This is because covering up makes the acupressure part of the massage more comfortable to receive.

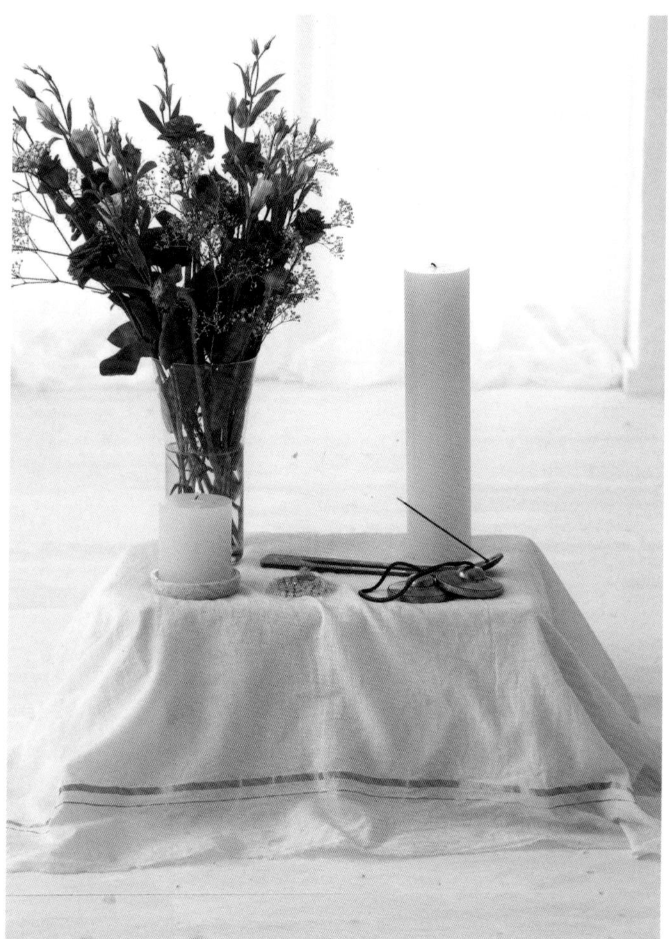

Above Making a shrine in the room where you give massage creates a sacred space. It is a personal place where you can honour elements that you feel are important to you within your practice.

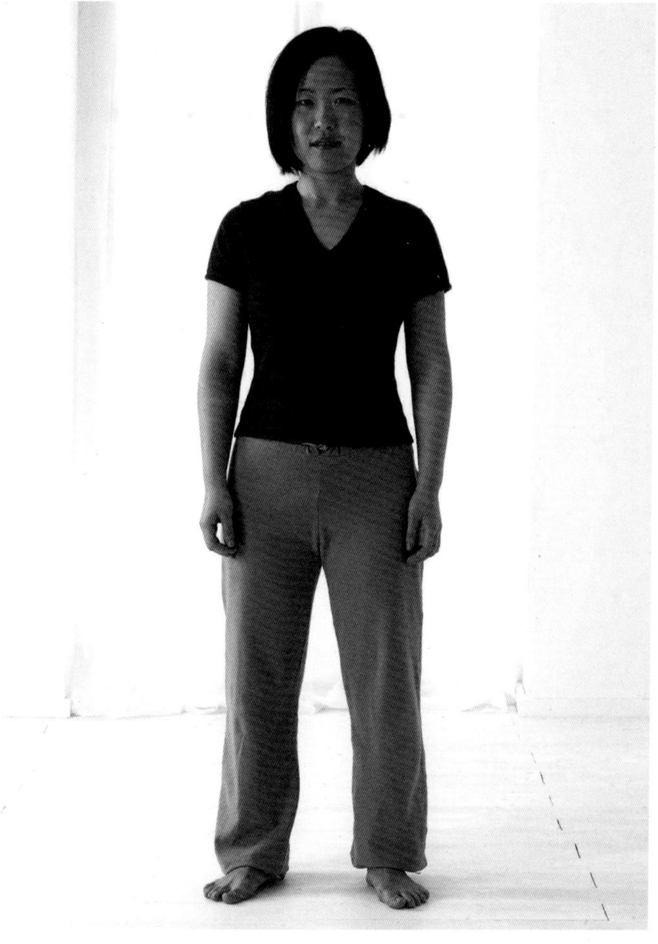

Above Wear something that is loose and comfortable for giving massage. Garments such as a simple t-shirt and stretchy tracksuit bottoms are perfectly adequate.

How to Use Your Body

Thai massage is a unique way of getting to know your body – whether you are giving or receiving. The beauty of this form of massage is that you are not restricted to the use of your hands alone. Thai massage uses the whole body, in soft, flowing movements, to create a kind of dance between giver and receiver.

Since Thai massage is a dynamic form of bodywork, it is important to focus on how to use the body safely and comfortably. The more at ease you, the giver, feel in your own body, the more relaxing the massage will be for the receiver. The following practical suggestions on posture will help to keep your body comfortable, so that the rhythmic, wavelike movements of the massage can flow freely and easily. Obviously, all the different exercises require different body positions, but it is useful to remember some general principles.

TERMS USED IN THIS BOOK

Throughout this book you will find specific terms that refer to ways of working in Thai massage.

- **Inside hand** As you face your partner, this is the hand that is closer to the midline of their body.
- **Outside hand** Facing your partner, this is the hand that is furthest from the midline of their body.
- **The fix** This describes the position of the part of your body that is securing a pose – this may be your hand, your foot, or any other part of your body.
- **Being square on to the body** When palming, thumbing or working an acupressure point, this means keeping your body at 90 degrees to your partner's. It makes efficient use of your body weight while protecting your own posture.
- **Keeping your body open to your partner's** A useful way of checking your body posture in any of the exercises is to make sure that your heart is open to your partner's heart, that your belly is open to their belly. These open positions support the principle of working with loving kindness.
- **Working with the breath** Exhale as you work into a stretch and inhale as you release away from it. As you work with the more dynamic stretches, try to coordinate your breathing rhythm with your partner's.

Caution

Some advanced positions appear in this book, to show the variety of poses that is possible, but you should only attempt them under the guidance of a professional teacher.

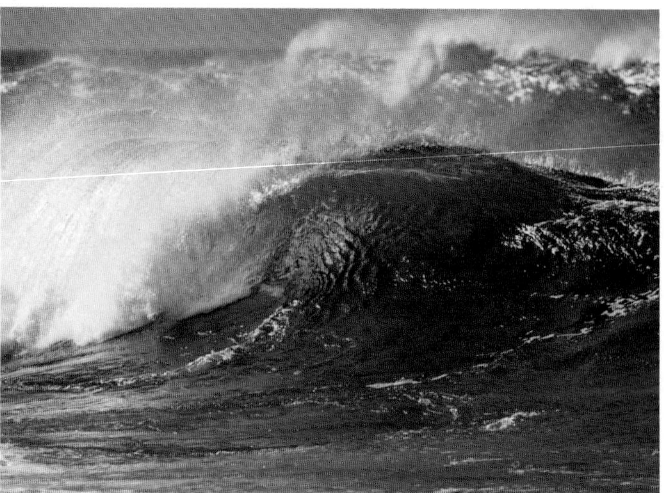

Above Like a wave ebbing and flowing, the rhythmic movement of leaning and releasing with the breath maintains a smooth and continuous flow throughout the massage, helping to unlock deeply held tensions within the body.

Getting it right

✗ Never press directly on to bone.

✓ Use your body weight, not your strength, and keep your back supported by a stable base. Bring your body weight up and over the area you are working, so that you can lean into your partner's body without any strain on your own.

✓ Get close to your partner. In order to use your body weight correctly you cannot give Thai massage at arm's length.

✓ Change your posture as often as you need to in order to stay comfortable. Be attentive to your own needs, too.

✓ Keep your movements economical: don't move your own or your partner's body unnecessarily. This helps you to see more clearly how exercises follow on from each other.

✓ Although you should work up and down the sen, the overall picture is of moving energy from the feet up towards the head.

✓ As a general rule, work in a measured and flowing way, with no sudden movements. Repeat each exercise about three times. Begin slowly and gently and work a little deeper with each repetition.

Wide-kneeling

Here, your base is wide and your centre of gravity is low. This is an extremely stable position that many people, especially beginners, find easy to use.

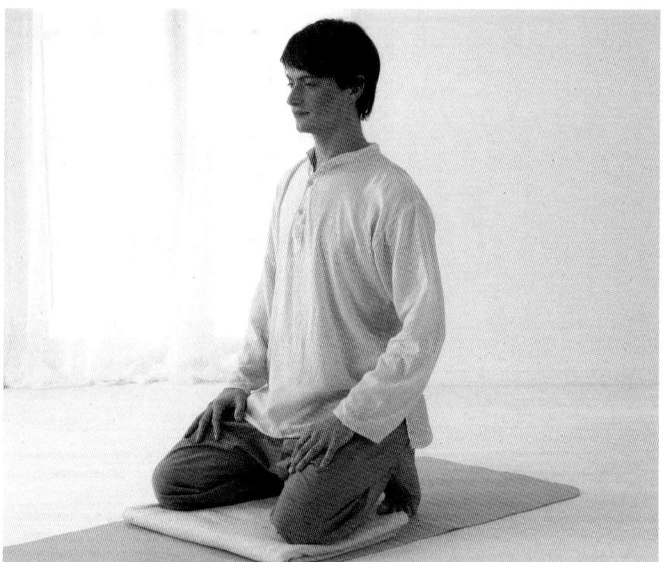

Above Keep your feet together and your knees apart. Remember to drop down through the tailbone, so you don't overextend into your lower back. You can alter your height very easily simply by tucking your toes under or sitting back on your heels.

Half-kneeling

This keeps your centre of gravity over the area you are working. The wide, stable base lets you overstep your partner without twisting your pelvis or back.

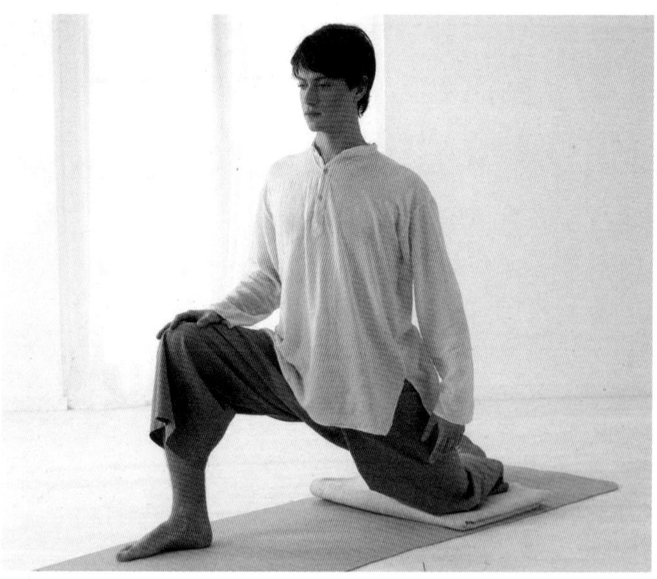

Above In this posture, focus on dropping down through the tip of your tailbone rather than lunging into the bent hip. Be prepared to change sides as often as you need to until, with increased practice, your hips open out more and your legs strengthen.

Palming

This technique applies general pressure to the sen and prepares the body for deeper energy work.

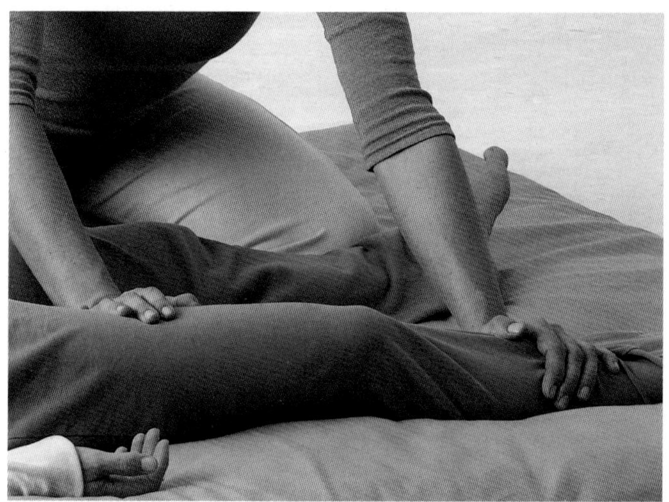

Above Use the padded part of the heel of your hand to apply most of the pressure and let your fingers relax around the body. Keep your arms straight, without locking the elbows. Relax your shoulders away from your ears. "Pour" your body weight down your arms so that the movement is slow and controlled. Gently rock your body weight from side to side, sinking into one palm then the other.

Thumbing

This technique is used for deeper energy work and for more focused pressure on the sen.

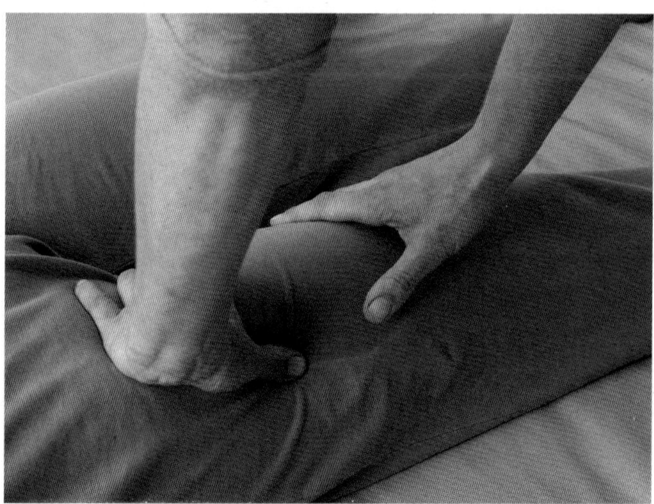

Above Use the soft, squashy part of your thumb rather than the point. To protect the thumb joint, spread the fingers wide for support and align the thumb with your wrist and elbow. Keep your arms straight but not locked and lean your body weight into one thumb and then the other, in a slow, rocking motion. Beginners may find that their thumbs ache, but practice should soon strengthen them.

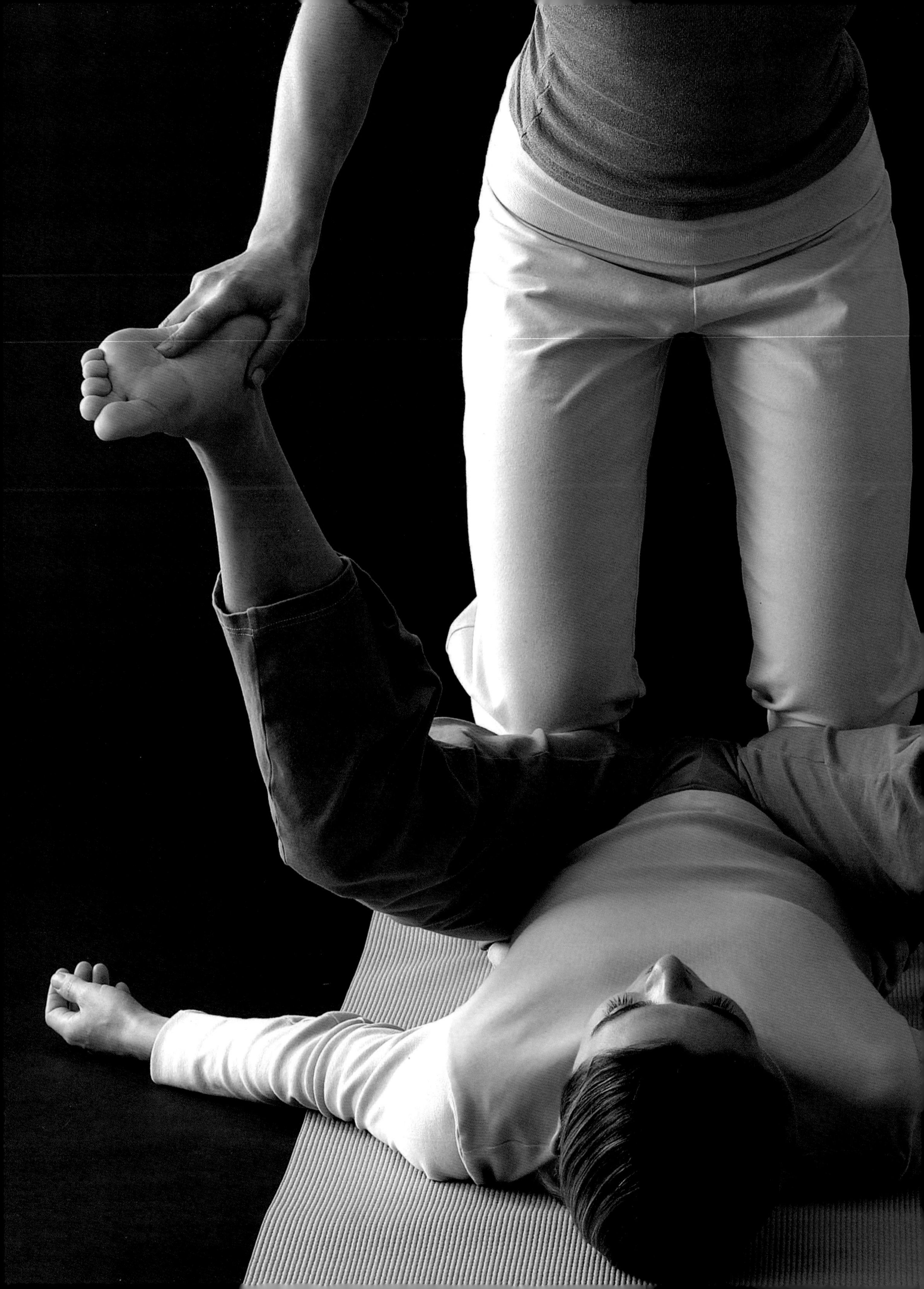

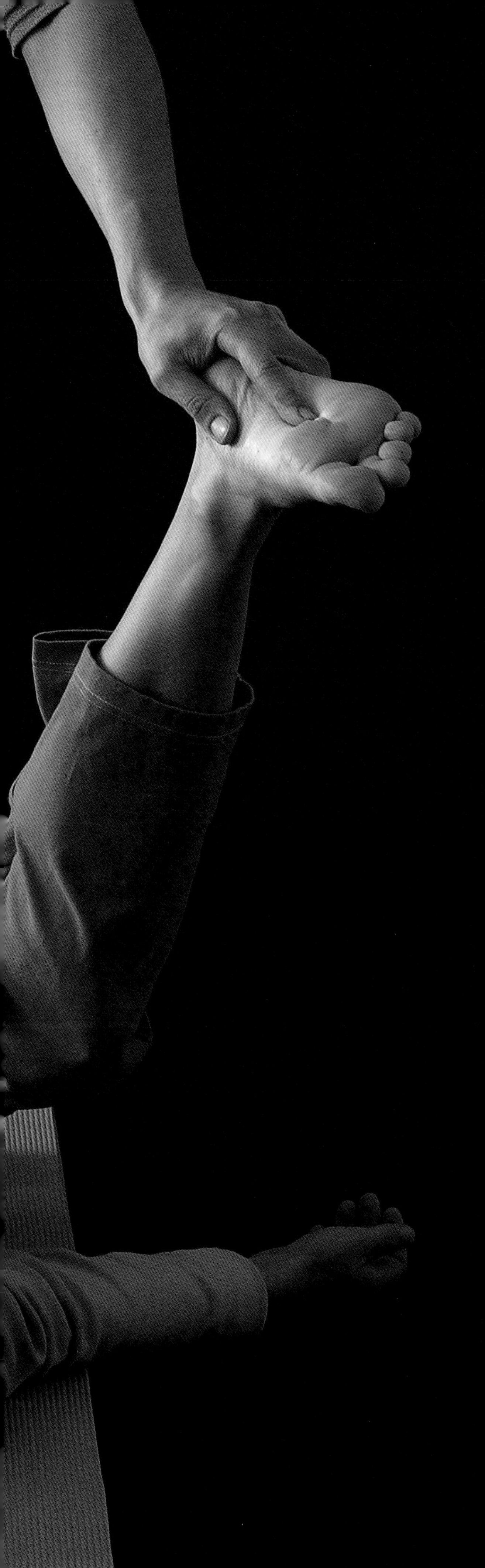

A Complete Body Routine

Traditionally, a full-body northern-style Thai massage lasts around two hours, flowing seamlessly from one part of the body to the next, moving energy from the feet towards the crown of the head. Nothing can replace this complete balancing of energy and the deep state of relaxation that follows. However, don't feel you always have to give a complete two-hour massage. A little goes a long way. Nor must you do all the exercises on every person – be guided by your partner's body type.

This chapter gives sequences for every part of the body and each ends with a visual summary – usually a selection of poses rather than a repeat of every one, to give an idea of the routine's overall flow. The sen on the artworks in this chapter are not multicolour-coded as at the start of the book, in order to focus on the main points being made. The chapter ends with routines for pregnancy and later life and for specific complaints.

Before You Start

This chapter will guide you through a complete full-body Thai massage. It focuses on one part of the body at a time, and it is suggested that you begin by practising each section separately. Take time to feel really comfortable and familiar with the work on each part of the body before trying to link all the sections together.

The sequence for each part of the body shows you how to open up the body gradually, moving from gentle exercises through to more dynamic stretches. The order of a Thai massage is not fixed: masseurs develop their own distinctive style and an experienced practitioner's treatments will vary from person to person. For a beginner, though, it is advisable to stick within the guidelines of this comprehensive structure, in order to give a complete and well-balanced massage.

COMMUNICATING WITH YOUR PARTNER

For a giver, the way to learn is to get feedback from your partner, so it is very important that you feel able to communicate freely during the massage. Although a significant aspect of Thai massage is the development of your intuitive skills and learning how to feel more sensitively with your hands, you are not a mind reader and you cannot expect to know how your partner is feeling. It is especially important when you are starting out as a masseur for you to ask your partner how the pressure and strength of the stretches feel for them.

As the giver, find out how much feedback is useful for you. Experiment and reach your own level – one that is helpful but that will not interfere with the experience of giving or receiving, and which allows space for silence and stillness within the massage. Take time at the end of each session to share what you enjoyed or didn't enjoy, so that you can learn from the experience.

ASSESSING YOUR PARTNER'S NEEDS

Thai massage is a powerful form of bodywork. It is a dynamic massage and involves passive stretching and mobilizing of the joints. You should be aware that not all the techniques in this book are suitable for everyone. So, before you start, it is essential to ask the right questions to find out about the state of your partner's health and how they are feeling. This will help you to decide on an appropriate and safe selection of exercises.

Massage is one of the oldest of the healing arts. If someone is in pain or suffering from illness or injury, its nurturing touch is a wonderfully supportive way of helping the body to heal itself. However, in the beginning, try to find a partner who is not suffering from any specific ailment, as it is easier and safer to explore the techniques on a healthy body. Remember, too, that you as the giver need to look after yourself throughout the treatment. There is no point in taking care of your partner's body if you take no care of your own.

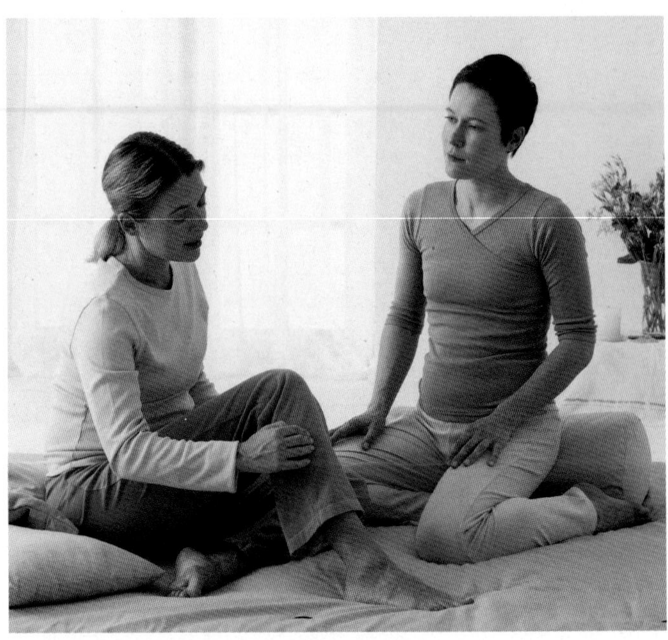

Above It's very important to ask the right questions to find out about your partner's health.

QUESTIONS TO ASK

The issue of contraindications is complex, and best assessed by a qualified practitioner with the skills and experience to judge what is and is not suitable for an individual. These general questions can help guide you but if you feel in any doubt about an exercise, don't do it. Specific dos and don'ts will be mentioned in each section.

- **Does your partner have any injuries?** You need to be particularly aware of spinal injuries and joint problems. Moving a damaged joint in the wrong way can be very dangerous. Avoid mobilizing any area of the body that is injured, inflamed or painful. Avoid pressing on bruises, cuts or recently healed wounds.

- **Is your partner muscle-bound?** Do they suffer from chronic tension? If your partner has very bound or tense muscles, don't press too hard or stretch too deeply as this will be counter-productive for them. It is more beneficial to do repeated energy line work and to introduce some easy stretches, so that you give your partner a feeling of release and ease.

- **Is your partner ill?** If their immune system is already working to combat illness, massage can sometimes be too much for the body to cope with.

- **Is your partner sensitive to pain?** Thai massage can be strong but should never be painful. Sometimes areas of the body that are unused to massage can feel highly sensitive to strong pressure. It can be very beneficial to work these areas provided you work within your partner's limits and encourage them to use their out-breath to help dissipate the strong sensations. If your partner is unable to do this, ease off the pressure and work more gently. The rule is that any feelings of "pain" should ease immediately after taking the pressure off the body.

- **Is your partner pregnant?** Many women find massage a wonderful means of relaxation throughout their pregnancy, but the routine shown in this book is not suitable for pregnancy. A full-body Thai massage for a pregnant woman must be given by a qualified professional. There is, however, a section at the end of this chapter highlighting some simple techniques that can be very beneficial and relaxing during pregnancy.

- **Does your partner have any specific medical conditions?** If your partner is suffering from any condition – and particularly if they need to take medication – they should consult their medical practitioner for advice before receiving massage.

The First Steps

You are now ready to start a Thai massage treatment. Give yourself plenty of time to enjoy these opening stages. You will soon discover that they are as important as the massage itself.

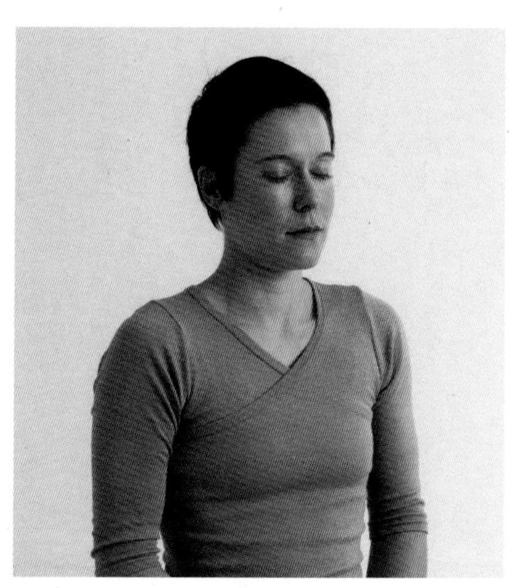

1 Quietening your mind Enjoy a moment of stillness with yourself. Listen closely to the coming and going of your breath. Allow your centre of gravity to settle. Relax. Notice how you are feeling in your body. Let yourself rest in this moment. Tuning into how you feel before you make contact with your partner can really help you to stay centred and grounded throughout the massage. It also gives space for your partner to settle into stillness.

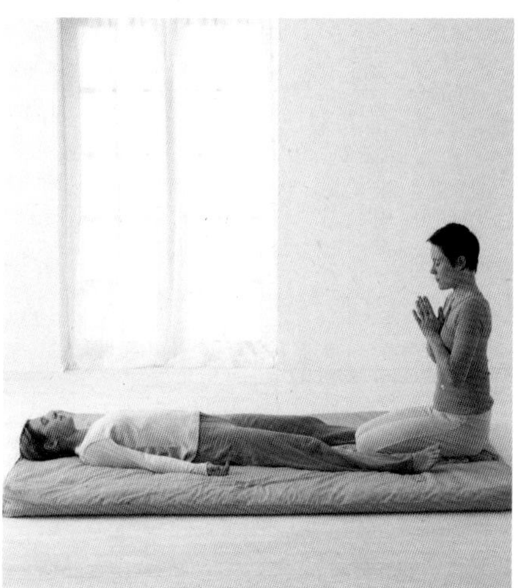

2 The opening prayer Traditionally, each Thai massage begins with a prayer to the founder of Thai medicine, Jivaka Kumar Bhaccha. This moment of prayer acknowledges the deep spiritual roots of Thai massage and helps you to open to what is beyond rational thought. It can also be used as a moment to invite a deeper healing potential into your work.

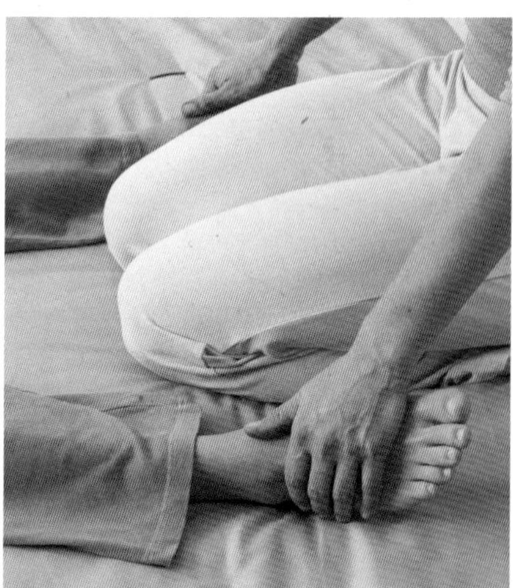

3 Making the first touch The quality of the first touch is important as it sets the tone of the whole massage. Your hands should be warm and dry and your touch should be firm but gentle, helping your partner to feel safe and relaxed.

The Feet

Our feet are our roots, our point of contact with the earth. They carry and support us in all our movements, so they play an enormous part in maintaining a healthy posture. Just like the foundations of a building, our feet provide a solid foundation for the body. Working on them is very grounding, helping to bring your partner out of their head and into their body. The majority of people enjoy having their feet massaged, so it is an excellent place to start for those who may be apprehensive about receiving a full-body massage treatment.

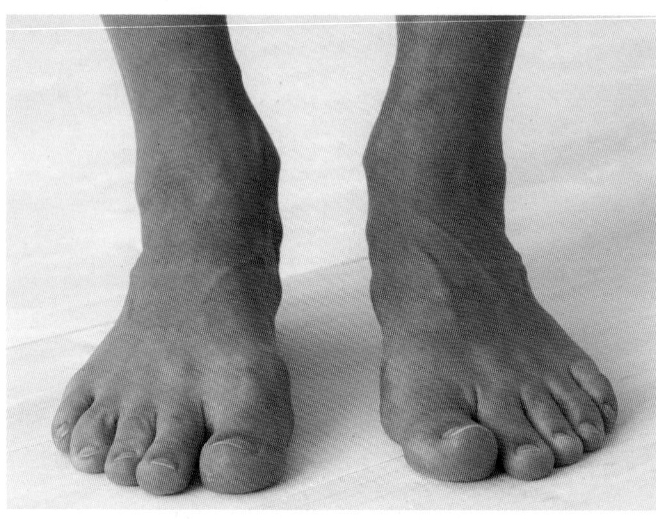

Above The feet are a vital part of our body, constantly carrying every movement and, quite literally, grounding us.

Getting it right

✗ Avoid pressing directly on cuts and bruises.

✓ Proceed with extreme caution if your partner has suffered any broken toes.

✗ If a joint is inflamed or painful because of arthritis, don't massage.

✓ Having some talc to hand for sticky hands and feet can make the foot massage more comfortable.

✓ Approach with a confident, firm touch, as some people can be ticklish or sensitive in the feet.

REFLEXOLOGY CHART

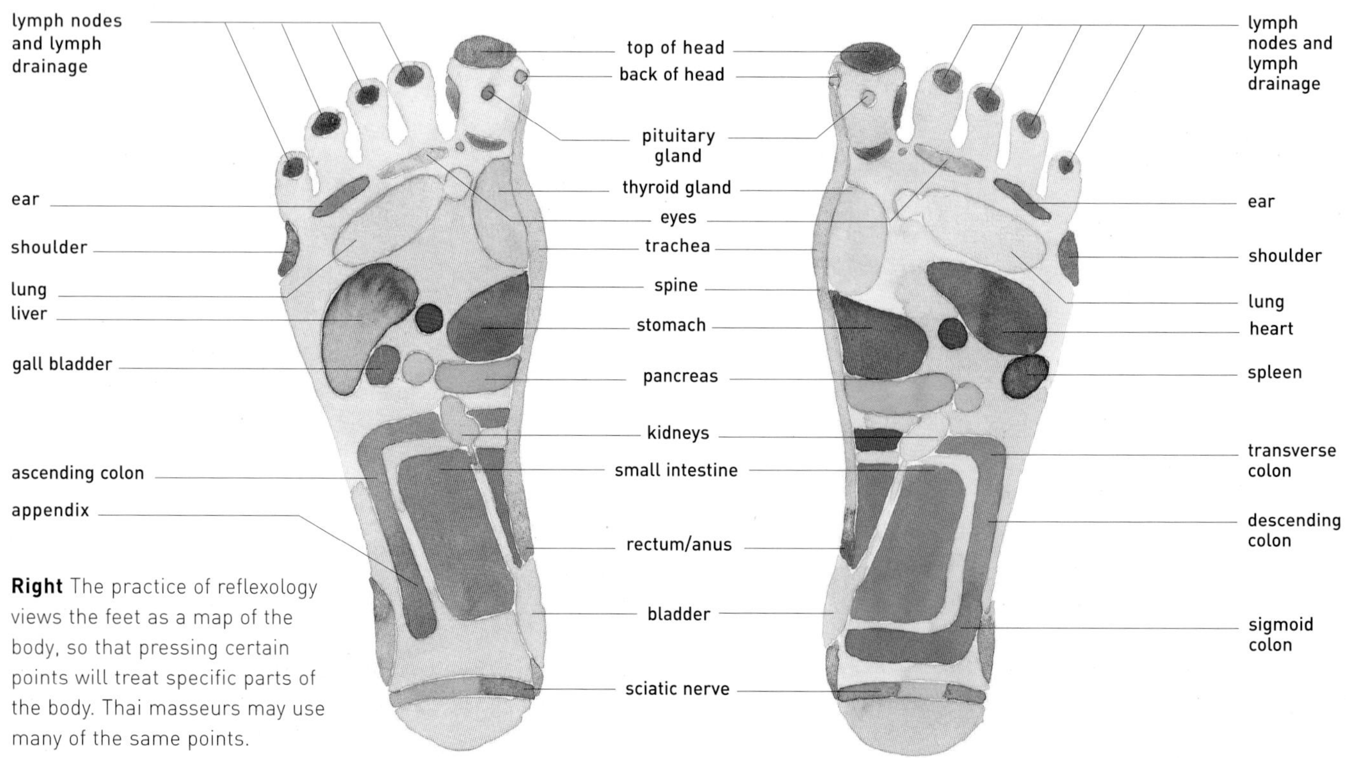

Right The practice of reflexology views the feet as a map of the body, so that pressing certain points will treat specific parts of the body. Thai masseurs may use many of the same points.

Preparing the Feet

These first four steps warm up the feet in preparation for deeper, more focused work. They also open up the ankles, which starts to open the hips gently. In this sequence work both feet simultaneously. Start near the ankle joint and work out towards the toes.

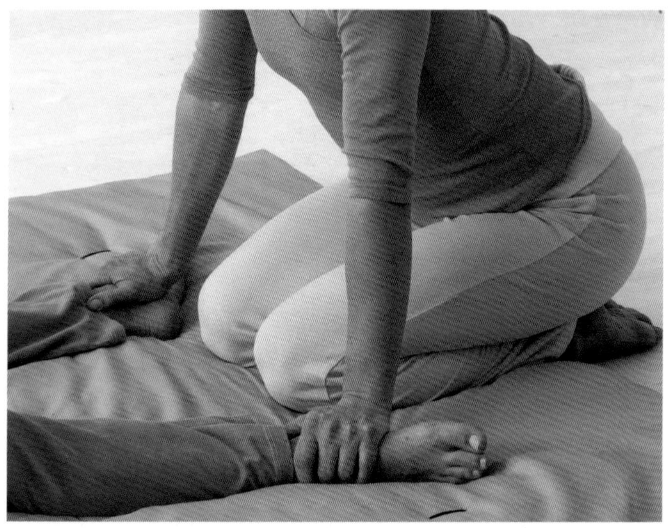

1 Warming up the instep Using the padded part of each hand, palm the whole instep up and down in a rhythmic rocking motion, leaning into and releasing out of the pressure. Begin near the heel and stop before you get to the ball of the big toe joint. Repeat several times until you feel the feet relax.

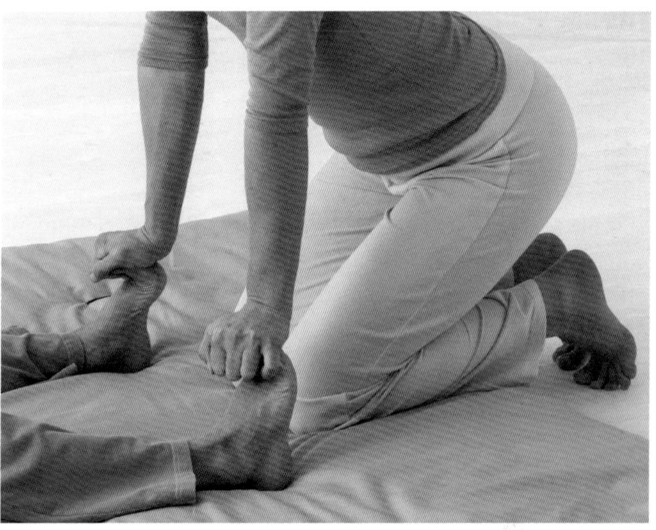

2 Opening the soles This stretch wakes up the foot. Place the heel of each hand, fingers pointing upwards, against the ball of your partner's foot, creating a point of resistance. Bend your elbows into your body and push against the sole of each foot so you see the whole leg move up into the hip socket. Maintain this resistance and slide your palms up until your fingers wrap over the toes. Now lean in and release. Repeat three times without changing your hand position. Use your body weight; your partner will tell you if it feels too much.

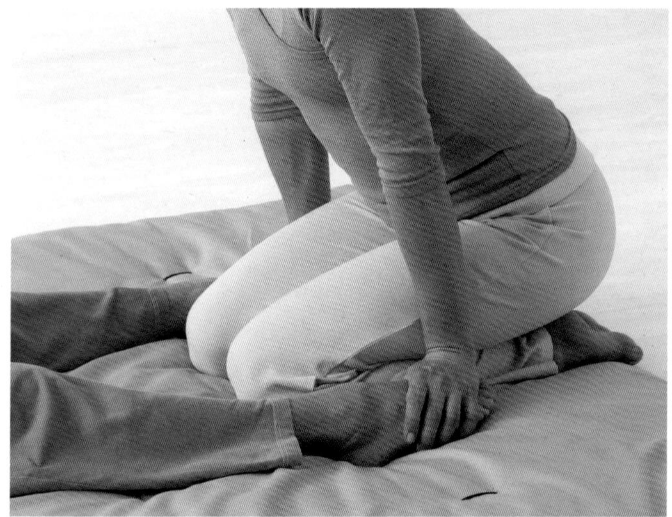

3 Lengthening the front of the feet This exercise will help to open up the front of the ankles while stimulating the energy lines that run through the top of the feet. Place your palms on top of your partner's feet, near the ankle joints. Lean down and slightly away, lengthening the front of each foot towards the ground. Now release and repeat, moving your hands down towards your partner's toes.

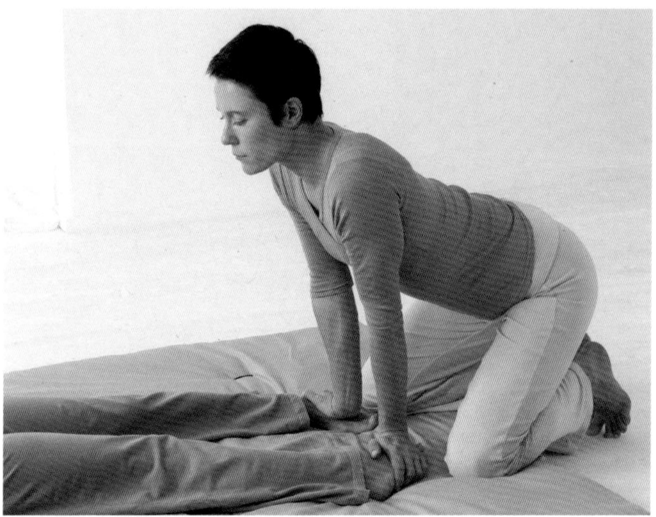

4 Opening the ankles and hips This is a wonderful position to open the hips while increasing mobility through the ankle joint. Cup your hands under the heels. Lift and lengthen the legs, turning the heels out and the feet in as you do so. Reposition your hands to fix on the tops of the feet, lean in with your body weight and lengthen the toes towards each other. See how the hips are affected.

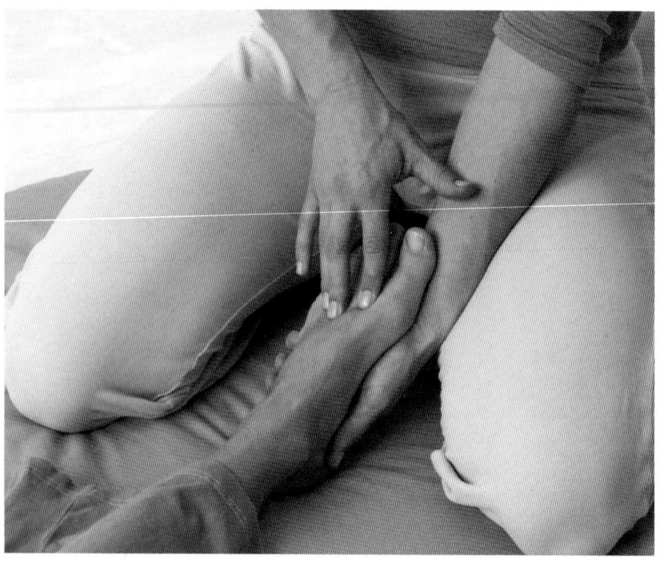

5 Working the top of the foot Keep the foot resting on the floor. Use one hand to support the sole and with the other work in between the tendons. You can use the flats of your fingers or your thumbs for a deeper pressure. This is an excellent way to work many valuable pressure points and create space throughout the front of the foot.

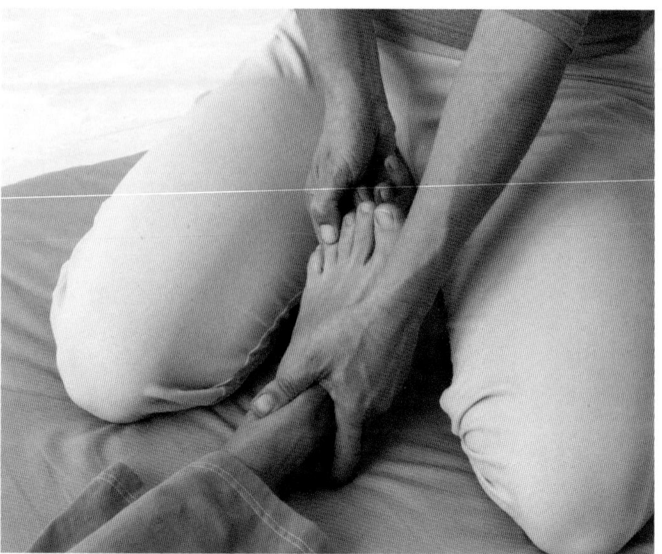

6 Squeezing the toes This produces a very satisfying feeling and lends a sense of completeness to the foot massage. Before you start, check for broken toes or arthritic joints and proceed with caution. Most arthritic joints benefit from mobilization as long as they are not currently inflamed.

Hold the foot firmly with one hand. With the other hand, work from the centre of the foot, squeezing and rubbing around all the joints of each toe. Work right to the tip of the toe and give the end a gentle pinch.

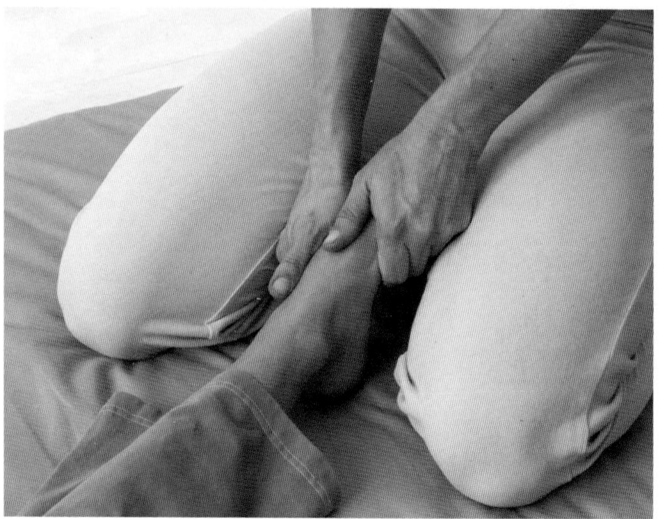

7 Kneading the foot This is wonderful way to relax the foot completely. The basic movement is a simple squeezing and releasing motion. Always start closest to the ankle joint and work out and away towards the toes. You can work both hands simultaneously or alternately. There is no fixed technique, so explore and enjoy.

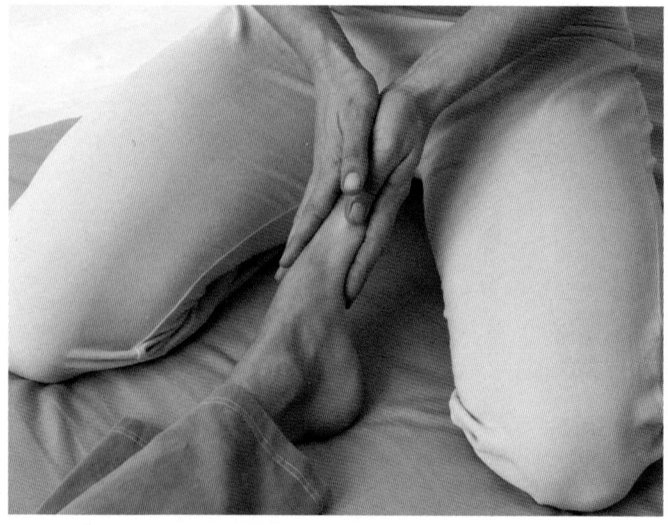

8 Sweeping off the foot Finish the foot massage by smoothing the skin with a swift brushing movement. Hold the foot firmly yet gently between your hands and sweep from the ankle joint to the tips of the toes. Repeat two or three times.

Review: the Feet

Now repeat the sequence on the other foot – use the pictures below as a reminder of all the steps. Remember to use your bodyweight as much as possible rather than your strength, keeping your shoulders relaxed and your breath even.

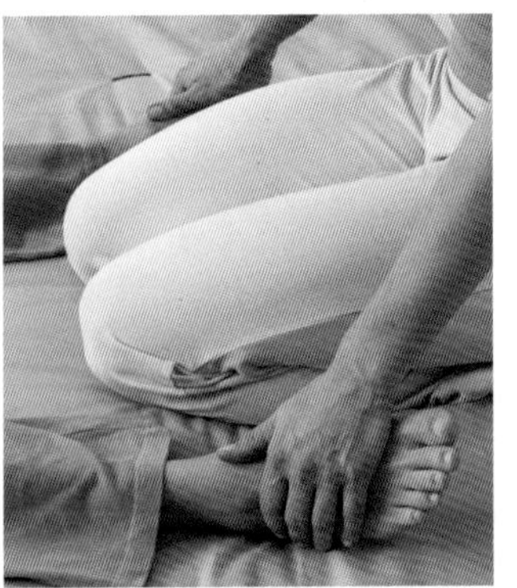

Making the first touch

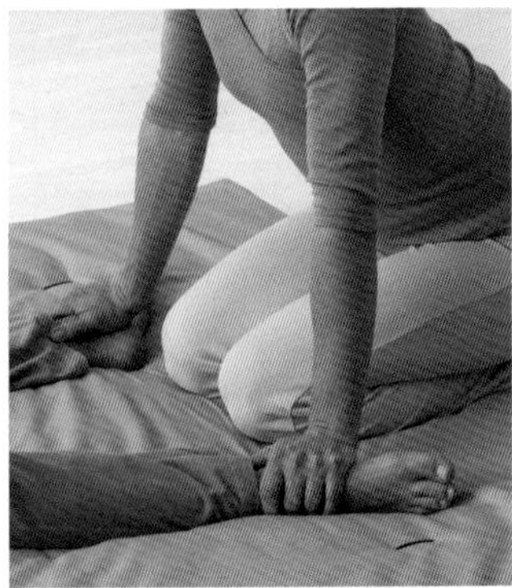

Warming up the instep

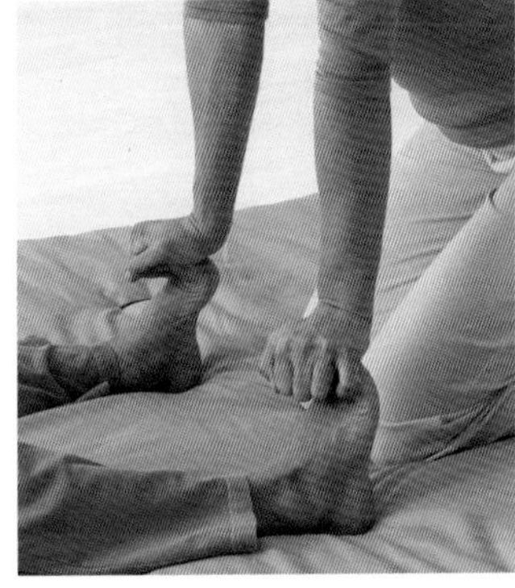

Opening the soles

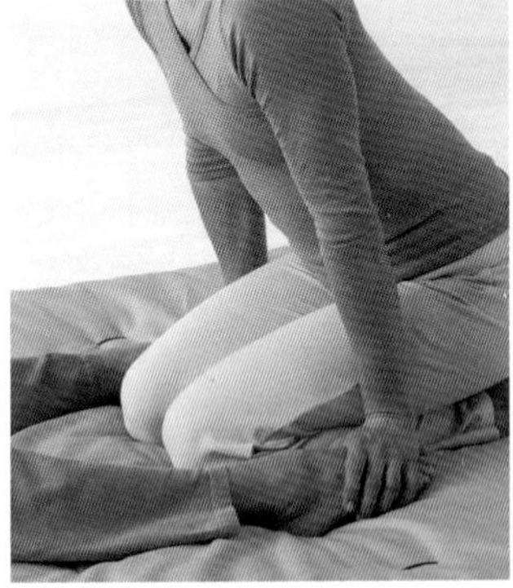

Lengthening the front

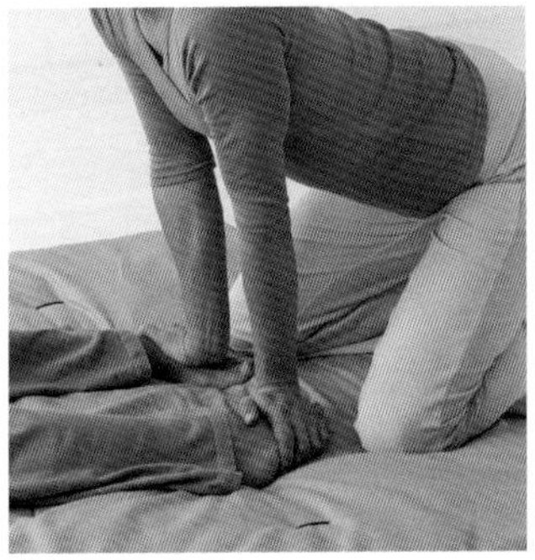

Opening the ankles and hips

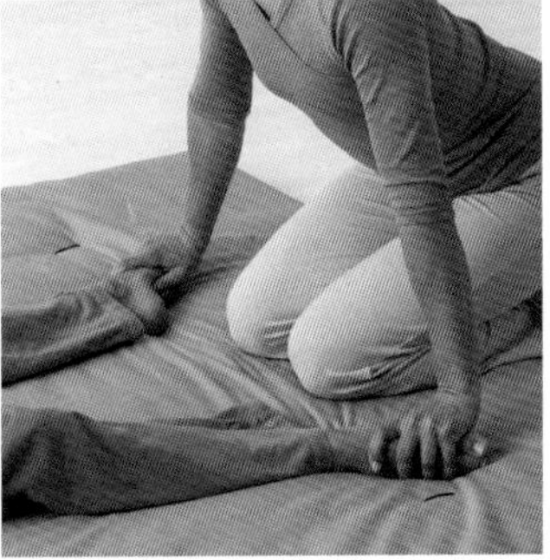

Thumbing

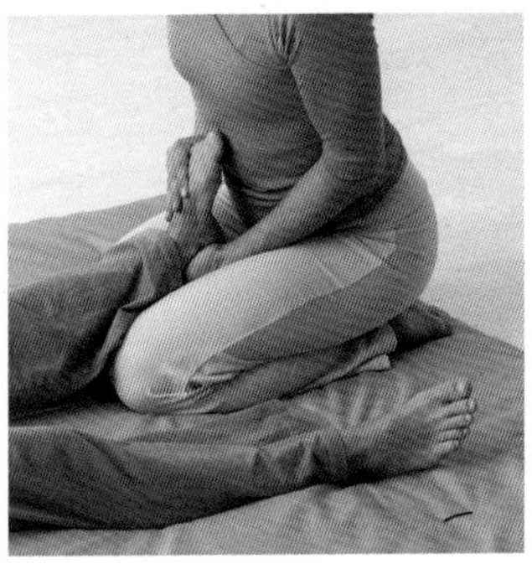

Ankle circles

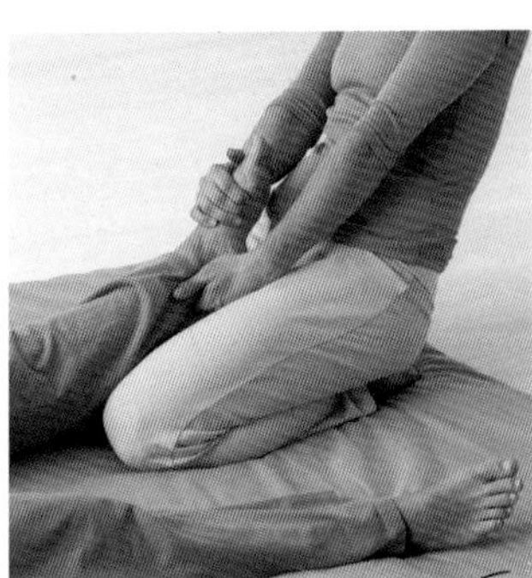

Twisting outwards

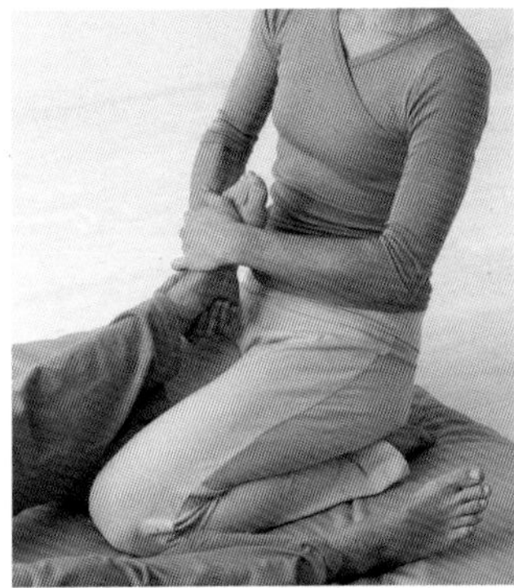

Twisting inwards

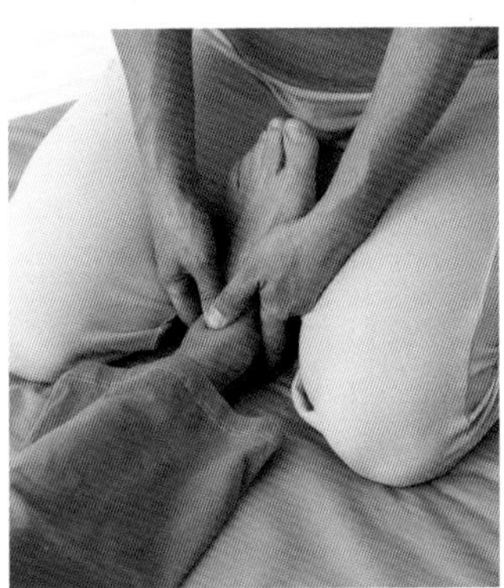

Knee pain point

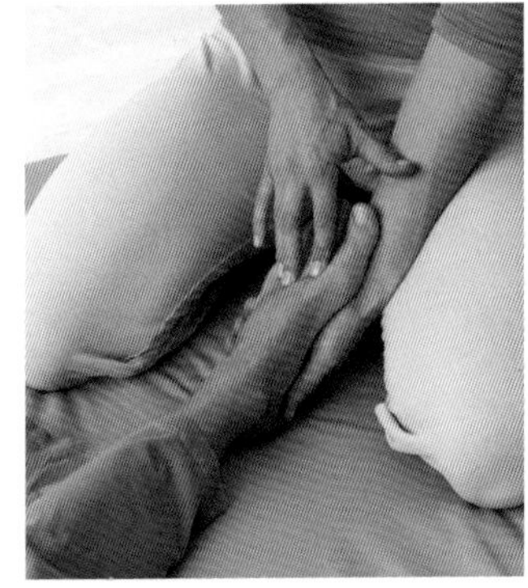

Working the top of the foot

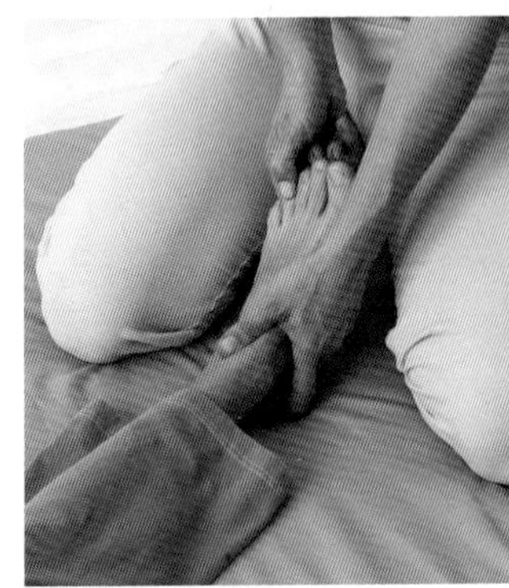

Squeezing the toes

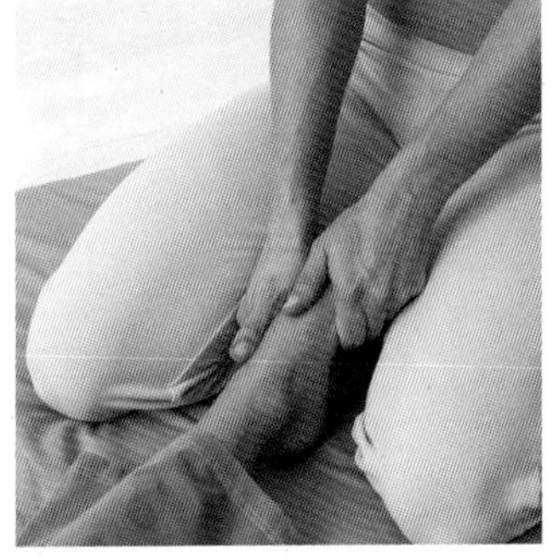

Kneading

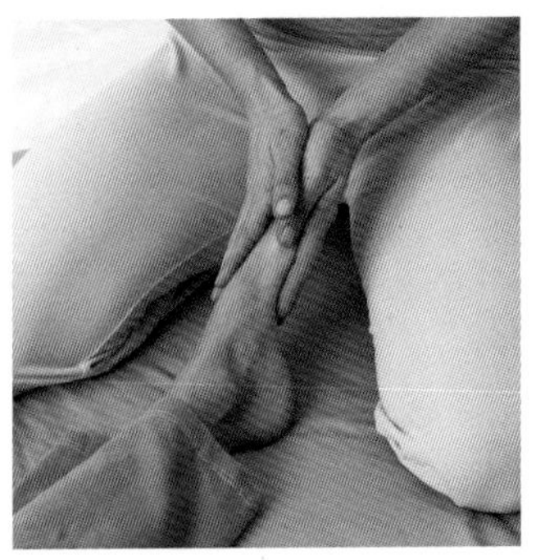

Sweeping off

Caution

People's feet take quite a pounding in everyday life and painful foot complaints of all kinds are very common, so always progress carefully prior to treatment. Examine your partner's feet thoroughly before you start and ask them about any problems. Can you see any cuts, bruises or swollen areas? Never press on these and avoid any joints affected by arthritis. Proceed with great care if any toes have been broken recently or in the past.

The Legs

Work on the energy lines of the legs stimulates the circulation of energy and blood. It eases tiredness and heaviness in the lower half of the body, giving renewed support for the legs and, in turn, for the rest of the body. It releases tension in the lower back and starts to open up the hips and pelvis for the deeper stretches. If worked slowly and rhythmically, the palming and thumbing of these lines can be deeply relaxing, laying the foundations for the rest of the massage.

Whichever side you chose to work first with the feet, start again on the same side for the legs. Always begin by working the inside of the leg: this will be on the leg that is furthest away from you. Palm all the lines on the inside leg first, then thumb all the lines and finish with another round of palming. When you have completed all the palming and thumbing here, repeat this pattern on the outside of the leg that is closest to you. Then, get up and move to the other side of your partner's body and repeat the sequence.

THE SEN OF THE LEGS

For demonstration purposes, the energy lines shown on the artwork (right) are numbered 1, 2 and 3 on the inside of the legs and 1 and 2 on the outside. There is a third line on the outside but it is more easily worked later, when your partner is lying on their side.

Inside leg

Line 1 runs from the anklebone along the underside of the shinbone to the knee. Above the knee, it begins at the lower edge of the kneecap and continues up the thigh to the groin. *Line 2* runs through the centre of the inside of the leg, from the depression below the anklebone into the soft, fleshy part of the calf and up to the knee. On the thigh it follows the more yielding groove of the muscle.
Line 3 begins at the back of the leg, on the Achilles tendon, and runs up the centre of the back of the calf, directly behind the knee. On the thigh, it continues just above the big tendon and runs up to the groin.

Outside leg

Line 1, from the masseur's point of view, starts at the knee pain point (see page 41) and continues – just outside the shinbone between the bone and the muscle – up to the knee. It then continues up the thigh from the outside edge of the kneecap; relax your hand to follow the line right up to the outside of the hip. *Line 2* is close to line 1. It starts just above the anklebone and runs up between the two bones of the shin, in the groove between the muscles. On the thigh, it starts a thumb's width lower than the first line and runs up to the head of the thighbone at the top of the leg.

WORKING THE LEG LINES

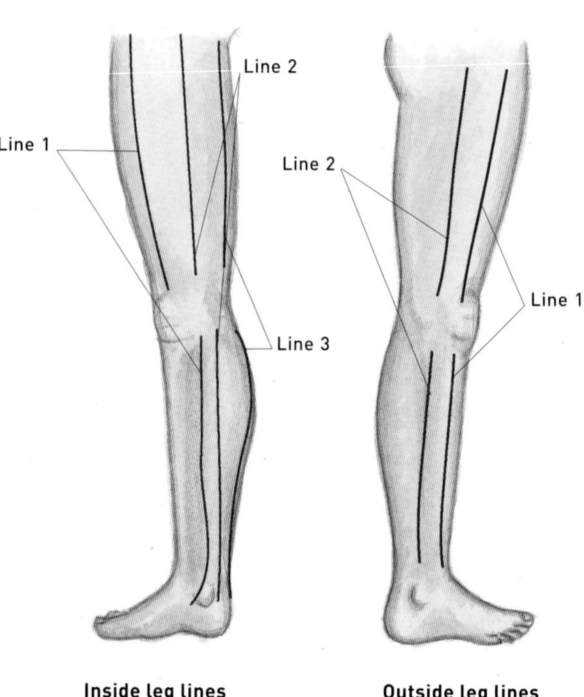

Above These two diagrams illustrate the path taken by the main sen energy lines in the legs – on the inner and outer leg.

Getting it right

✗ Do not press directly on to:
- bone
- any varicose vein (work only above the area under pressure)
- the knee (work gently either side of it)
- the groin area (this is painful and intrusive)

✓ Check the pressure and work sensitively. Each person has different levels of sensitivity and the pressure should be deep but never painful. If it feels strong, encourage your partner to focus on their breathing and to enjoy the new sensation of an energy workout for the legs.

✓ Remember to check for bruises and cuts; if the legs are covered you may not see them.

✓ Take care of your own posture. If you find yourself twisting to reach up and down the leg, move your body until you are square on to your partner's leg.

Palming and Thumbing the Legs

Steps 1–4 form a short distinct sequence that you can do first on one leg and then on the other. Different legs are seen being worked below, to show the poses from the clearest angles. Find a comfortable position and feel free to adjust it as you work.

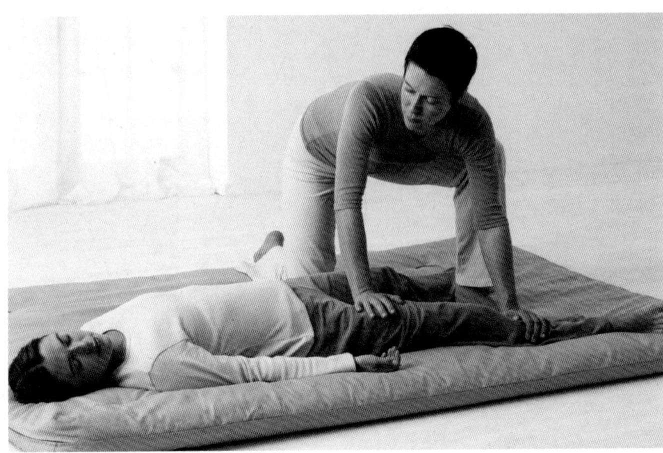

1 Palming the inside leg Begin with one hand near the ankle and one on the thigh just above the knee. Shift your body weight from side to side in a slow, rhythmic rocking motion, palming your hands up and down line 1. Repeat with lines 2 and 3.

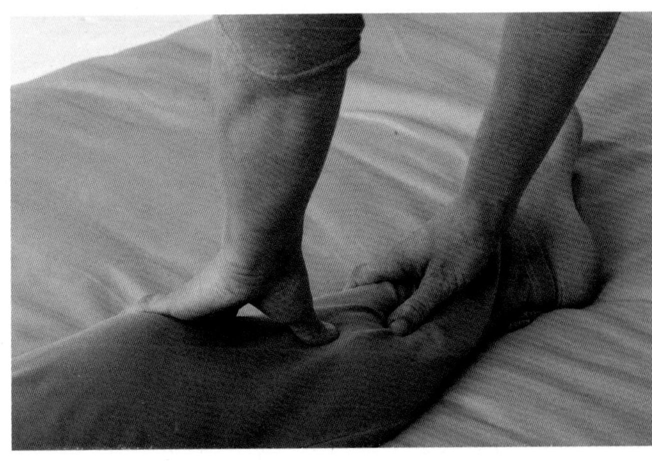

2 Thumbing the inside leg As the pressure is deeper here, check that it is comfortable for your partner. Start with one thumb at the ankle joint and the other about a thumb's length away. Walk the thumbs up and down line 1. Repeat with lines 2 and 3.

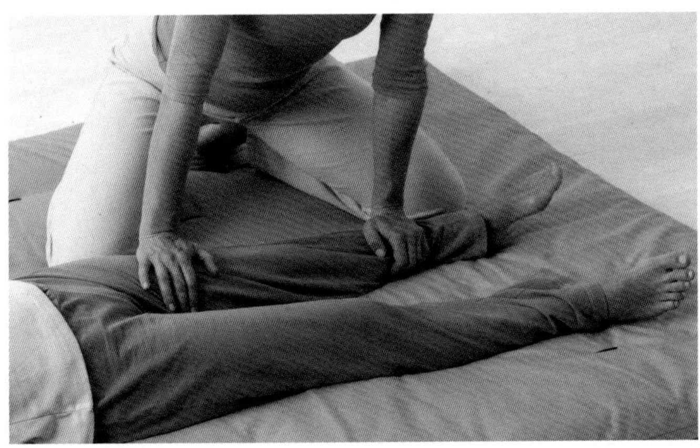

3 Palming and thumbing the outside leg Palm, and then thumb, lines 1 and 2 of the outside leg. (You may find that you want to change your body posture when you work the outside.)

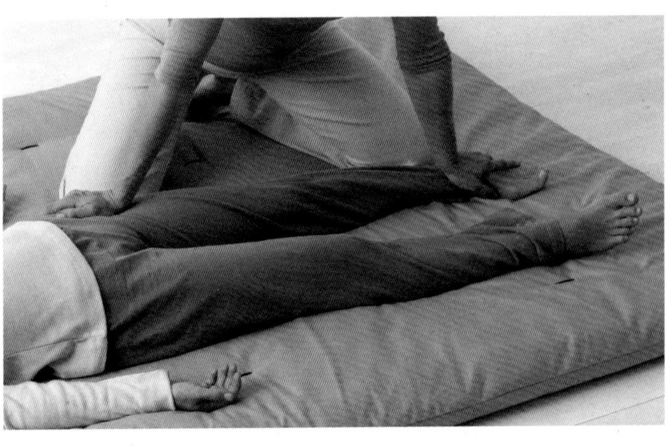

4 Stretching the outside of the leg To complete the work on one side of the body, lengthen and stretch the outside of the leg before moving around to the other side of your partner's body to repeat the palming and thumbing from the other side. Fix one hand on the outside of the hip and the other on top of the foot. Now lean in and release. Repeat two or three times.

Getting into the flow
When palming, keep your breathing even, free and smooth. One way to develop a good rhythm is to sing to yourself. For example, the carol *Silent Night* has the rocking rhythm of a lullaby, mirroring the sinking and releasing that gives energy line work its relaxing quality.

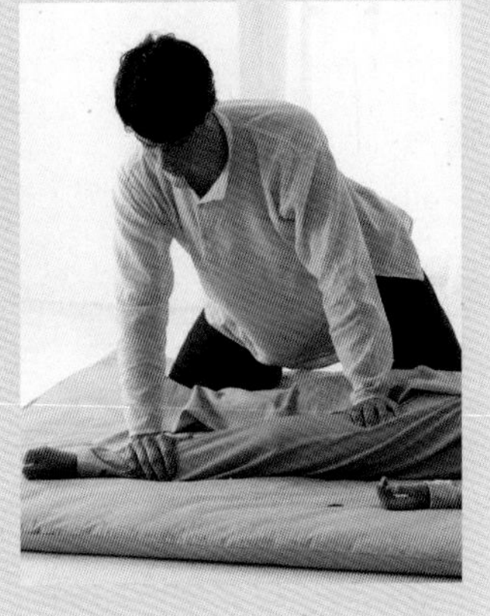

Technique tips
To palm, keep the lower hand on the calf, and the upper one on the thigh. Use the same smooth rocking motion for both palming and thumbing.

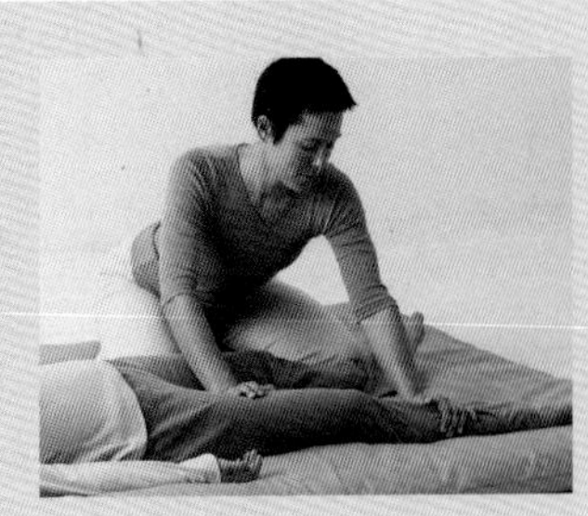

Single Leg Exercises

Like the feet, our legs help to ground and connect us to the earth. Northern-style Thai massage places a strong emphasis on working the legs. This sequence releases blocked energy and deeply held tension in the joints of the legs and the pelvis, bringing about deep feelings of release. Run through all the exercises on one leg and then repeat the sequence on the other leg.

As you work, keep your body movements economical and use your body weight to achieve the full depth of every stretch and line workout. If you have done the foot exercises prior to these single leg exercises, then start with the leg that is on the same side of the body. So, if you began your foot routine with the left foot, then work the left leg first.

Getting it right

✓ Check with your partner for any joint injuries, especially to the knee. Work with sensitivity and awareness and if in doubt leave it out.

✓ Keep communicating: as you are progressing to more dynamic stretches, it is important that your partner gives you plenty of feedback.

✓ Try to keep the movement flowing between each posture so that the sequence begins to feel like one continuous movement.

Relaxing the Leg

This sequence is beneficial for stiffness in the lower back, immobile hip joints and tightness in the legs. The energy line work on the thighs will not only relax that part of the legs, but will also rejuvenate tired knees.

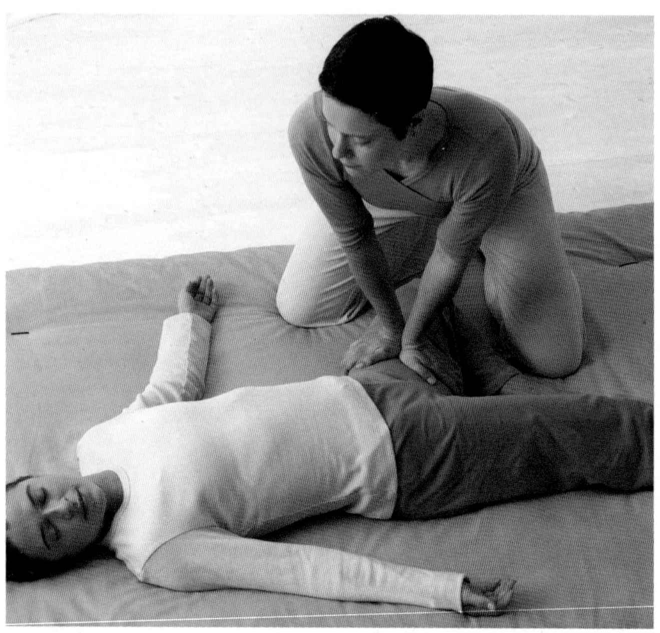

1 The tree Bend your partner's leg so that their knee falls out to the side. If the knee does not easily reach the ground, support it with a cushion. Align your body with your partner's knee. Place the heels of your hands in the centre of the thigh, close to the hip joint, and lean your body weight in and out. Adjust your hand position, working up and down the thigh. Avoid working too close to the knee joint.

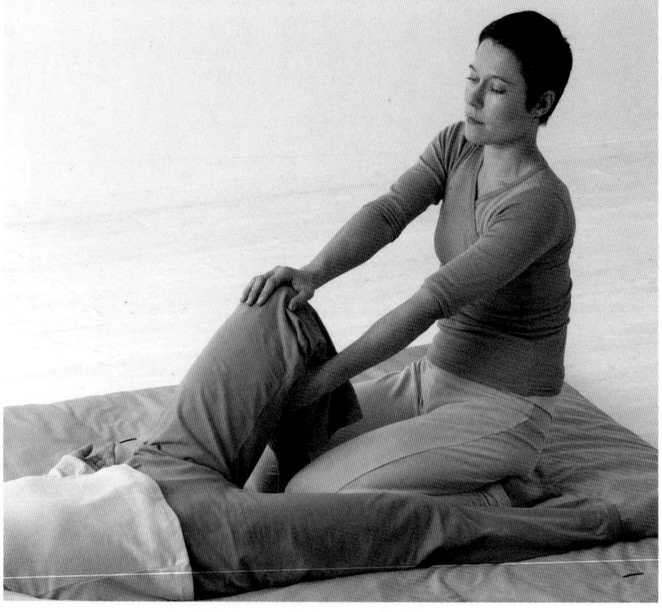

2 Relax the calf Bring your partner's knee upright, placing their foot on the floor and securing it between your knees. Support the knee with one hand and clasp the other around the bulk of the calf muscle, scooping it away from the bone and leaning back at the same time. Change the fixing of your hands and work the calf from the other side. Make three or four scoops up and down the calf muscle.

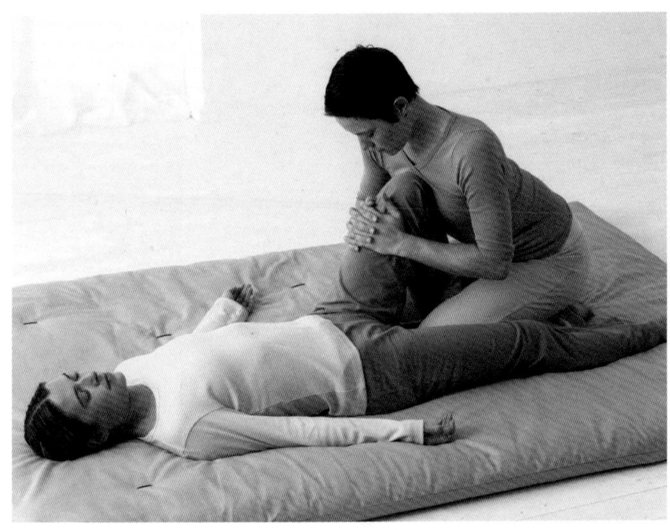

3 Butterfly squeeze: palming Keeping the knee upright, move closer so that your breastbone rests upon it. Clasp your hands together like butterfly wings and then place the heels of your hands on inside line 1 and outside line 1. Let your elbows drop and then gently squeeze your palms together. Work up and down the thigh two or three times.

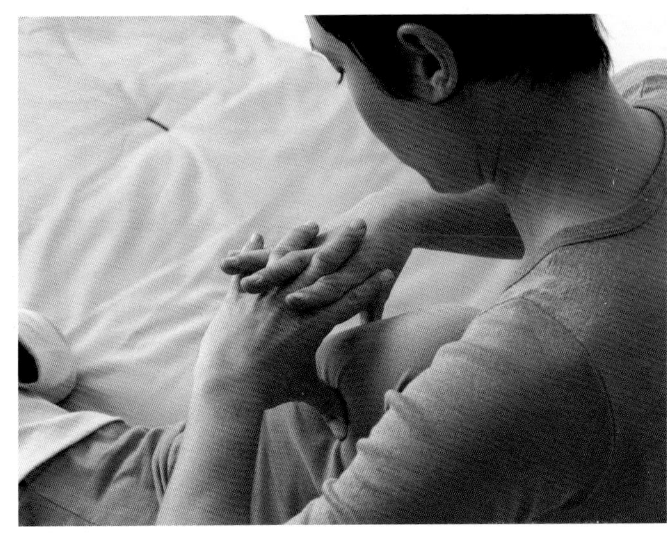

4 Butterfly squeeze: thumbing This exerts deeper pressure on the lines of the thighs. Unclasp your fingers a little and place your thumbs along the inside and outside lines of the thigh. Using your elbows as levers, gently squeeze your thumbs, working up and down the leg as before.

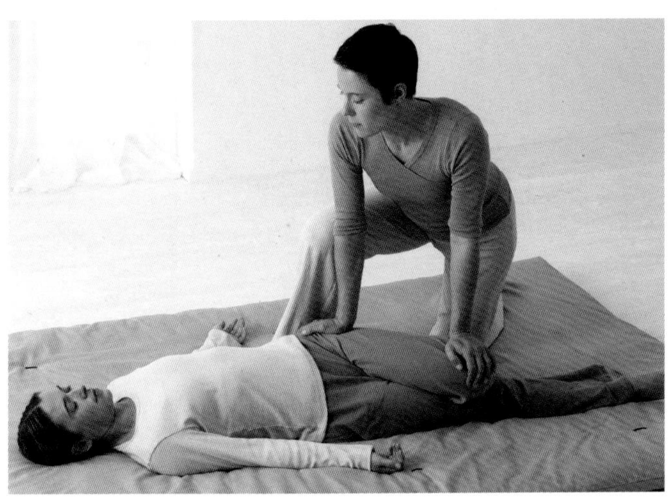

5 Cross hip stretch This exercise opens up the outside of the hip. Keep the foot where it is and let the knee drop across the outstretched leg. It is important to fix the knee in place with one hand, as any movement in this joint feels very uncomfortable. With your free hand, palm around your partner's hip and down the outside of the thigh. Start close to the hip joint and work towards the knee. Repeat three times.

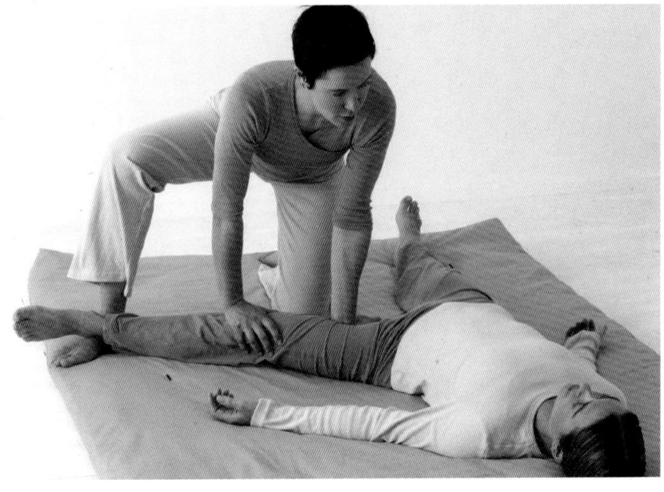

6 Open leg stretch This opens the inner thigh and groin. Straighten your partner's leg and move their foot out to the side. Be aware of any strain behind the knee and don't take the leg to the edge of their stretch. To fix the leg, place one hand gently over your partner's knee. With the other hand, starting close to the hip, palm up and down the third inside line of the thigh. Do not press too close to the knee joint.

Step 5 tip

If the knee will not drop across easily for the cross hip stretch, place a cushion between the knee and lower leg to support it.

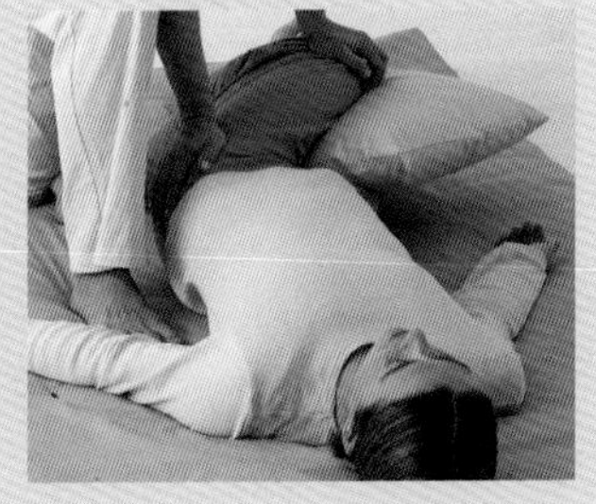

Step 6 tip

Support your partner's foot by placing their Achilles tendon against your knee pain point. This keeps their leg elevated slightly off the ground.

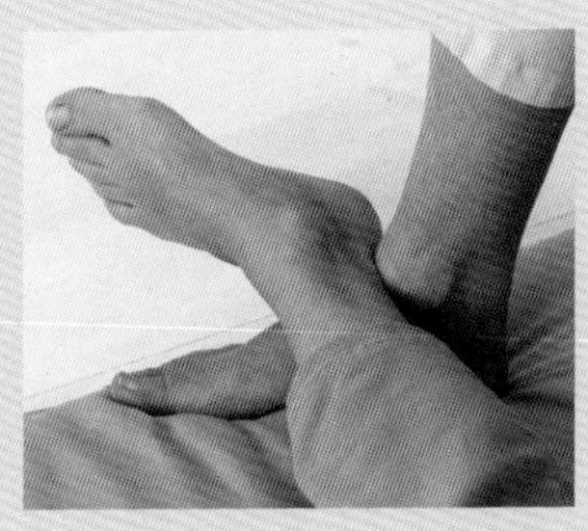

Opening the Hips and Groin

The following exercises are wonderful for all body types. They help to release energy held in the hips and groin and also start the process of stimulating the energy flow up into the lower back.

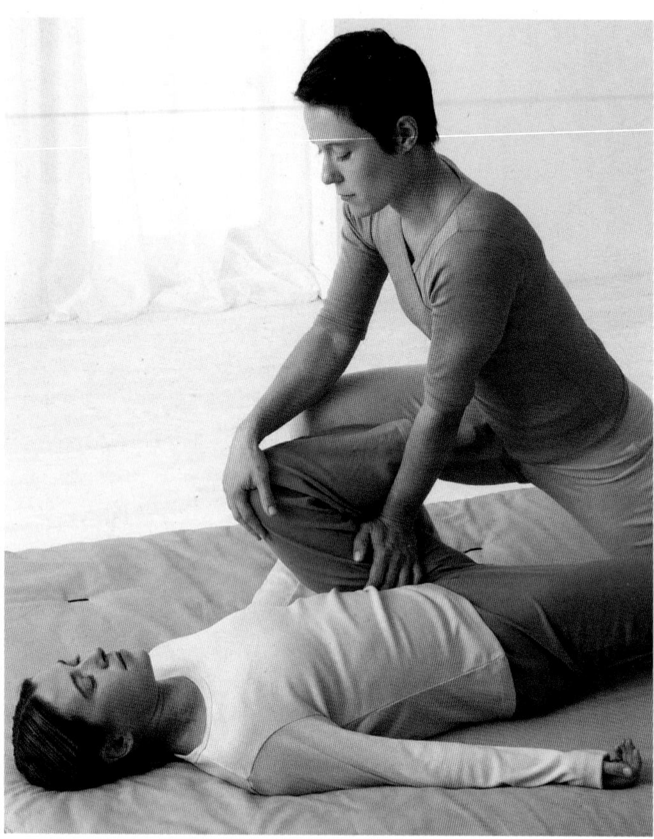

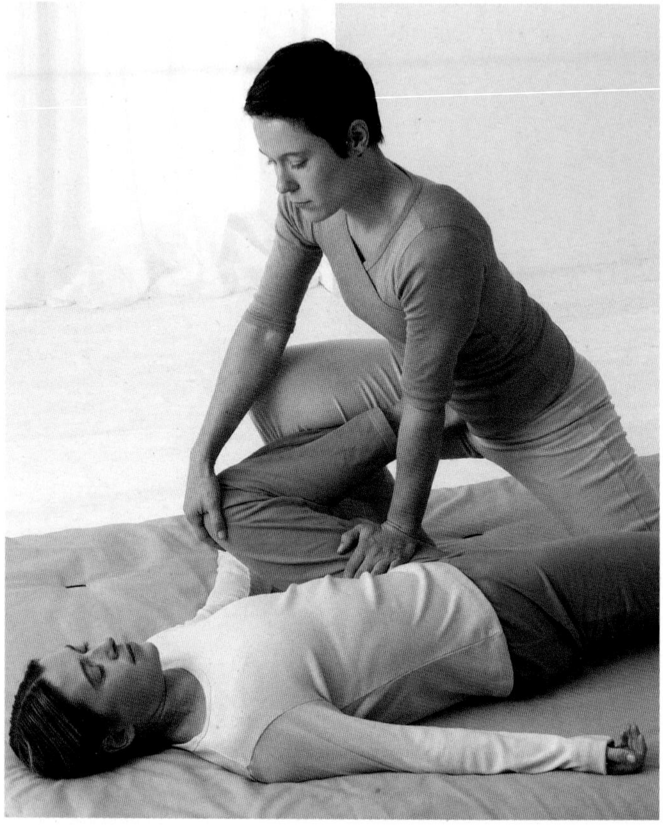

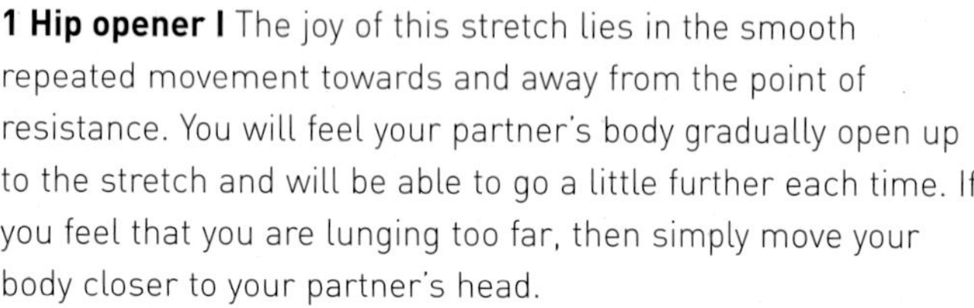

1 Hip opener I The joy of this stretch lies in the smooth repeated movement towards and away from the point of resistance. You will feel your partner's body gradually open up to the stretch and will be able to go a little further each time. If you feel that you are lunging too far, then simply move your body closer to your partner's head.

From the last position, support your partner's knee and heel with your hands and bring the instep of their foot up into the crease of your bent leg. Angle their knee so that it is pointing straight up towards their shoulder. Place your outside hand on the knee and, with your inside hand, palm the thigh as you sink into the stretch. Repeat a few times, working with your breath. Exhale as you gently lunge forward until you reach the point of resistance, then ease out. There is no effort required, since all the power comes from your centre of gravity.

2 Hip opener II This stretch is deeper than the previous one, and is often more satisfying for flexible people. Stay in the same position as for Hip opener 1, but move your supporting hand and leg away from your partner's body and let their hip drop out to the side. Work in the same way as before, exhaling into the stretch and inhaling as you release. Follow the natural direction of the leg up and out towards your partner's shoulder: you may find that it moves in an almost semicircular direction.

Caution

Avoid this stretch if your partner suffers from a hernia.

Getting a flavour of the dance

With the hip, groin and back-of-leg sequences shown on these and the following pages, you as the giver can really begin to appreciate and enjoy involving the whole of your body in your massage technique. The use of your body weight, along with the combination of working with your hands and feet together, will start to give you a flavour of a very special rhythm. It is this rhythm that leads many people to refer to Thai massage as a kind of "dance" – your movements become a rhythmic dance and you also engage in a dance with your partner.

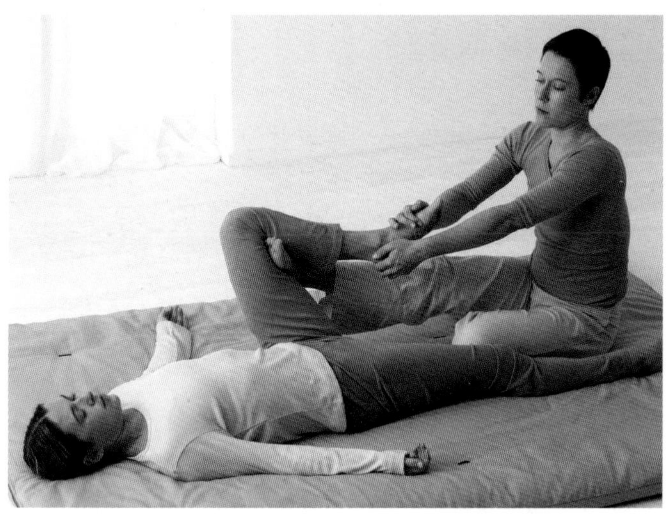

3 Kung fu foot This is a "transition" pose, leading you into the next step. Sit back but keep your partner's knee upright. Once you are sitting, take hold of their foot and place the outer edge of your foot (with toes pointing in and heel pointing out) at the back of their knee. Use your foot to guide their knee slowly out and down to the floor. You are now ready for the step 4 position.

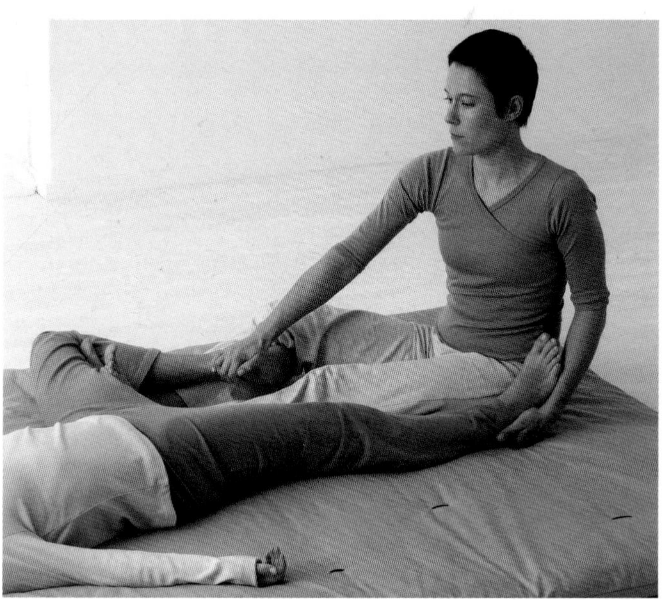

4 Paddle boat This is a wonderful exercise that releases deep into the groin and lower back. Use the instep, not the heel, of your inside foot to paddle up and down the thigh. Start near to the groin and work to the knee and back, being careful of the area around the knee. Begin with your knee bent and extend fully into the foot for a complete stretch. You can vary the strength of the stretch by moving closer or further away.

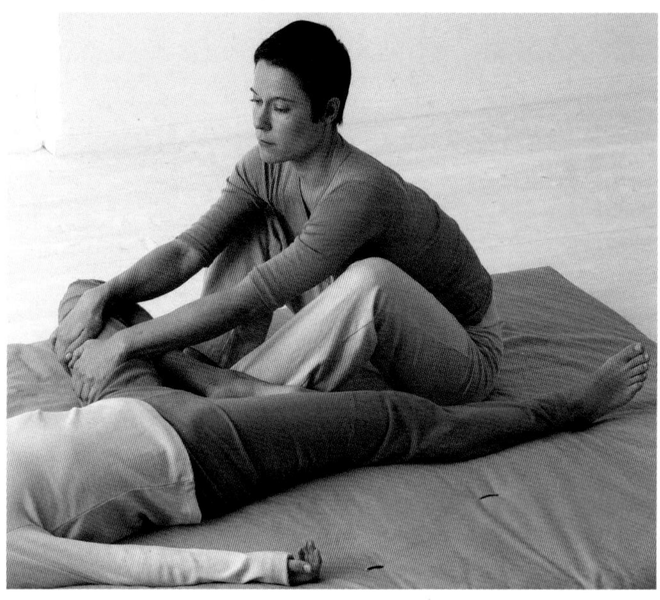

5 Foot sandwich This exercise relaxes the front of the thigh. Keep the knee where it is and sandwich your feet between the calf and the thigh. Shift your body closer to your partner so that you can reach between your knees to scoop around the back of the thigh. Work with alternate hands, leaning away slightly for a deeper pressure.

A close fit for step 4
Make sure that your partner's foot is tucked snugly behind your knee; hold their heel in place with one hand. With your other hand bring their outstretched leg close into your body and hold under that heel too. This snug fit gives the pose its stability.

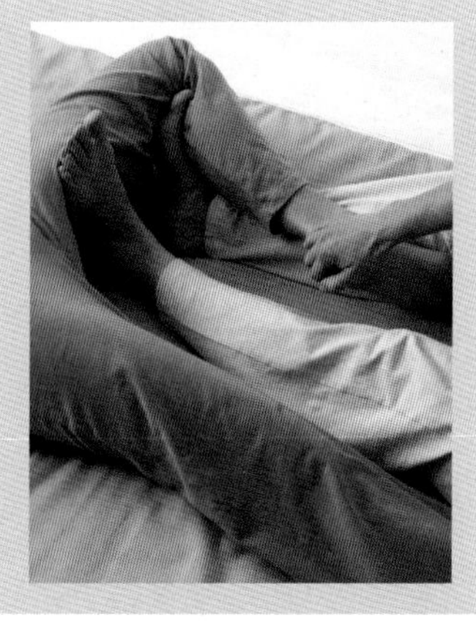

Making room in step 5
When tucking your feet in the bend of your partner's leg, you can try gently rolling your partner's calf muscle out of the way to make more room for your feet. If both of your feet still don't fit comfortably, then just take your outside foot away.

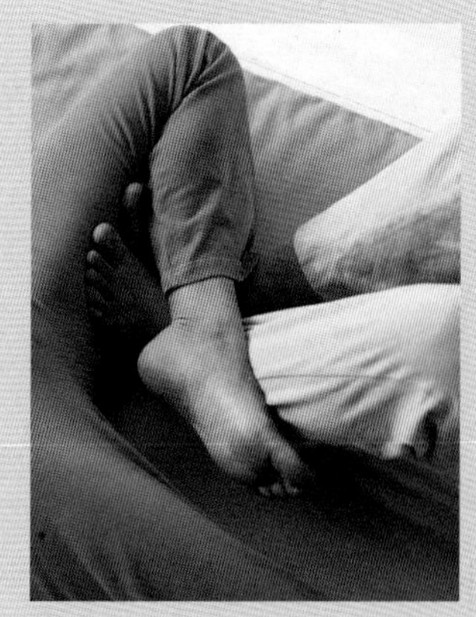

Opening the Back of the Leg

Staying with the same leg as for the previous exercises, we now finish the single-leg sequence. These steps stimulate energy flow up the back of the legs and into the lower back and hips. If your partner has tight hamstrings, work with sensitivity.

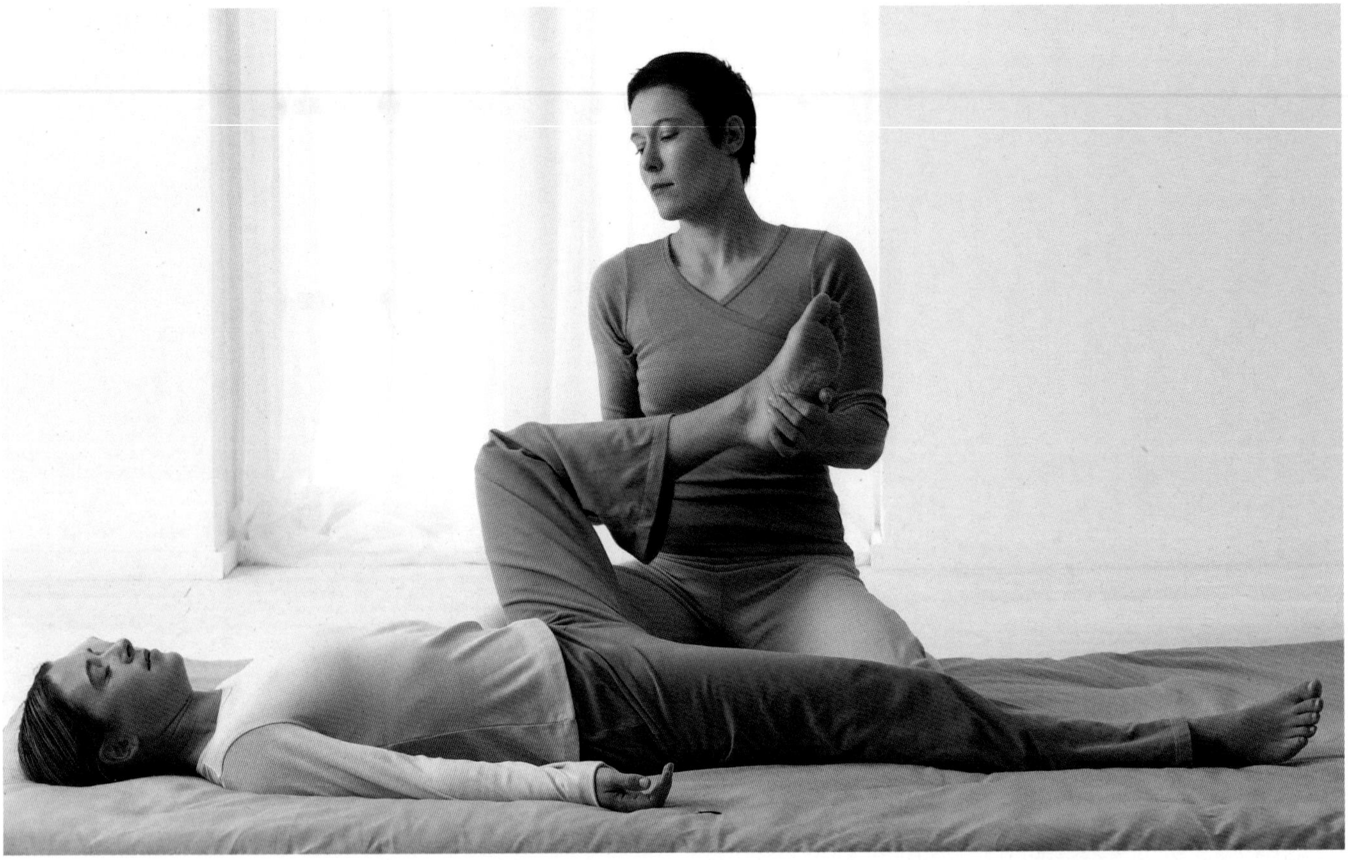

1 Leg circles This is a wonderful exercise for all body types. It encourages a deep feeling of letting go in the hip joint and can be used at any point in this sequence.

Before you start, make sure that your posture is comfortable and stable. Cup one hand under your partner's heel and your other hand under their knee. Keep their lower leg parallel with the floor. Now circle their knee, exploring the full range of movement as you do so. The movement can be big or small, fast or slow, whatever suits your partner. Circle the leg several times in both directions.

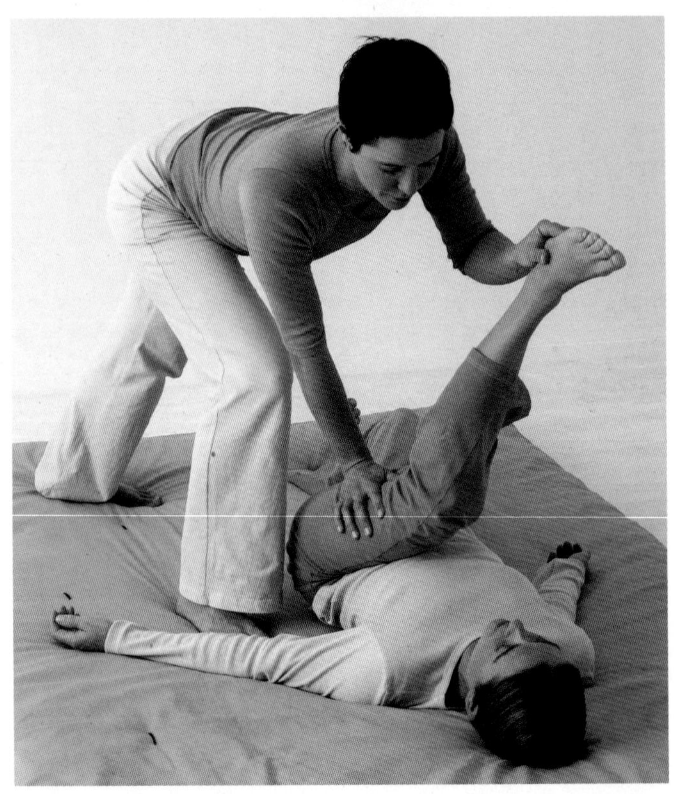

2 Hamstring yawn This exercise opens and energizes the leg from the hip to the heel. Keeping your body open to your partner's, stand with a wide stance. Bend your partner's knee across their body so that it is angled towards the opposite shoulder. Align yourself with the leg. Cup the heel with your inside hand, and with your outside hand palm the outside edge of the thigh. Encourage your partner to breathe with you. As you exhale, rock your weight on to your front foot, palming the thigh and pushing the heel in a smooth arc over the head. As you inhale, release the heel and thigh and rock back on to your back leg. Repeat three times.

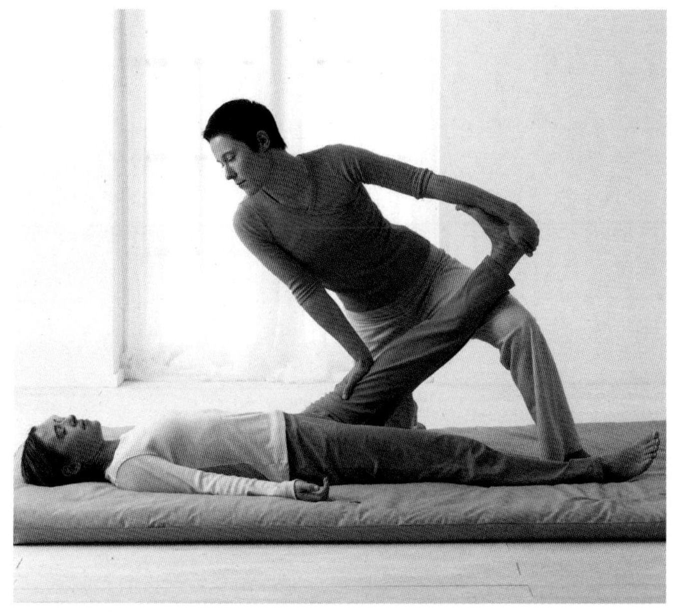

3 Pour the tea As its name suggests, this movement is a tilting motion; the weight is "poured" forward on to the thigh, opening up the back of the calf and heel.

From standing, drop down to half-kneeling, straightening your partner's leg and letting it rest on your thigh. Create a lever by cupping your fingers under the heel, making sure the toes are resting against your forearm. Rest your other hand on your partner's thigh, keeping away from the knee joint. Lean into the stretch as you exhale, and then release. Repeat three times, gradually working more deeply, but carefully sensing and controlling the strength of the stretch behind the knee.

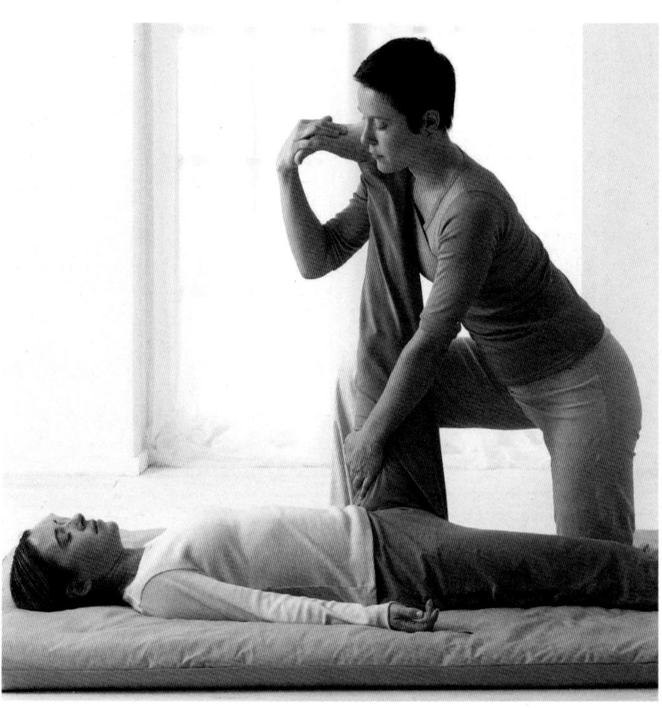

4 Double bass This stretches and stimulates the energy lines along the length of the leg. Not everyone can straighten their leg at 90 degrees, so if this feels a struggle for your partner, work at a more shallow angle where the leg can remain straight.

Drop down on to your other knee so that you are square on to your partner, with your body open to theirs. Take the leg up towards the vertical and let the foot rest on your outside shoulder. Fix one hand on the front of the thigh and the other on the ball of the foot. Use the top hand as a lever to gently open up the back of the leg. Encourage your partner to exhale as you lean down on to the ball of the foot. (This movement is quite small.) Once you have reached the point of resistance, release. Repeat several times, deepening the stretch as tension is released.

Variation to the Double Bass

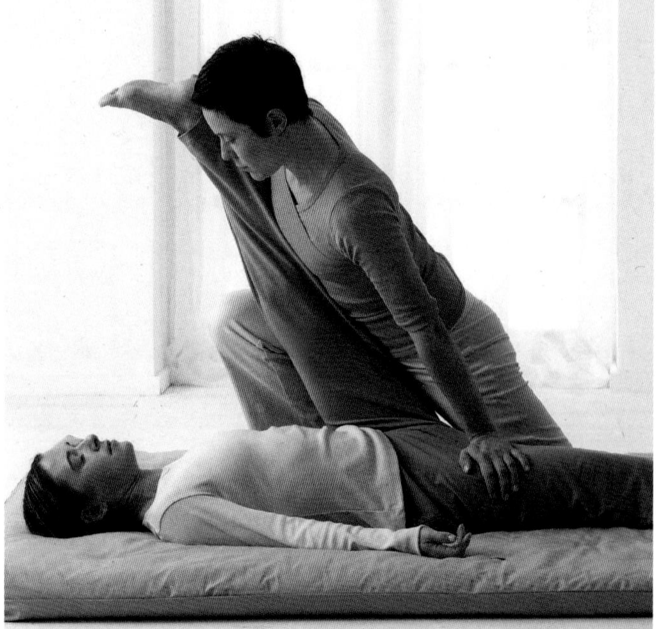

Above If your partner is a very flexible person, then you may want to try a version of the Double Bass that features a more dynamic stretch. Cup your partner's heel in your hand and tuck your arm close into your body. Fix your other hand on the thigh of the outstretched leg and sink your body weight forwards, taking the heel towards their head, to open more deeply through the groin.

Spinal Twist

Twists are invigorating as they help to stimulate the circulation and functioning of the internal organs. This twist releases tension throughout the mid spine, helping to create space in the ribcage and so encourage deeper breathing.

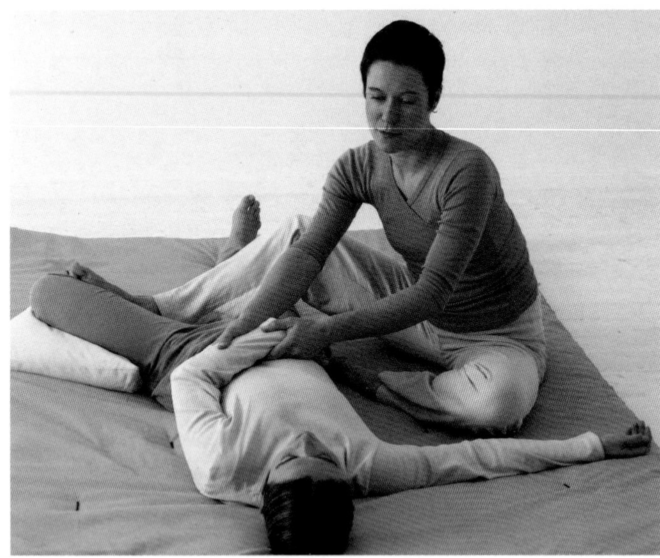

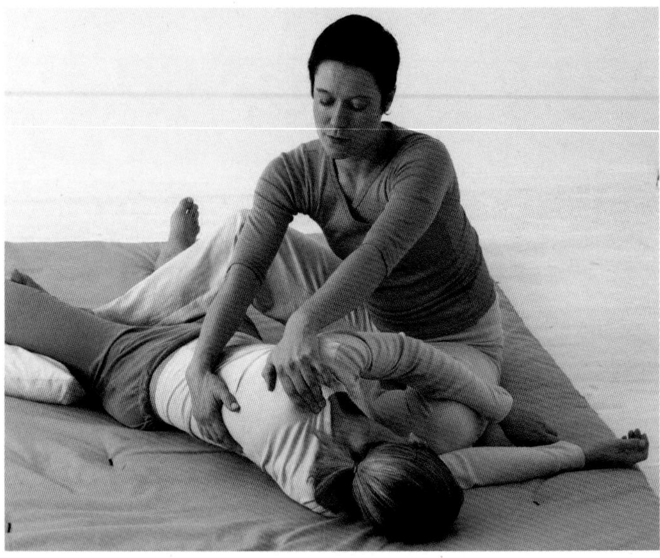

1 Put your partner's leg back into the tree pose (page 46). For most people a cushion under the knee is a good idea. Sit on the opposite side to the bent leg. You will need to move the arm closest to you out of the way. Fix the sole of your foot gently over the bent knee to give stability in the final stretch. Reach across the body and take hold of the other arm above the wrist.

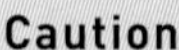

Caution
People with spinal injuries or disc problems should avoid this movement.

2 Ask your partner to inhale. As they begin to exhale, pull the arm towards you, walking your hands up towards the armpit. Clasp behind the shoulder blade with one hand and with the other palm up and down the back of the ribs and waist. Ease off a little for the inhalation, giving your partner room to breathe in, and work more deeply into the twist on the exhalation. To release, let go of the arm completely. Always work with the breath in twists, as the spine is able to undo itself more freely on the exhalation. Repetition is not necessary – one twist is sufficient.

Technique improver

To begin with, the single leg sequence can seem quite overwhelming, as there are many different exercises all flowing into one another. To familiarize yourself with the sequence and the feeling of continual movement, it is a good idea to simulate it on your own body. The more that you are able to experience the techniques in your body, rather than just trying to remember them with your head, the sooner the exercises will make sense to you.

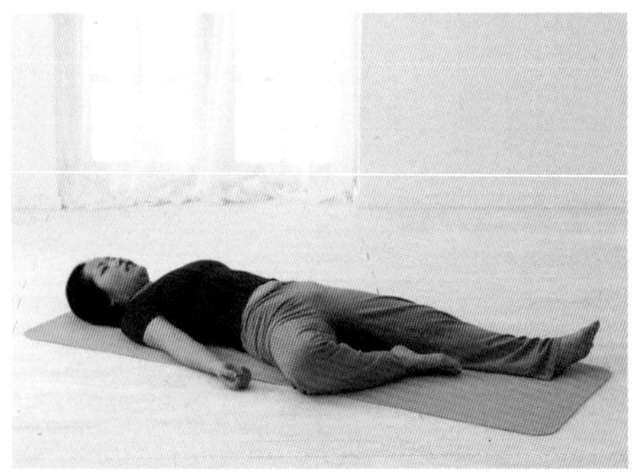

Tree pose

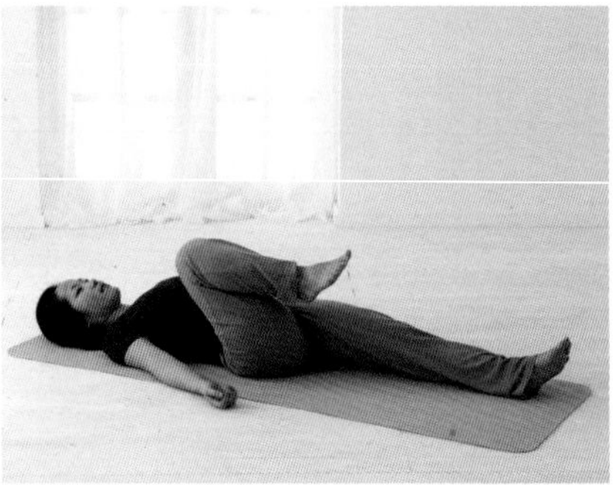

Hip opener

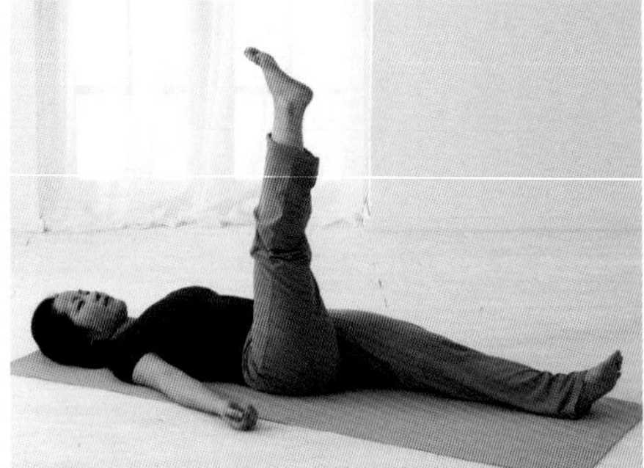

Double bass

Review: Single Leg Exercises

You are now ready to repeat the whole single leg sequence on the other leg. Use the pictures below as a reminder of the sequence. Take plenty of time to feel comfortable with the steps for each body section before moving on to the next one.

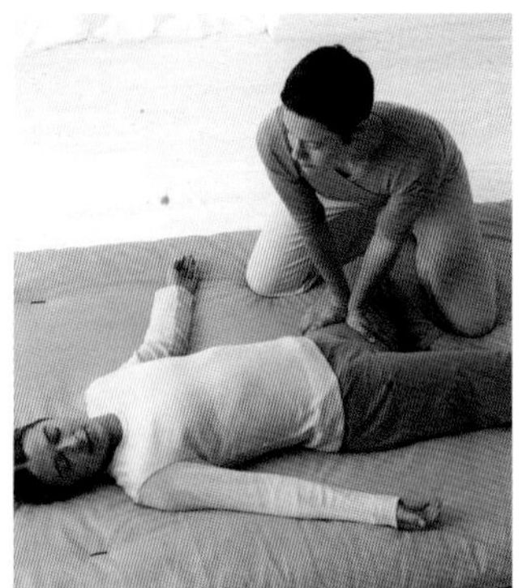
The tree

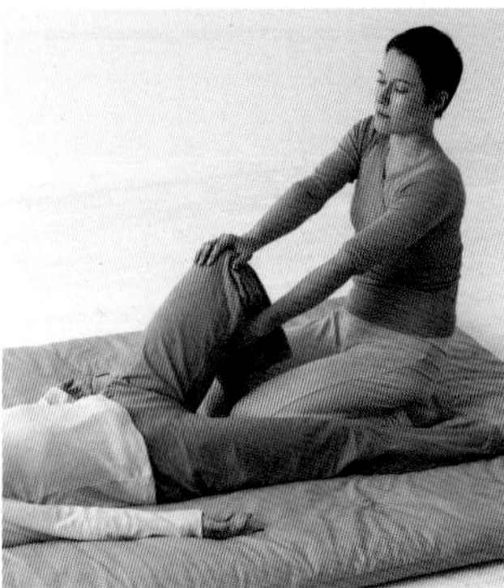
Relax the calf

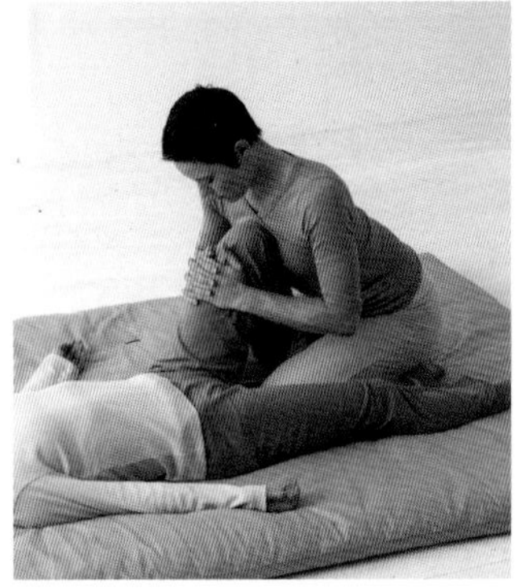
Butterfly squeeze: palming

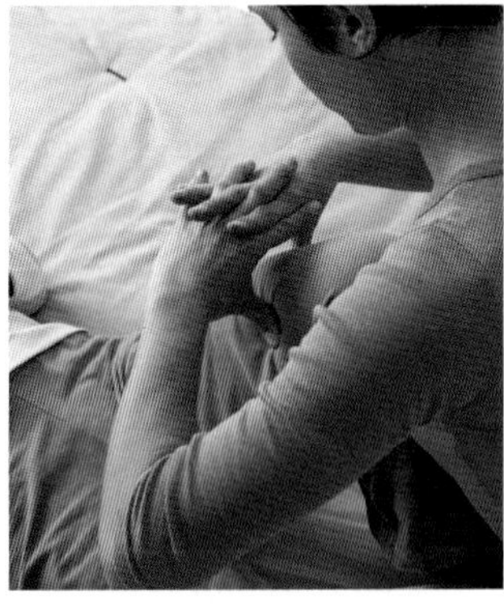
Butterfly squeeze: thumbing

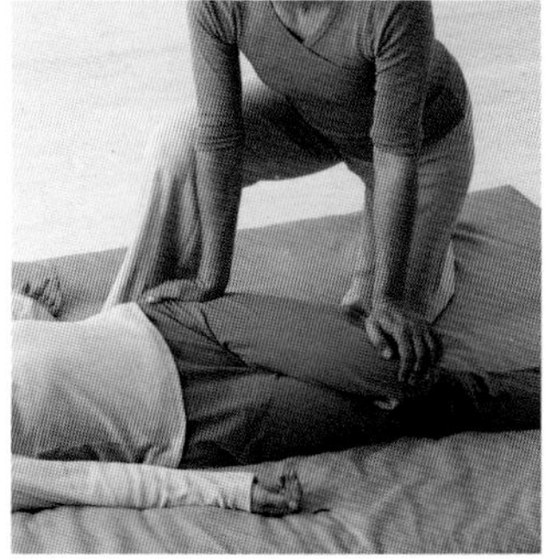
Cross hip stretch

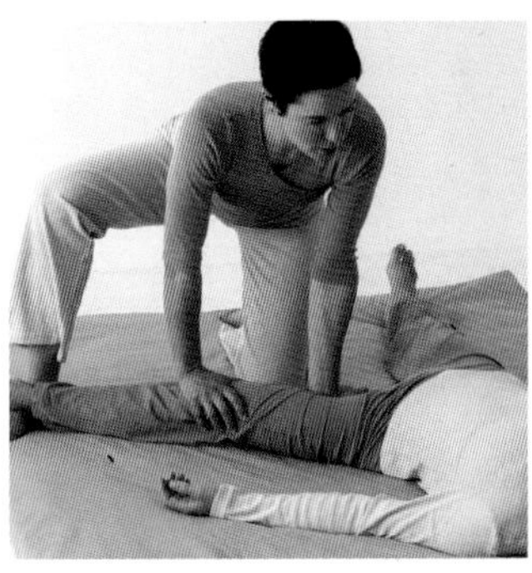
Wide leg stretch

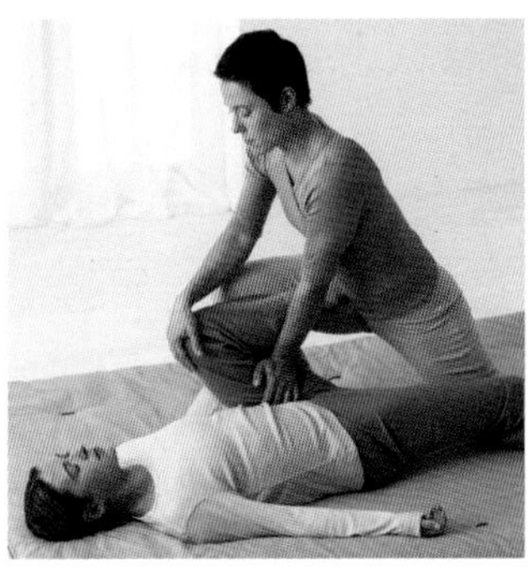
Hip opener I

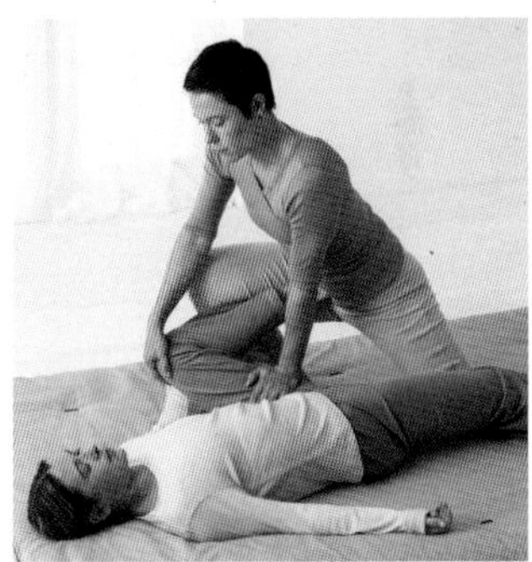
Hip opener II

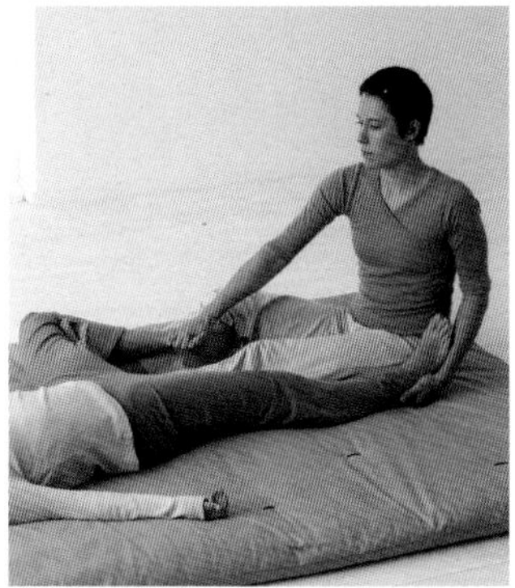
Paddle boat

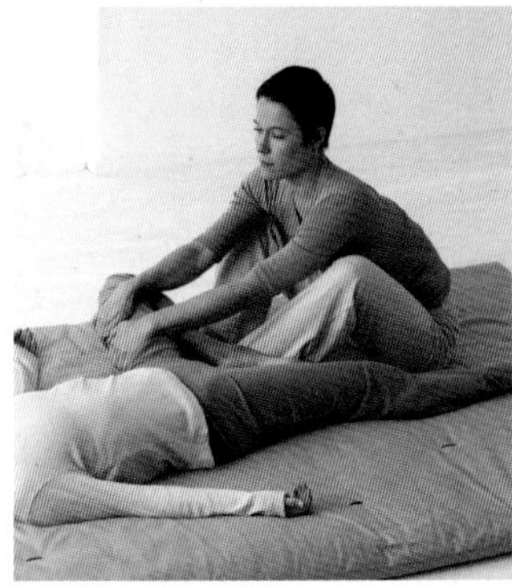
Foot sandwich

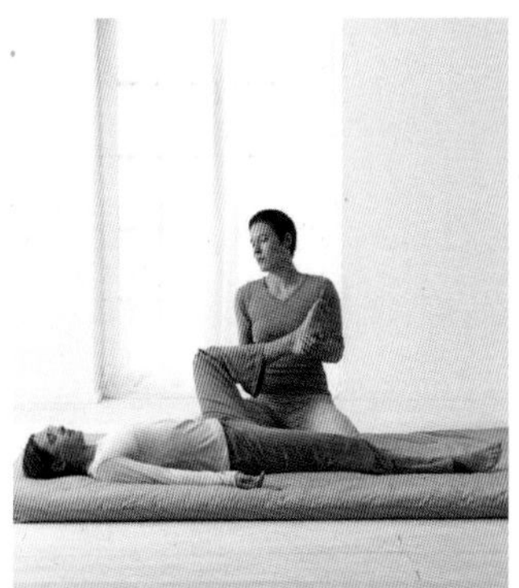
Leg circles

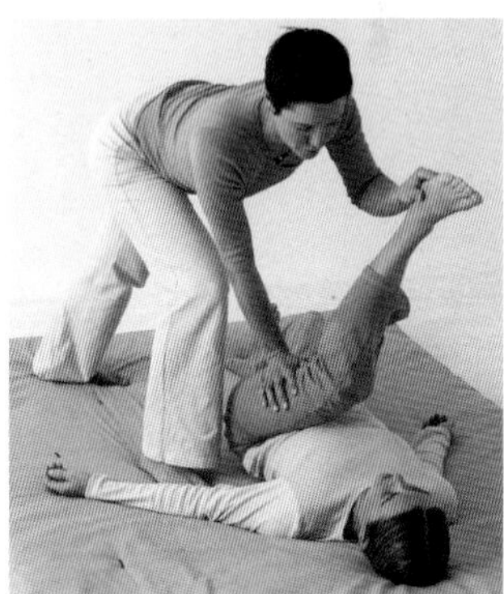
Hamstring yawn

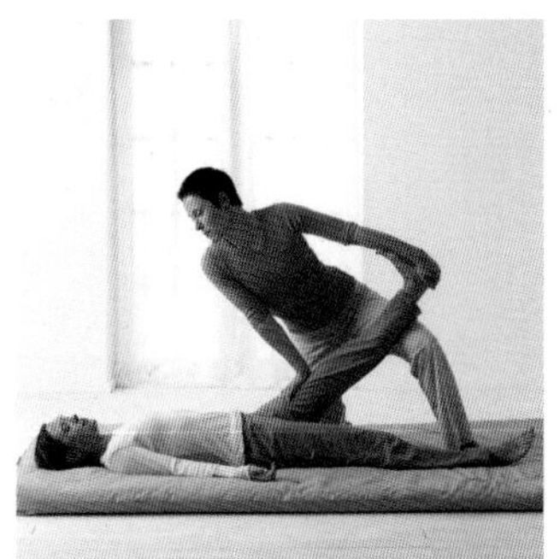
Pour the tea

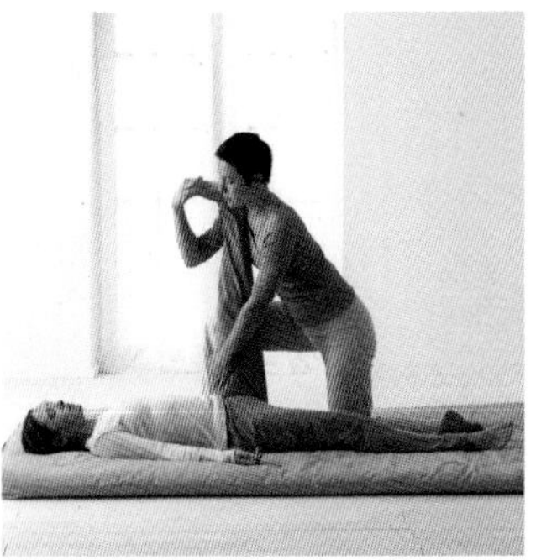
Double bass

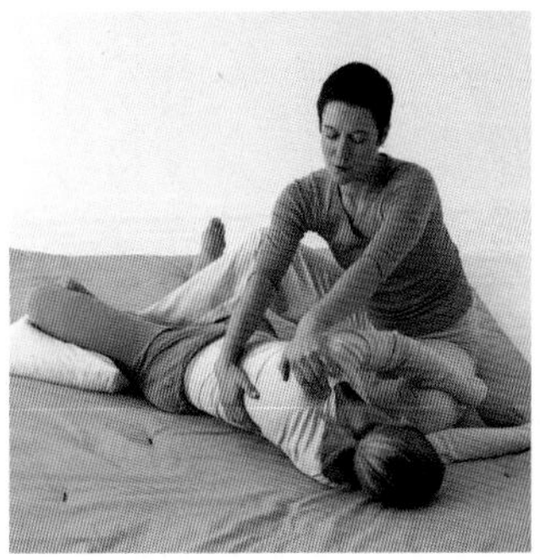
Spinal twist

Caution

Once again, check for cuts and bruises before starting and ask your partner about any joint problems. Their legs may be covered up and so areas to avoid may not be readily apparent.

Double Leg Exercises

This dynamic sequence works both legs simultaneously and focuses on opening the lower back and the hips. It introduces the body to inversions, back bends and forward bends, and is stimulating and invigorating for the whole system. The exercises are particularly helpful for those with low blood pressure or a sluggish digestive system.

There is enough variety in this sequence to find something to suit all kinds of body types, so do not feel that you have to try every exercise on every person. As some of these exercises involve deep stretches, it is important to establish good communication with your partner so that they can tell you when they have reached their limit.

Knees to Chest

A useful counter-stretch or relaxation pose, this is great for most body types. Your own posture is important here: place your feet apart as shown to create a stable base.

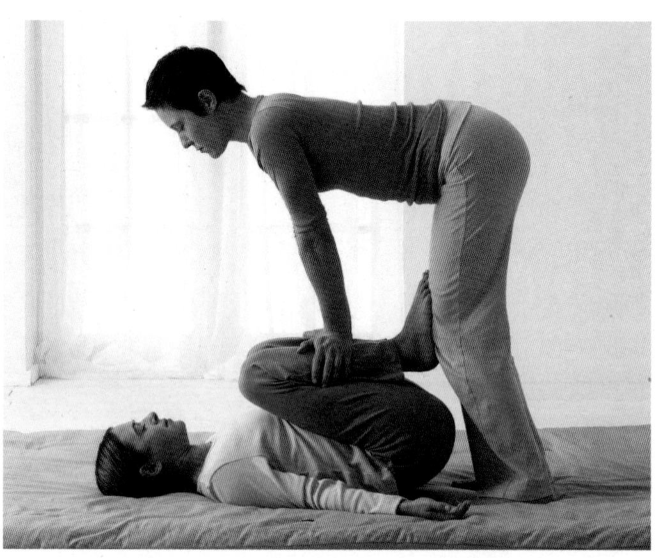

Above Place the soles of your partner's feet against your kneecaps, keeping your knees together and slightly bent. Place your hands on the outside of their shinbones and, as you sink your body weight into your knees, simultaneously lean your weight down into your palms. Ease in and out several times. If your partner is tight in the front of their hips or has over-developed thigh muscles, you may have to let the knees open slightly.

Crossed Leg Stretch

This works into the back and hips. Align your body with the direction in which you are working. The focus should be felt in the bent leg. Repeat the exercise on both legs before moving on.

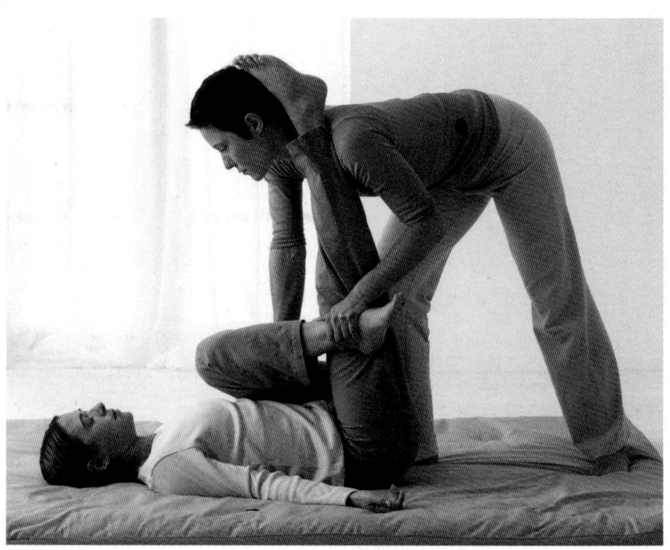

Above Ask your partner to bend one leg and straighten the other. Let the heel of the straight leg rest on your inside shoulder. Fix one hand on the ankle of the bent leg and the other on the thigh, just below the knee. Reposition yourselves so that the direction of the stretch is towards the opposite shoulder. With your feet wide, rock on to your front foot, palming up and down the outside of the thigh. Release and repeat three times.

Getting it right

✓ Watch your posture: work with a free spine, using the power in your legs, rather than your back.

✓ When practising the sequence, try to avoid putting your partner's legs down completely between the postures, which will make you tire very quickly.

✗ Don't use inversions for menstruating women, or those with high blood pressure, detached retinas or heart disease.

✓ As these poses are more dynamic, coordinate your breathing with your movements. Always move into a stretch on the exhalation and release on the inhalation.

The Plough

This stretch is an excellent one for toning and releasing tension in the abdominal organs. It stimulates the sen sumana energy line and the spinal column in general.

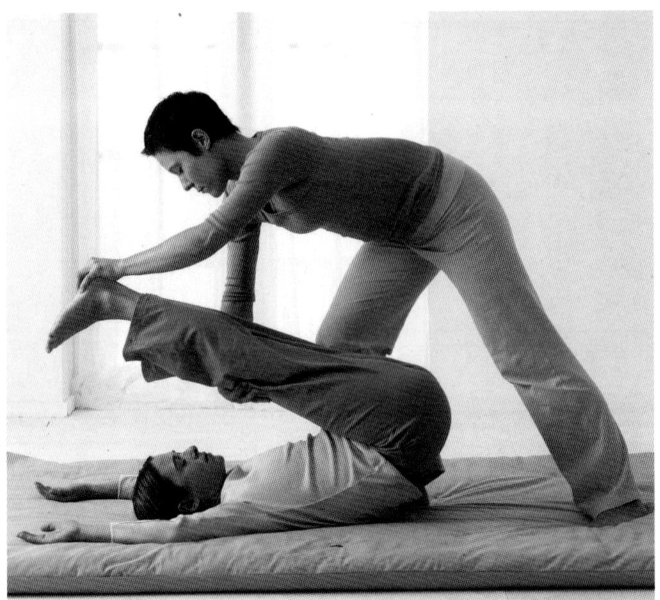

Left Hold both feet in your hands and reposition yourself so that your back leg is directly behind your partner's sacrum. Watch your posture: keep your feet wide for stability. Cup one hand behind your partner's heels, keeping the feet together, and support the fronts of the shins with the other hand to keep their body straight.

Exhaling, rock on to your front leg and take your partner's feet in an arc above their head. Encourage your partner to exhale as you move into the pose, as this will give a deeper feeling of release in the spine. Their lower back will naturally come off the ground at this point. Keep their hips in line with the rest of the body – don't let them swing out to the side. As you inhale, release your partner's hips back down to the ground. Work slowly in and out three times, gradually increasing the depth of the stretch.

Easy and advanced variations to the plough

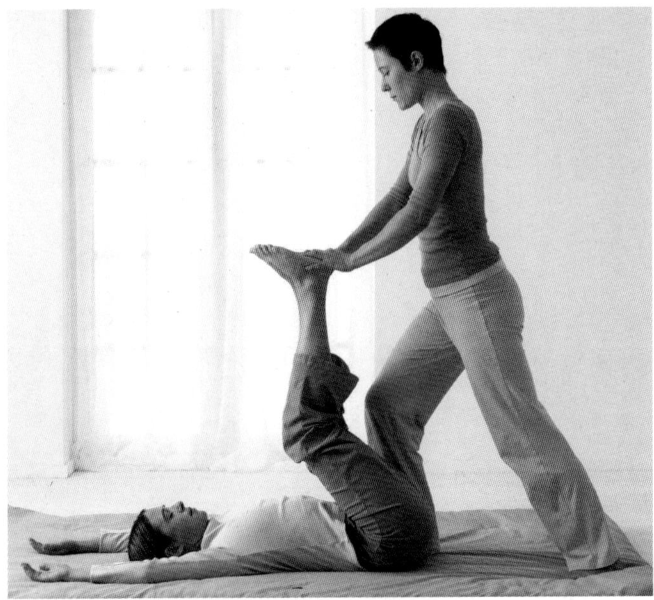

Above If your partner finds the regular plough pose too strong in the back of the legs, or if you notice a shaking in the legs, ask them to bend their knees a little to take the pressure off the hamstrings and bring the focus of the stretch into the back.

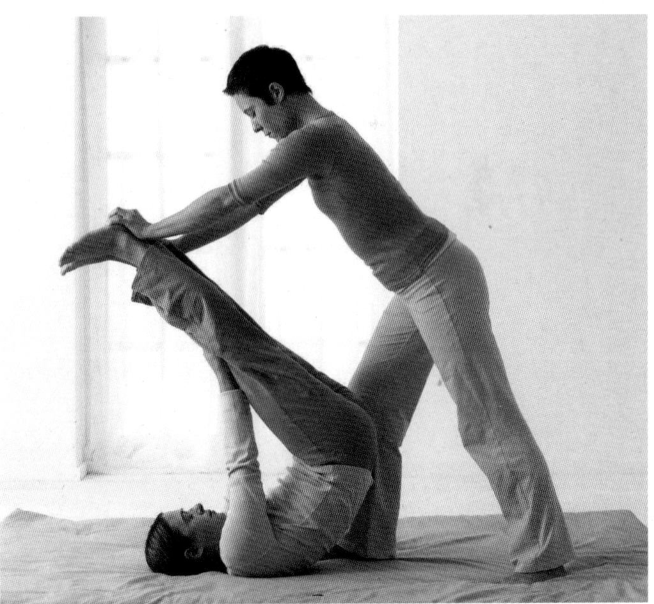

Above The shoulder stand is an advanced pose that is an extension of the assisted plough. It involves an additional release for the shoulders and neck. This gives an indication of the kind of pose you may be able to attempt once you know more about Thai massage. It is better to work this pose with a fully qualified teacher and a supple recipient.

Caution

Avoid the full plough stretch in cases of neck injury, detached retina or heart disease, for people with high blood pressure or for women during menstruation.

The Frog

This is a deep stretch to open the middle and lower back. It is not suitable for those with knee problems or injuries to the groin or spine. Make sure that you are working with the breath in this exercise.

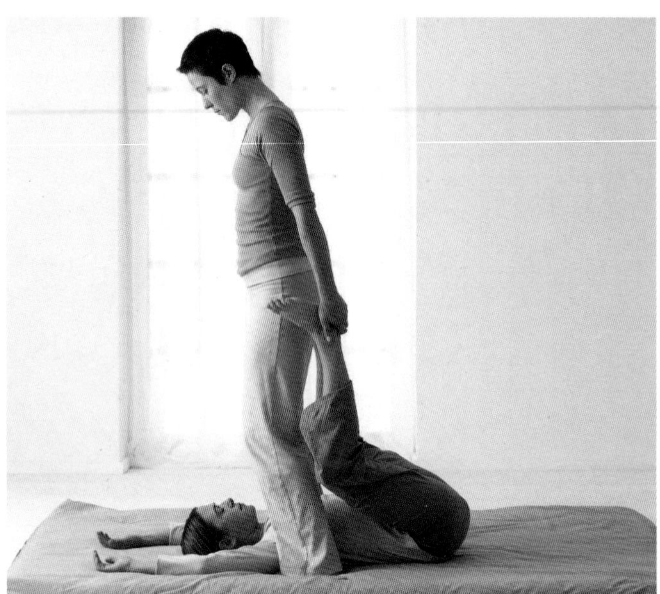

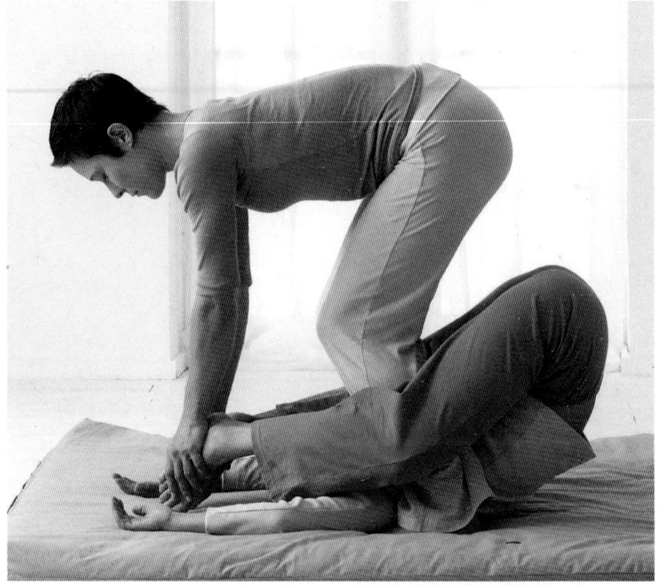

1 Hold one heel in each hand and encourage your partner to let the weight of their legs hang from your hands, with knees bent and hips relaxed. Ask them to place their arms above their head. Step in between their legs and stand as high up into their armpits as you can. Inhaling, lift their feet up and bring them round in front of your body so that the soles of the feet are together. It is normal for the hips to come off the ground.

2 Once the feet are together, settle them lower so that they are level with your pubic bone. Now, exhaling, push your partner's feet in a gentle arc over their head, extending your arms fully. Take the feet as far as they can go but do not force the body. When you reach your partner's point of resistance, release a little and repeat three times, without coming fully out of the posture each time.

The Butterfly

This time the direction of the stretch is straight down towards your partner's face. The pose focuses on opening the hips and groin. It is not appropriate for very stiff people or those with knee problems or injuries to the groin or spine.

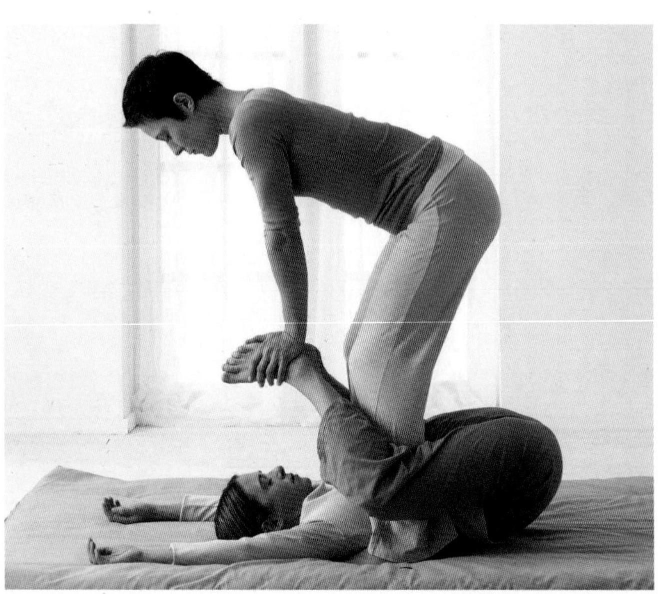

Left From the previous pose simply step away from the armpits until you are level with your partner's ribcage. Keep their feet together. You may feel some natural resistance, so check the pressure with your partner and then continue to sink your body weight down through your arms.

Undo the pose slowly. Move your partner's feet apart and, holding their heels, step back through their legs. Now rest for a moment, in the knees to chest pose featured previously.

Close-up on the fix

To fix this pose, place one of your hands over the other on the recipient's feet and lean your body weight down on to the feet.

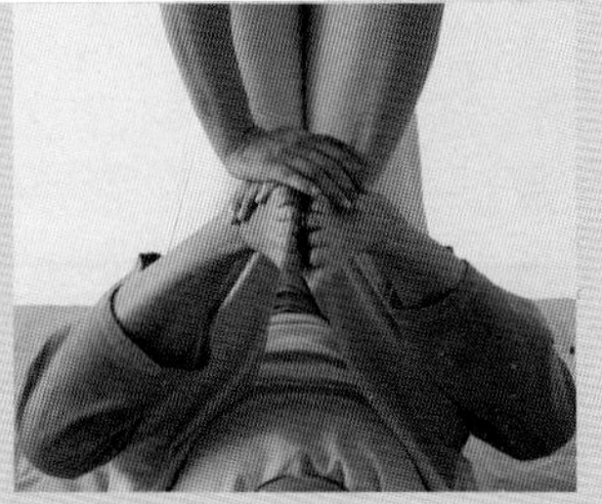

The Bridge

Do not be daunted by this pose. It benefits all body types (but avoid in cases of spinal injury). It opens the chest and the front of the hips, invites deeper breathing and stimulates the spine and sen sumana. It also boosts kidney function, helping to detoxify the body.

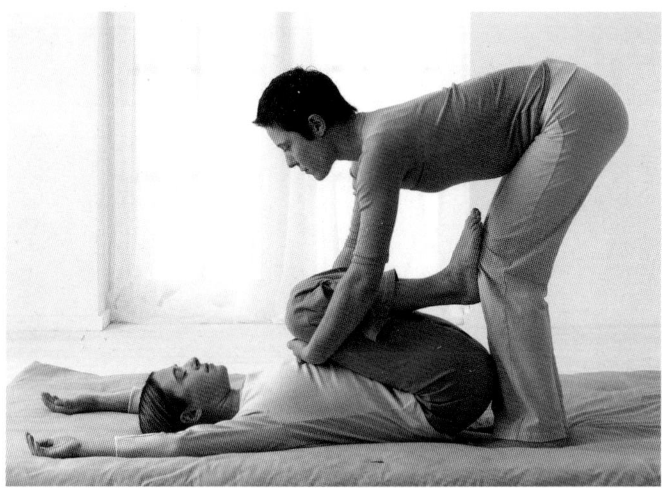

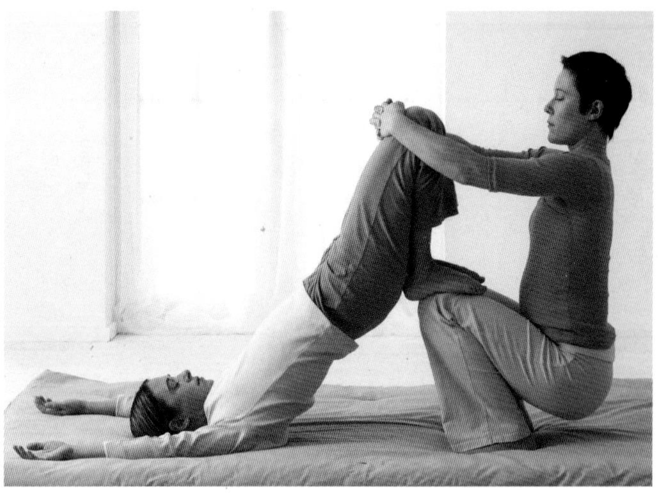

1 Position yourself as in the knees to chest pose and walk your feet as close as possible to your partner's buttocks. Make sure your knees are together and your feet are wide, creating a strong, pyramid-shaped base. Clasp your hands firmly around the fronts of their knees. This is your hold. Remember that you are using your body weight rather than your strength. Work with your breath to support your movements.

2 Sink your knees into your partner's feet and draw their knees up and over towards you as you squat down. Encourage your partner to go with the movement, without actually being active in it, by exhaling as they come up. Remember to squat rather than sit, otherwise you won't be able to stand up again. Enjoy the position. Check that your shoulders are relaxed and your chest is open. If you wobble, continue to hold the knees and don't let go. To release, ask your partner to drop their hips as you straighten up: this will give you the momentum to stand. Repeat three times.

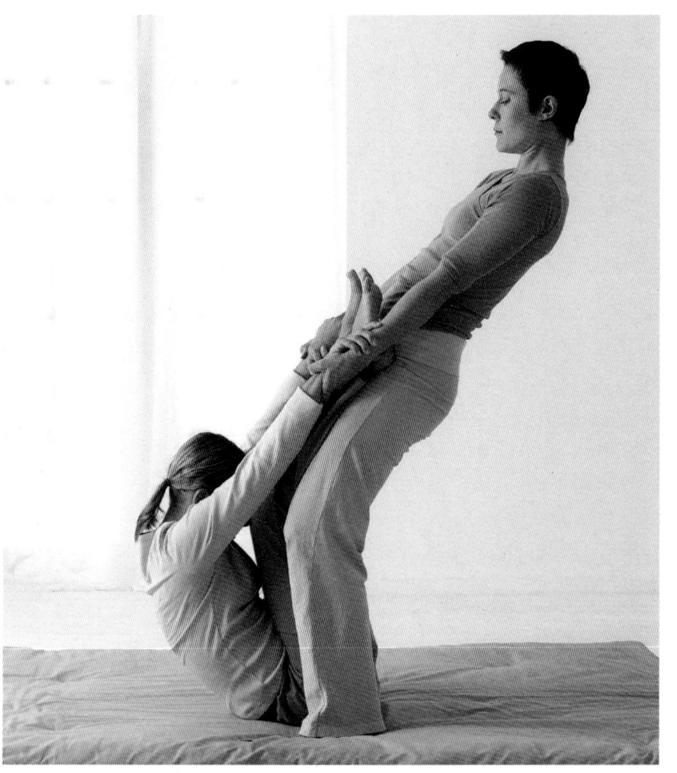

Forward Fold

This is a lovely counter-pose for all the deep stretches and back bends and is suitable for most body types. To protect your posture, use the power in your legs, rather than your back.

Left Rest your partner's legs up against your lower body. Depending on your height, their legs will stay together or will rest either side of your hips. Clasp each other's wrists. Bend your knees and, exhaling, straighten your legs and lean back, drawing your partner's upper body towards you. Their hips should stay on the floor. If they feel stiff in the backs of their legs, ask them to bend the knees slightly. Release their weight back down to the mat and repeat the pose three times.

Technique improver

This double leg sequence shows the direct relationship between the yoga tradition and the passive stretches used in Thai massage. Doing this will show you how your own body responds in these postures, which in turn will help you move your partner's body with more sensitivity and awareness. Try a variety of poses for yourself to feel how different shapes affect your body. Notice how moving with the breath can increase the feeling of release in your body.

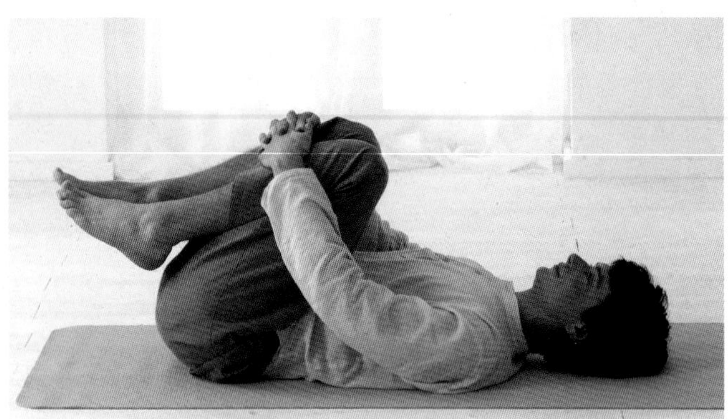

1 Knees to chest pose Lie flat on the floor with your knees bent. Bring your feet off the floor, allowing your knees to fall towards your chest. Try to keep the whole length of your spine in contact with the mat, using the weight of your arms and hands to draw your knees closer in towards you. Now relax your thighs completely and breathe. Take time to enjoy the feeling of your lower back and pelvis gradually broadening and sinking into the ground.

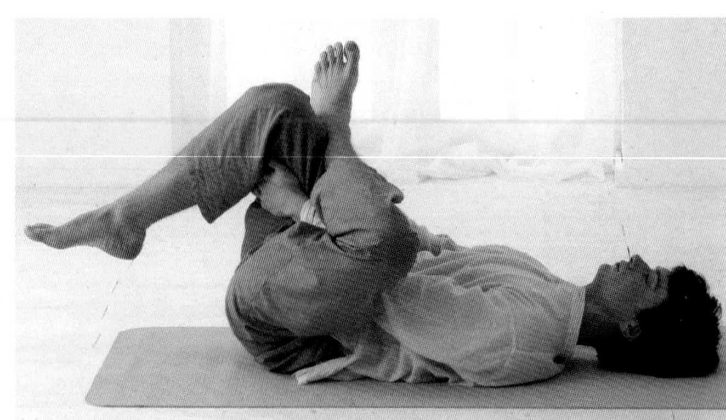

2 Crossed leg stretch From the previous position, place one foot down on the mat and let the other foot rest across your bent knee. Allow your knee to drop out to the side. Inhale and reach your hands up through the gap in your legs to clasp around the back of your bent knee. Now exhale and relax your upper body back down on to the floor. You should feel a stretch along the back of the crossed thigh and buttock. For a deeper stretch, use your elbow as a lever to encourage your knee to drop out further. Do not force anything. Hold the stretch for a few breaths, then release the leg and repeat on the other side.

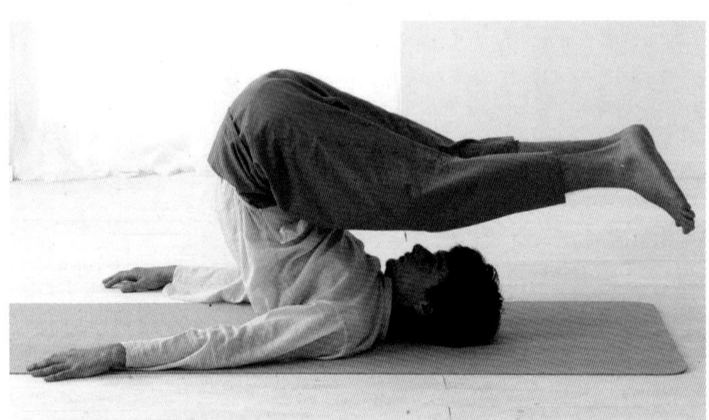

3 Halasana: the plough Start with your knees bent and your feet flat on the floor. Your arms should be alongside your body, palms down. Now bring your knees in towards your chest. Press your palms down into the floor and extend your legs up and over your head. If they start to shake, bend them a little. Once in position, let the weight rest on your shoulders, not on your neck. To release, unfurl the spine slowly back on to the floor. Don't attempt this pose if you have a spinal injury, disc problems or neck problems.

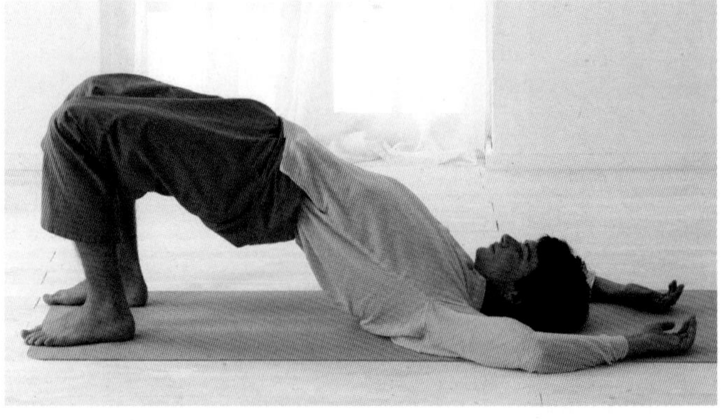

4 Setu bandhasana: the bridge Begin with your knees bent and feet flat on the floor, hip-width apart. Place your arms above your head, with your elbows slightly bent, feeling the whole of the back of each arm fully in contact with the floor.

Work in harmony with your breath, using it to give the pelvis the momentum to lift slightly off the floor. Exhaling, sink the soles of your feet into the ground and feel your knees move slightly away from you. On the next exhalation, use the power in your legs to elevate your pelvis a little higher off the ground. Be careful not to push or pull too much in the buttocks or front of the hips. Keep your feet, knees and hips in alignment.

To release, slowly sink your weight back down to the ground and rest before repeating the exercise two or three times.

Advanced pose – the assisted bridge position

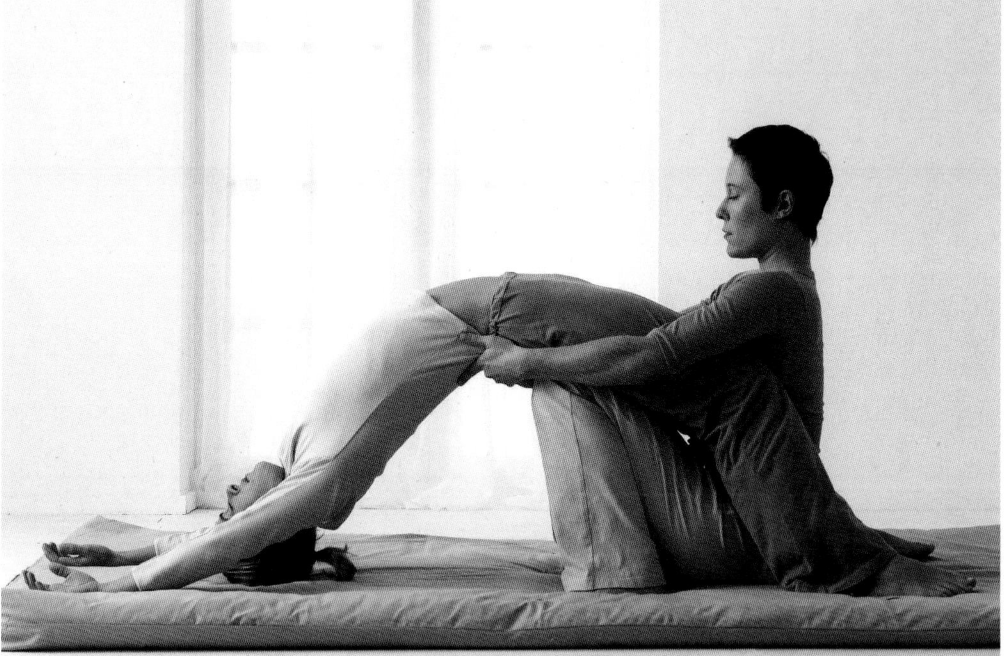

Right The assisted bridge pose is an advanced exercise that illustrates how Thai massage correlates directly with yoga asanas. The fish pose provides a deep opening for the front of the hips and a sense of expansiveness through the chest and upper back. Given passively, as part of a Thai massage, it gives the receiver a wonderful sense of freedom throughout their body. Remember, you will only be able to attempt poses like this once you are well-versed, and following the guidance of an experienced teacher.

Review: Double Leg Exercises

Use the pictures below as a reminder of all the exercises featured in the double leg sequence. Remember that not all of the exercises are suitable for every kind of body type, so allow yourself to be selective, according to your partner's individual needs.

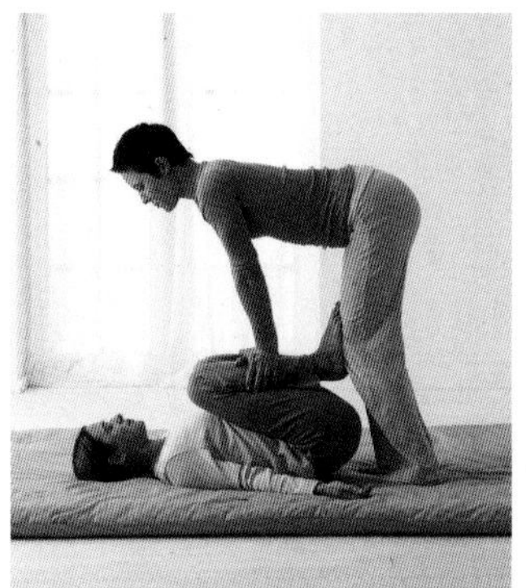

Knees to chest

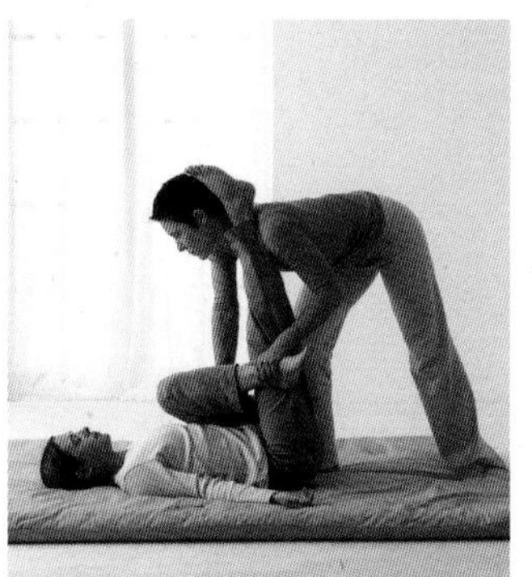

Crossed leg stretch

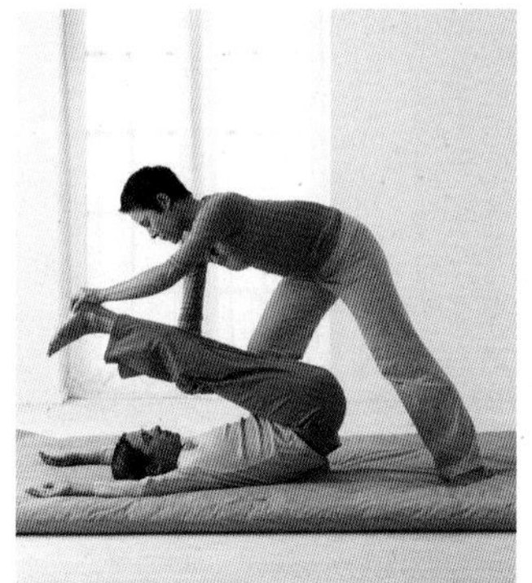

The plough

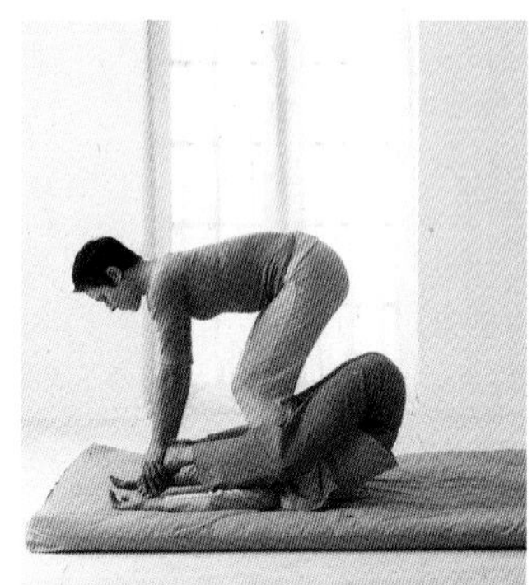

The frog

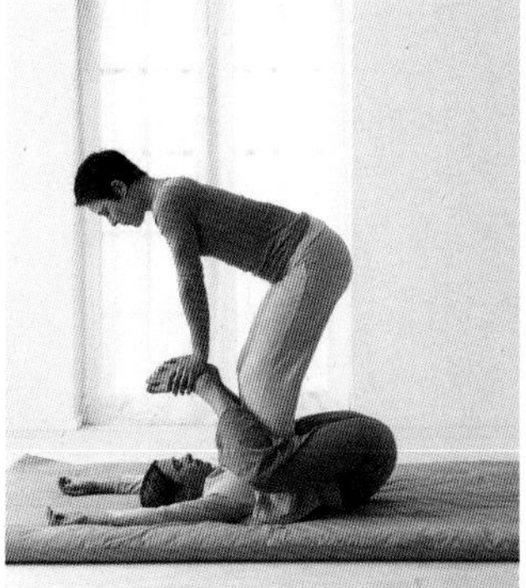

The butterfly

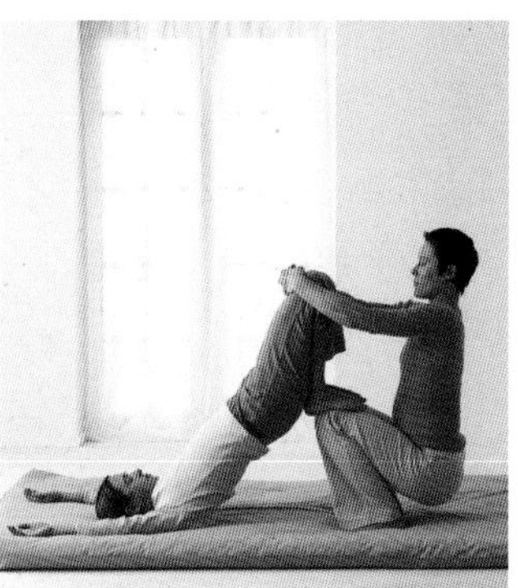

The bridge

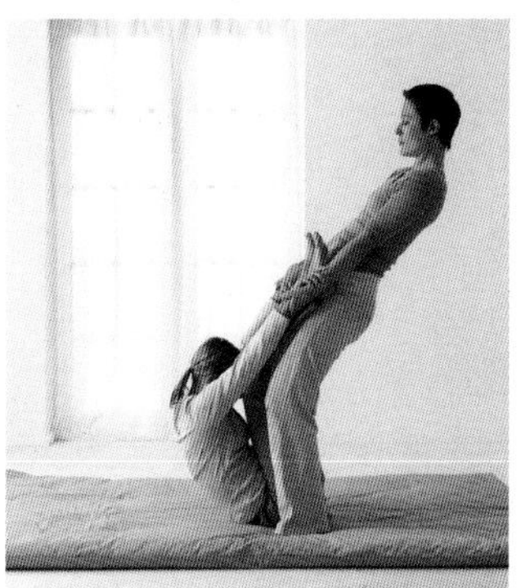

Forward fold

Caution
When giving double leg exercises, always be very careful to protect your back in order to avoid any strain. Remember that you should use the power in your legs, rather than your back, and keep your spine relaxed and free.

The Abdomen

As all ten sen pass through the abdomen, this is the energetic centre of the body. It is also the centre where we digest and process not only the food that we eat but also all of our experiences and emotions. The abdomen is extremely responsive to changes in our emotional state, so we can assess how relaxed we are by tuning into our belly, learning to sense if it feels soft and yielding or hard and resistant. The more we can release tension here, the more we can let go of tension throughout the whole of the body.

Working the abdomen stimulates a sluggish digestion and eases constipation. It encourages deeper breathing into the lower part of the lungs, helps to quieten and relax the entire body. It releases stiffness and tension into the lower back, ideal for back pain sufferers who find it too uncomfortable to lie on their front to receive a back massage. Repeated energy work to the abdomen can provide much-needed relief to the lower back.

Getting it right

✓ Work with the rhythm of your partner's breathing. If you have difficulty hearing or feeling it, ask them to breathe more deeply and audibly, but without forcing the breath.

✓ Many people are unused to having their abdomen massaged and may be sensitive. Approach with care and ask your partner to tell you what feels comfortable.

✗ If there is any abdominal pain or if your partner has had any abdominal surgery in the last two years.

✗ Don't work on a full stomach: it is advisable to wait at least two hours after a meal.

Technique improver

Feeling the movement of the breath in your own body will help you to gain another level of sensitivity for giving abdominal massage. It is also a very effective way to relax your whole being, both physically and mentally. As you breathe in and out the belly expands and contracts. When massaging the abdomen, you are simply following the natural rise and fall of the belly, helping to accentuate this movement for deeper relaxation. Repeat this exercise a few times until you feel familiar with how working with the breath can release tension in the belly.

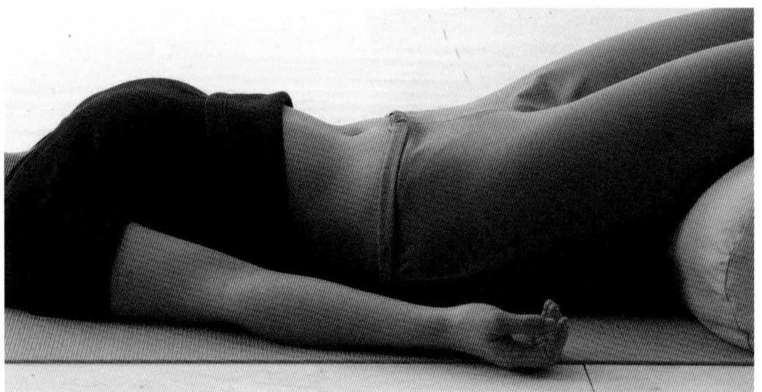

1 Lie on the floor with your knees bent; you may want them supported in some way. Close your eyes and listen quietly to the flow of your in- and out-breath. Rest one hand on your belly and notice how your hand moves up and down as you breathe in and out. Don't worry if you can't feel anything at first: tuning into the breath can take a little time.

Inhale normally and, as you exhale, draw your belly muscles in towards your spine, so that your abdomen is completely sucked in. Suck it as far in as it will go and empty your lungs completely.

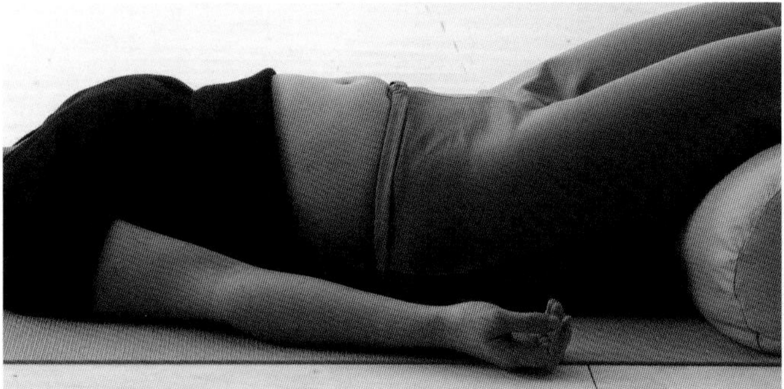

2 Pause slightly at the end of the exhalation. When you need to inhale, do nothing except let go of your belly muscles. The belly will inflate of its own accord, like a balloon, and the in-breath will be sucked into the body, filling the lungs completely.

Repeat for at least five breaths, then relax. Let yourself breathe normally, noticing any differences in your body.

Relaxing the Abdomen

Make yourself really comfortable here, or your partner will pick up on the tension through your hands. Sounds from your partner's belly are to be welcomed, as they indicate movement of energy and a release of tension.

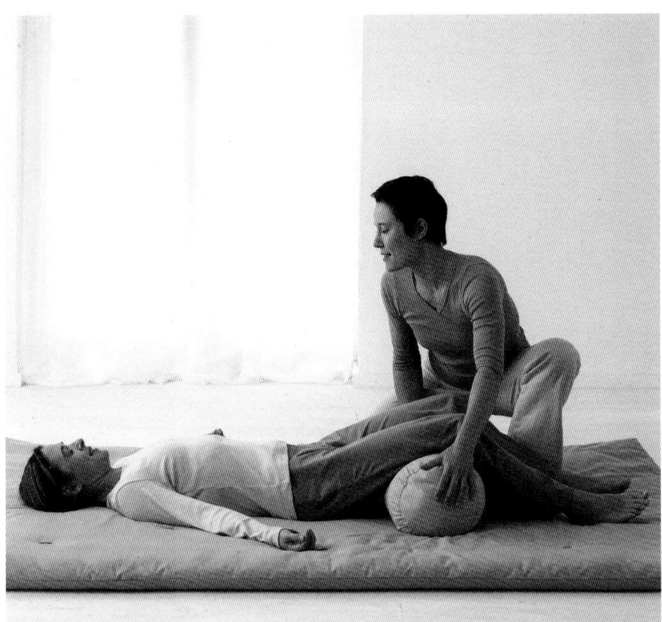

1 Getting comfortable The position of your partner is very important. As a rule, the knees should be bent up, to help the front of the body to relax more fully. This is especially important for women as it also protects the ovaries. Put a couple of pillows, a rolled-up blanket or a yoga bolster under the knees.

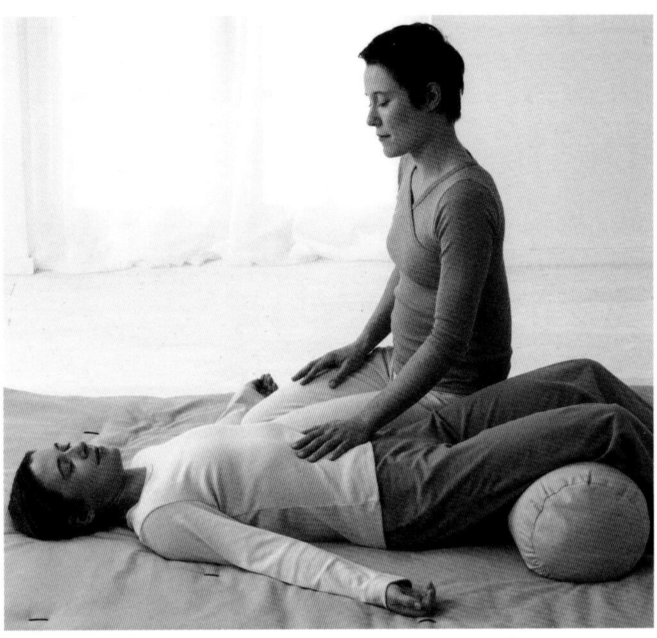

2 Tuning in Sit close in to the side of your partner. In this position you can listen to your partner's breath, noticing how fast or slow, deep or shallow it is. Allow your body to settle and become aware of your own breathing. Now place a relaxed hand on the belly. Let the weight of your hand rest without actively applying any extra pressure.

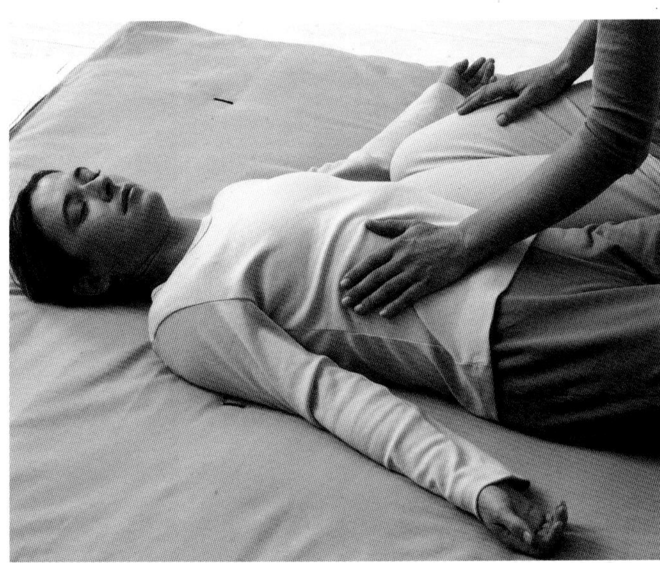

3 Relaxing circles This initial movement is superficial. Simply make circular clockwise motions across the surface of the abdomen. Work slowly and smoothly, with broad general strokes.

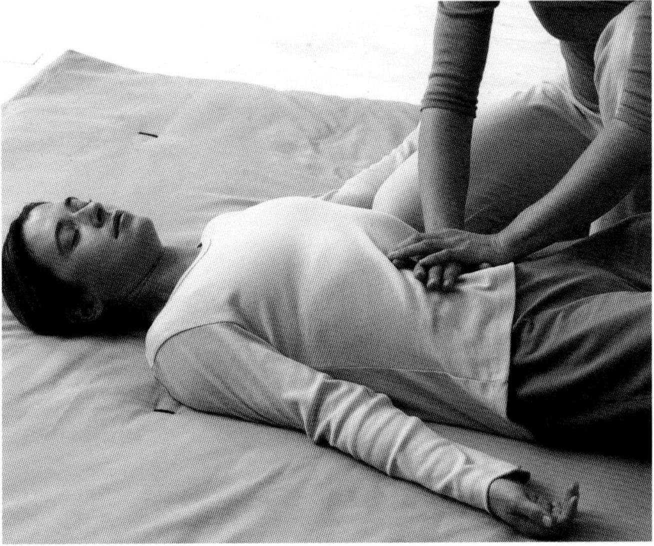

4 Making waves This movement is a little deeper. It's very relaxing and can be used at any point in the abdominal massage. Place hand over hand and work into the soft fleshy area between the ribcage and the hip. The heel of your hand and the flats of your fingers should move in an undulating wavelike motion across the belly.

Working the Abdomen

Traditional Thai massage work on the abdominal area involves working with energetic pressure points. The skill that you are aiming to develop here is to coordinate the pressure that you exert with your partner's breath. The idea is that you sink in as they exhale and then release as they inhale.

When working this part of the body, one good approach is to start with a round of palming, and then follow this with a round of deeper pressure, using the flats of your fingers. Finish off by palming the points again. If the belly is extremely sensitive or tense, your partner may not feel able to take the deeper pressure – if this is the case, then simply repeat the palming.

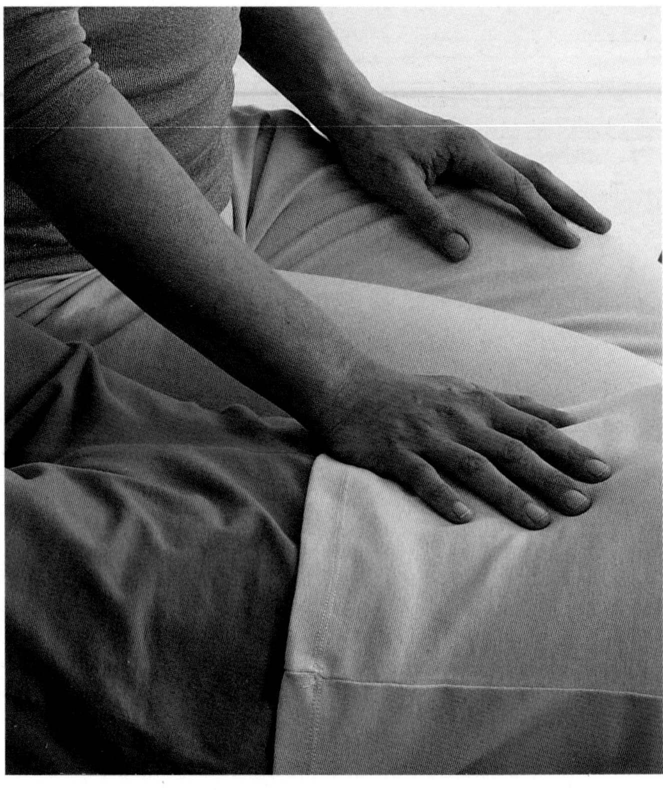

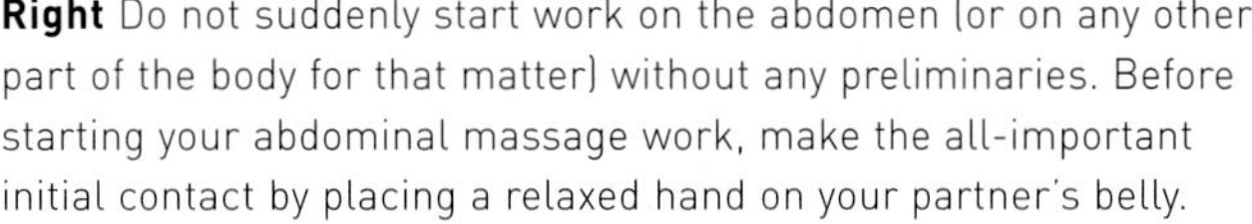

Right Do not suddenly start work on the abdomen (or on any other part of the body for that matter) without any preliminaries. Before starting your abdominal massage work, make the all-important initial contact by placing a relaxed hand on your partner's belly.

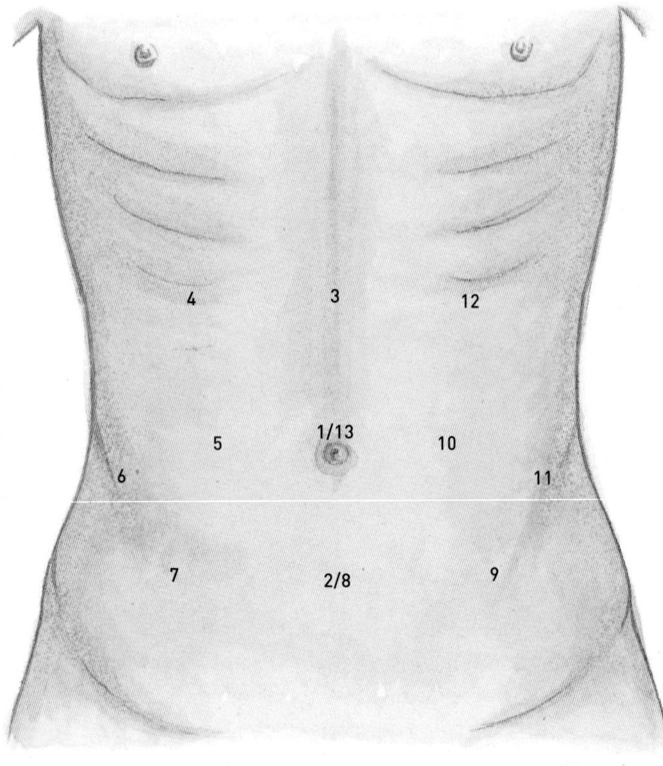

USING PRESSURE POINTS ON THE ABDOMEN

Key to the pressure points
1/13 navel and intestines
2/8, **5**, **7**, **9**, **10** intestines
3 stomach and solar plexus
4 liver
6 and 11 kidneys
12 spleen and stomach

Left This artwork shows the pressure points to be worked for an abdominal massage. For sluggish digestion or constipation, work clockwise, as this follows the natural direction of the digestive system and encouraging this movement will help to stimulate elimination. Use the flats of your fingers in a circular rubbing motion and work the points in this clockwise order: 1, 2, 7, 6, 5, 4, 3, 12, 10, 11, 9.

For a general relaxing stomach massage, begin at point 1, then go to point 3, and then follow the numbers round, but this time working anticlockwise.

Palming and Thumbing the Abdomen

Remember when pressing to use the flats of your fingers – don't dig in sharply with your fingertips. Communication with your partner is especially important here as this can be a very sensitive area of the body for many people.

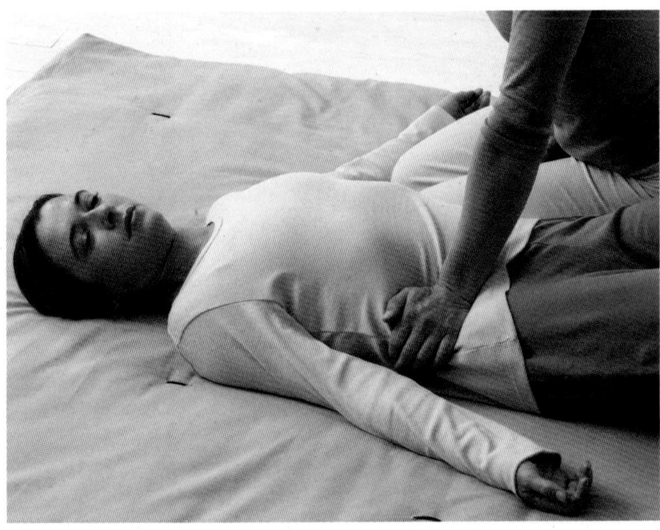

1 Palming Check that your arms are straight, but not locked, and your shoulders are relaxed. Sink your body weight down through the heel of your hand. If the belly yields, don't be afraid to sink all the way in; just check that the pressure suits your partner. If the abdomen is feeling very sensitive, work more lightly.

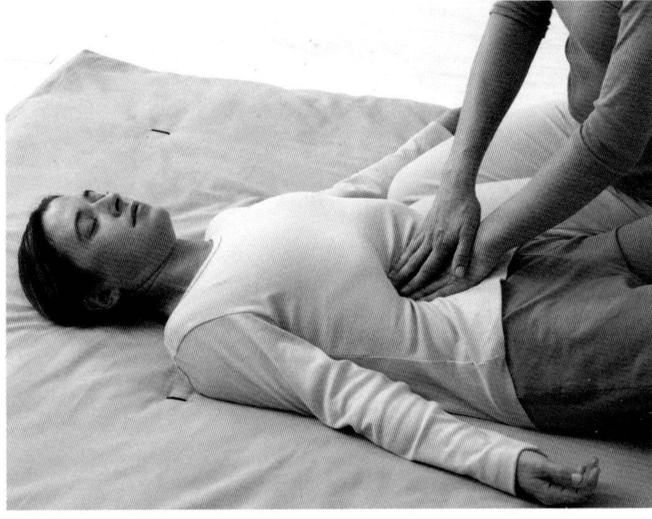

2 Finger pressing For a more focused pressure, use the flats of your fingers. For greater control and a deeper workout, place one hand on top of the other. Work in the same way as for the palming, sinking your body weight down through the flats of the fingers.

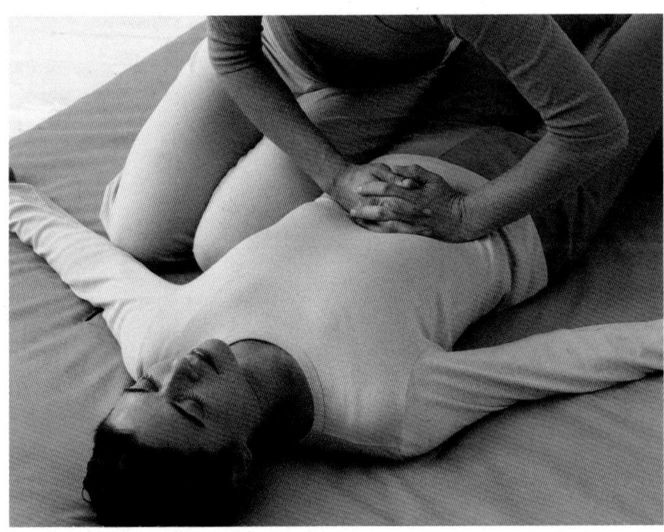

3 Wind release This is an optional exercise that is very effective for releasing trapped gases in the abdomen. Clasp your fingers together and take your elbows wide. The action is a scooping movement. Begin just below the ribs and work down with several scoops until you can feel the pubic bone against the sides of your fingers.

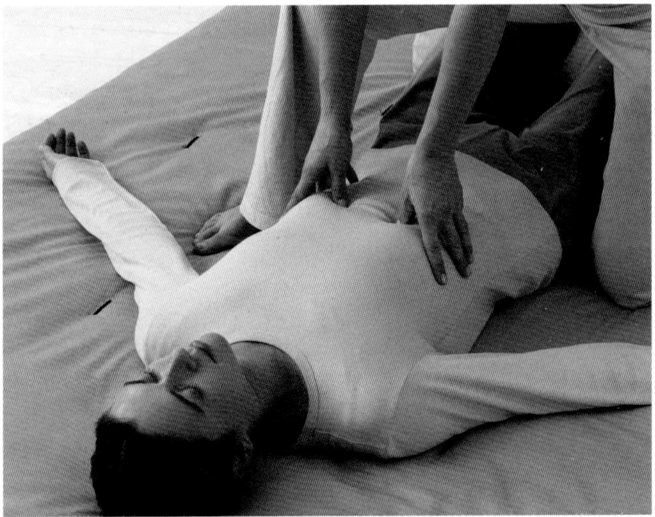

4 Thumb points For this exercise, overstep the body in a half-kneeling position. Focus on the six points that run either side of the belly button. Work points 4 and 12 simultaneously, then points 5 and 10, then points 7 and 9. On your partner's exhalation, sink your thumbs in slowly, pause for the inhalation and work slightly deeper on the next exhalation. You can work surprisingly deeply, so long as you maintain a slow, smooth rhythm in and out. Take time for at least three breaths in each position. Complete with some gentle belly circles.

The Chest

The routine shown here works with your partner's natural breathing rhythm, helping to open the lung cavity and encourage deeper breathing. It also directly stimulates sen sumana – the central energy line that runs up through the core of the body, incorporating the spinal column and all the chakras. This line not only affects the mechanical workings of the ribcage and lungs but also links directly with the energetic heart centre of the body. Be aware that although the techniques are simple, they can have a powerful effect on your partner.

Chest Routine

These exercises help to protect against coughs, colds and lung and throat infections, as well as stimulating the immune system as a whole.

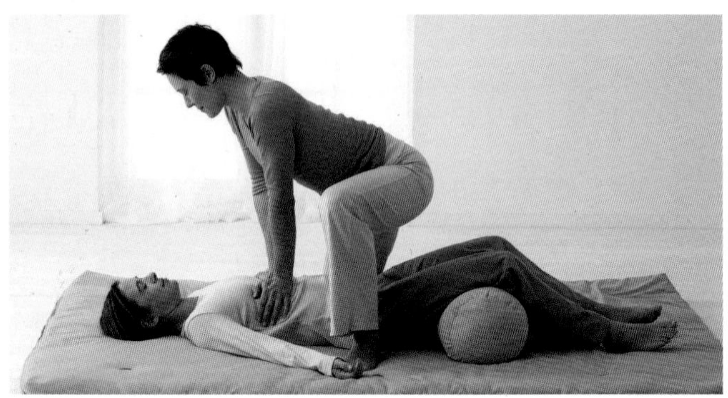

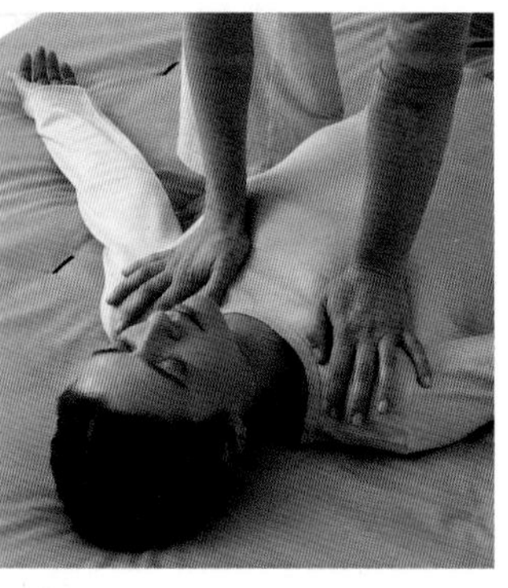

1 Palming the chest Overstep your partner's body and make sure that you can drop your weight down directly over the ribcage. Keep your arms straight and your shoulders relaxed. Place your hands on the ribs well below the nipples. Allow your partner's ribs to expand as they inhale; when they begin to exhale, sink into the ribcage, following the breath out as far as your partner will allow. Now repeat the exercise about two or three times.

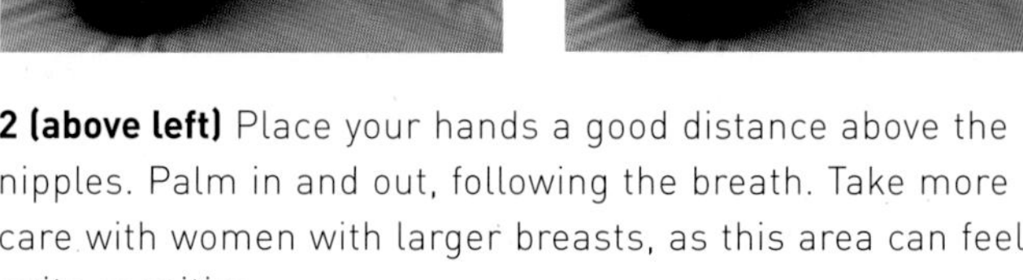

2 (above left) Place your hands a good distance above the nipples. Palm in and out, following the breath. Take more care with women with larger breasts, as this area can feel quite sensitive.

3 Shoulder nest (above right) Find the "nest" (bowl-shaped dip) just inside each shoulder joint. Place the heel of the hand gently into this dip and sink in and out two to three times.

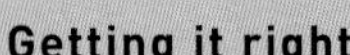

Getting it right

✗ Don't press directly on the area around the nipple.

✗ Never push or force the breath out, or hold beyond your partner's natural limit. The chest and ribcage area can hold a lot of tension, so approach it with sensitivity.

✓ Work slowly and smoothly: it is important to maintain an even rhythm as you move in and out of the postures.

✓ Make sure that you are comfortable as a comfortable posture for your own body will enable you to listen with greater sensitivity to the responses of your partner's body.

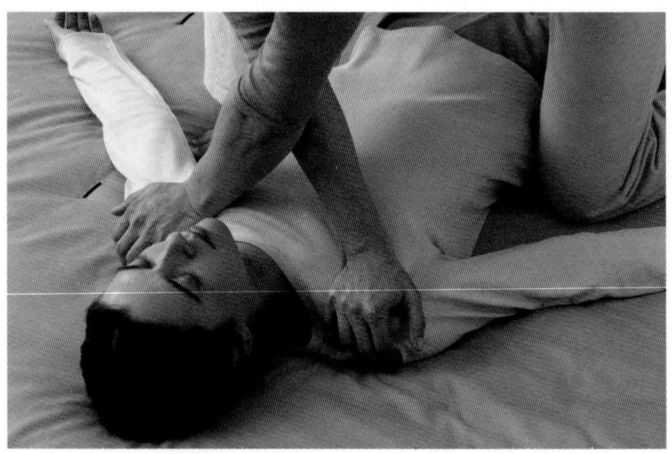

4 Crossing the shoulders Now cross your arms so that the opposite hand sits in the nest. As you sink your body weight in, sense a feeling of opening up the chest widthways.

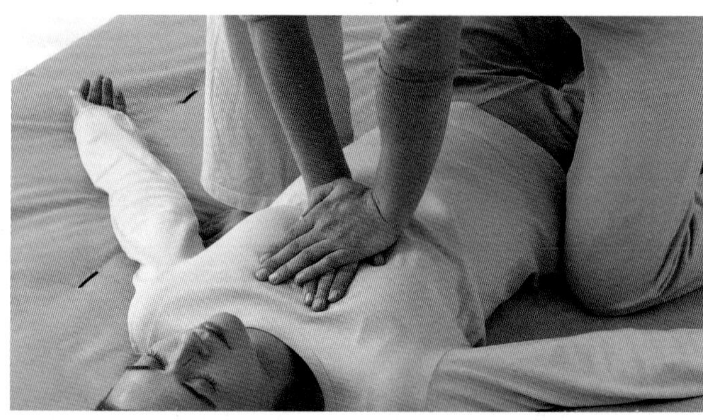

5 Sternum press Place hand over hand across the centre of the sternum (breastbone). Make sure that your fingers are slightly out to the side so they don't press against the throat. Be equally careful not to press too low, as there is a fragile piece of cartilage at the base of the breastbone. Work with the breath. Repeat three times.

Variation to sternum press – sternum circles

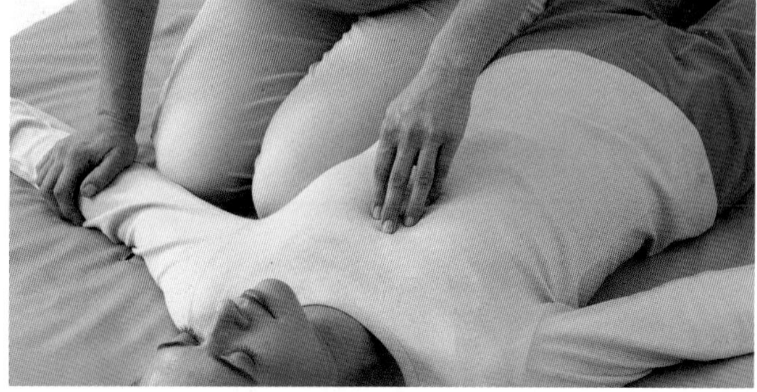

Above If step 5 feels too strong, use circles as an alternative. Position your first three fingers so the middle one presses on the sternum and the outer two work into the small pockets between the ribs, close to the bone. Make firm circles with the flats of your fingers, working from the base of the sternum up towards the throat.

Review: Abdomen and Chest

Use the pictures below as a reminder of the abdomen and chest exercises. Take time to feel comfortable with the steps for each body section before linking sequences for different sections together.

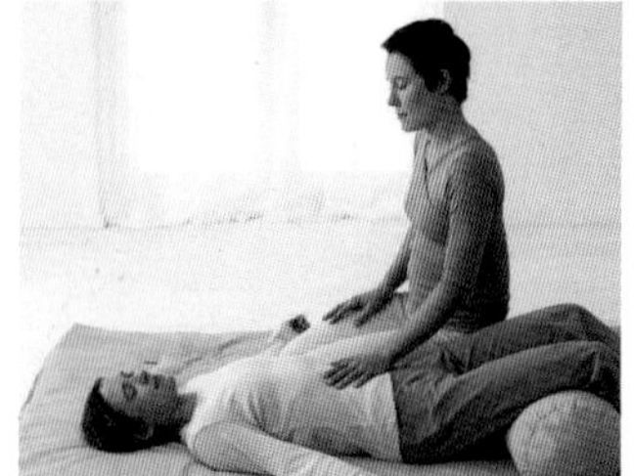

Tuning in

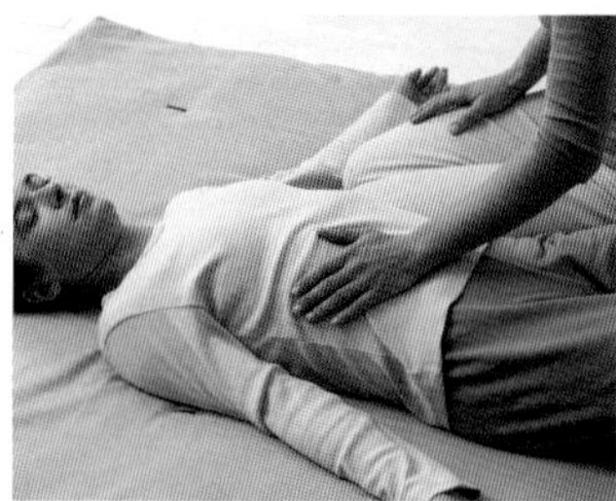

Relaxing circles

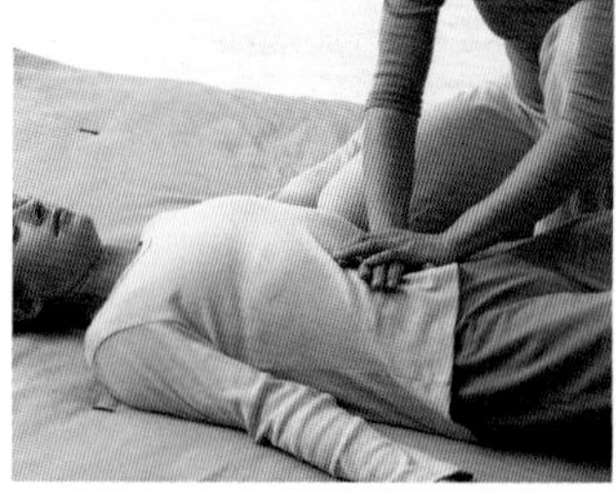

Making waves

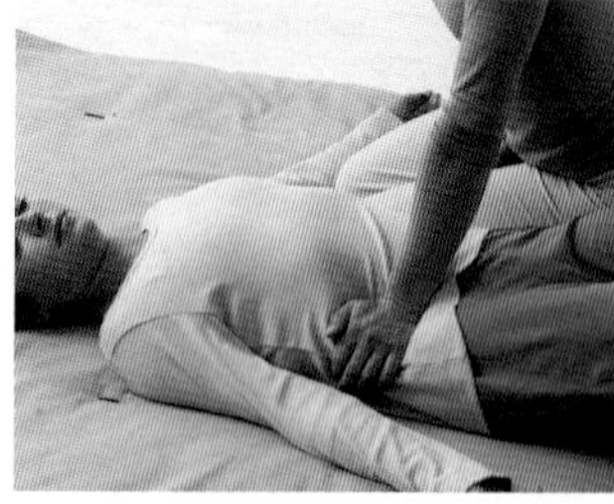

Palming the belly

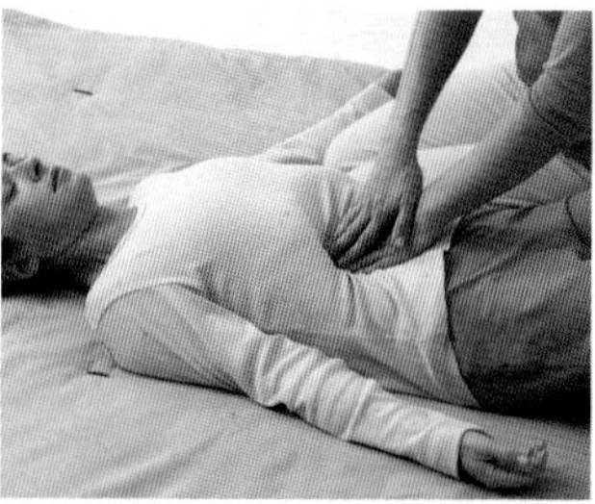

Pressing the belly

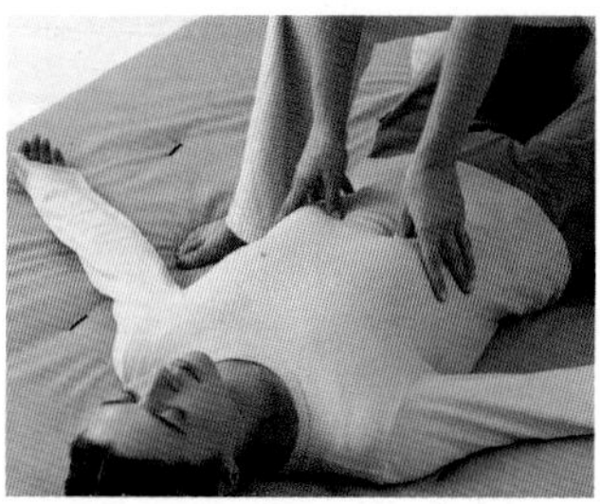

Thumb points

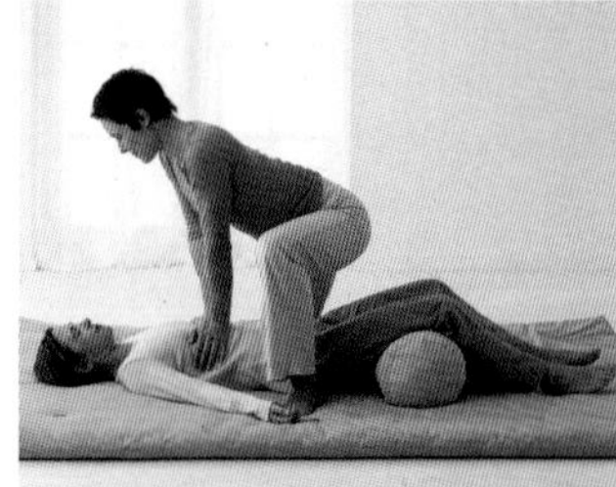

Palming the chest

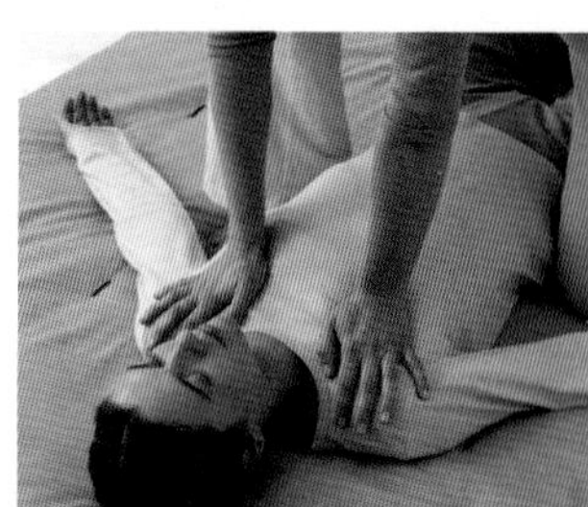

Palming the chest

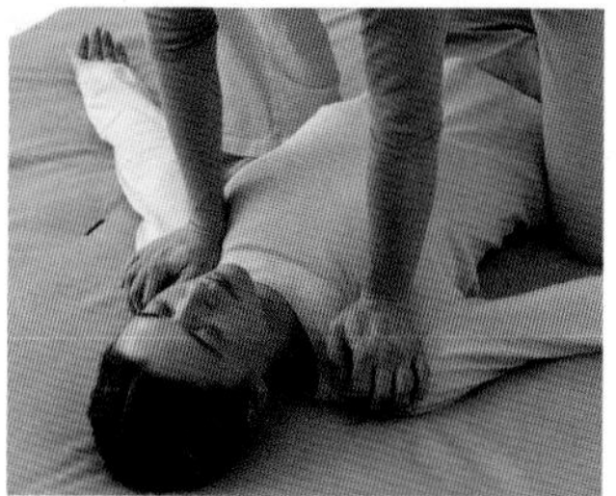

Shoulder nest

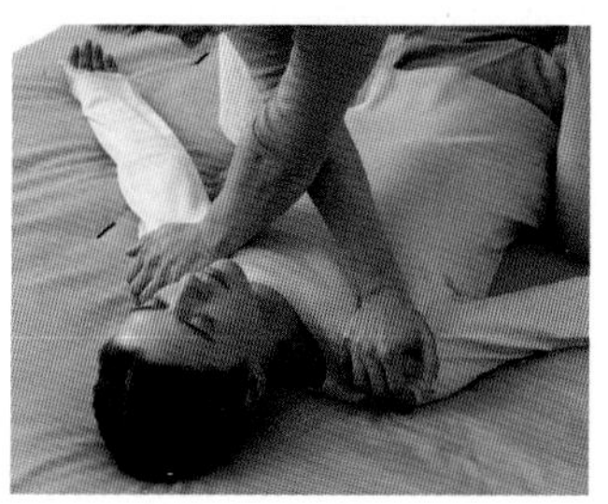

Crossing the shoulders

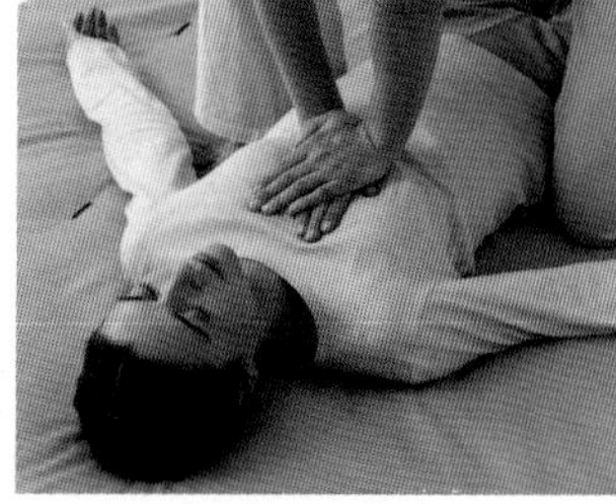

Sternum press

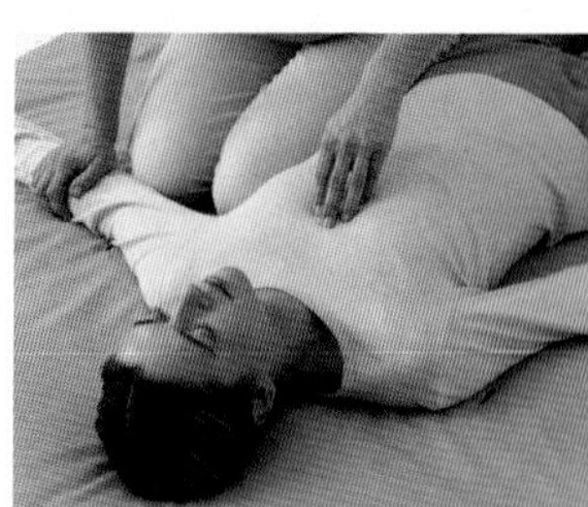

Sternum circles

The Arms

We use our arms to express what we want in life. We reach out and draw towards us what we love, or we hold back and push away things that are harmful to us.

Having stimulated the energy flow up through the abdomen and chest, you can now continue to unblock the flow along the arms, providing an enormous sense of release in the upper body.

After what can be emotional work on the abdomen and chest, working the arms (and the hands, which we will come to soon) can prove to be a fundamentally grounding experience for the receiver.

SEN KALATHARI

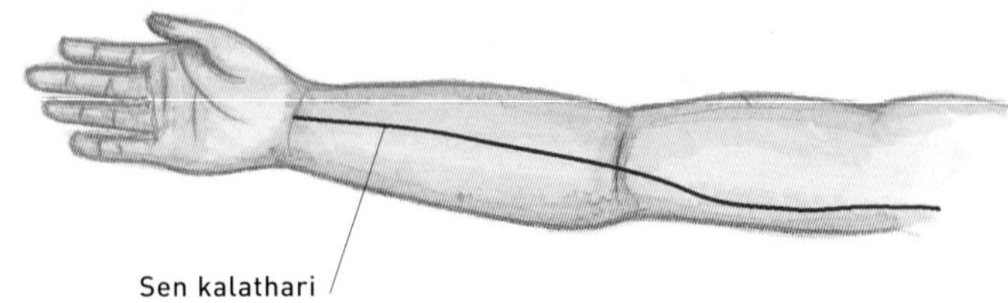

Above There are three sen that run through the arms. For beginners, it is best to focus on the central line, sen kalathari, which is shown here. Working this line has the most relaxing effect.

Working the Arm Lines

With this sequence of exercises, work the dominant arm and hand of your partner first, then move round to the other side of their body and repeat the whole sequence on their other arm.

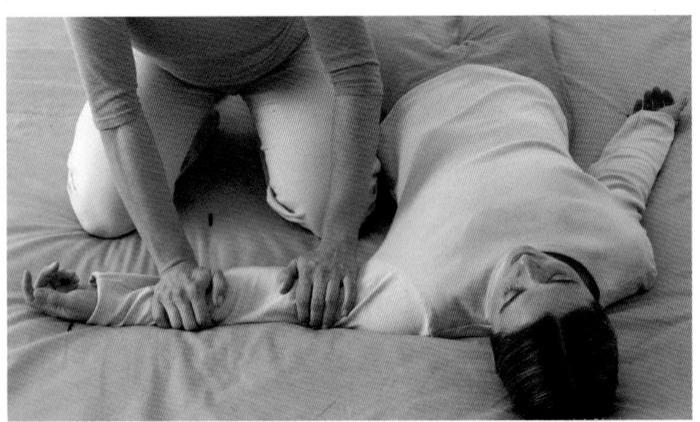

1 Palming the arm line Extend your partner's arm out to the side and palm up and down the inside of the arm, starting with one hand near the wrist and the other above the elbow. Palm in the same rhythmic fashion as with the leg lines, smoothly rocking the weight from one hand to the other. Check that your posture is relaxed and steady. Do one round of palming, then a round of thumbing. Palm the whole arm up and down to finish.

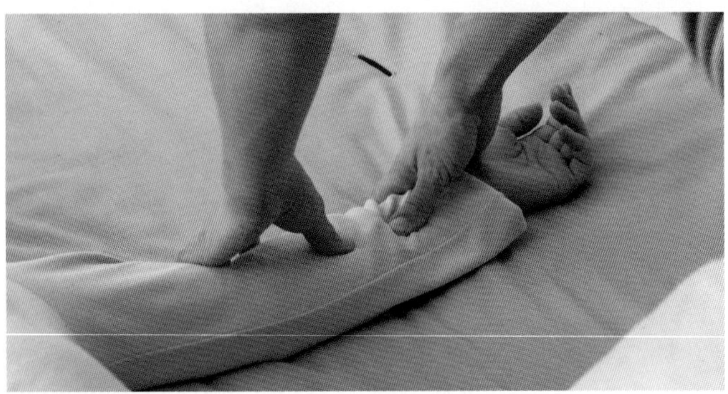

2 Thumbing the arm Thumb the lower and upper arm separately as they require slightly different techniques. Begin between the tendons just above the wrist and walk the thumbs alternately up to the elbow joint and back down again.

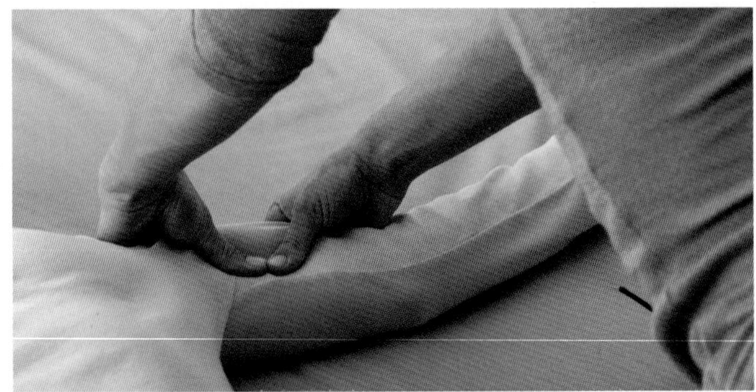

3 Thumbing the upper arm Use both thumbs simultaneously instead of the usual alternate pressure. Place the tips of your thumbs together and roll and squeeze the bicep muscle up, away from the bone. Use your fingers to give counter-pressure on the back of the arm. Start with your thumbs above the elbow and work up towards the armpit.

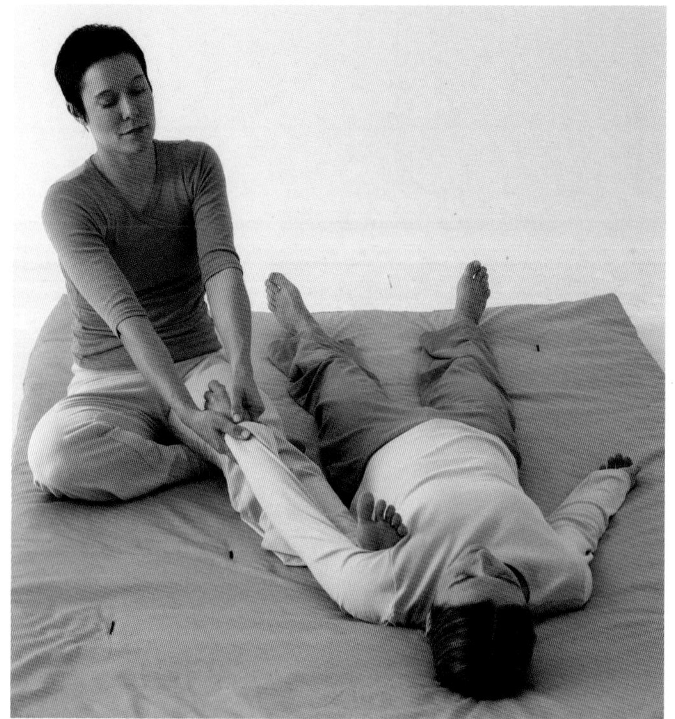

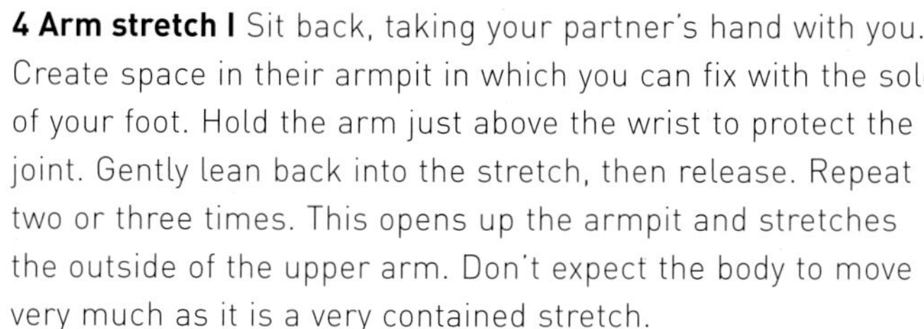

4 Arm stretch I Sit back, taking your partner's hand with you. Create space in their armpit in which you can fix with the sole of your foot. Hold the arm just above the wrist to protect the joint. Gently lean back into the stretch, then release. Repeat two or three times. This opens up the armpit and stretches the outside of the upper arm. Don't expect the body to move very much as it is a very contained stretch.

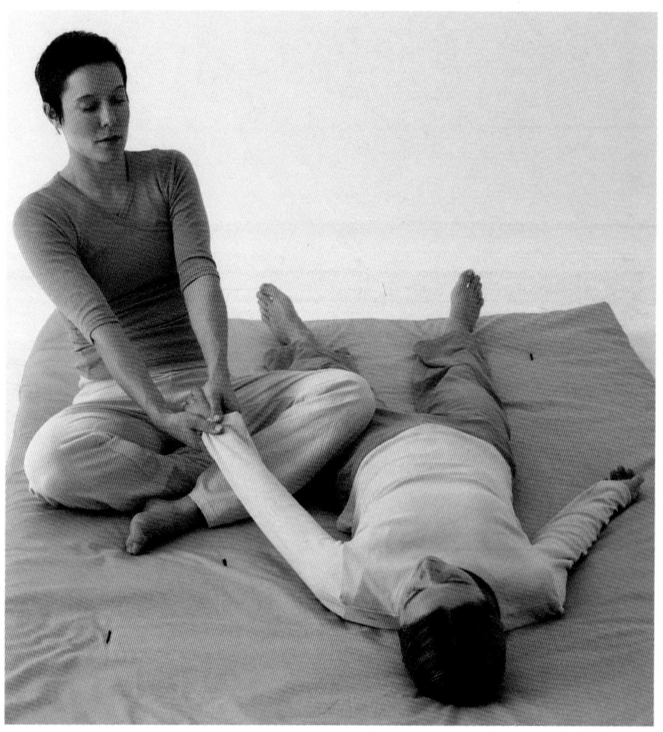

5 Arm stretch II This second stretch focuses on creating space between the shoulder and the ear, gently stretching the neck. Clasp firmly above your partner's wrist and lean away until you see their head roll slightly. Release the stretch slowly and let the head roll back. Repeat two or three times.

Technique improver

Of all the senses, our sense of sight is probably the most developed. When we are learning massage we often rely on what a pose looks like to judge whether or not we are getting it right. However, it is the quality of your touch that is important, so developing your sense of touch will add depth to your massage.

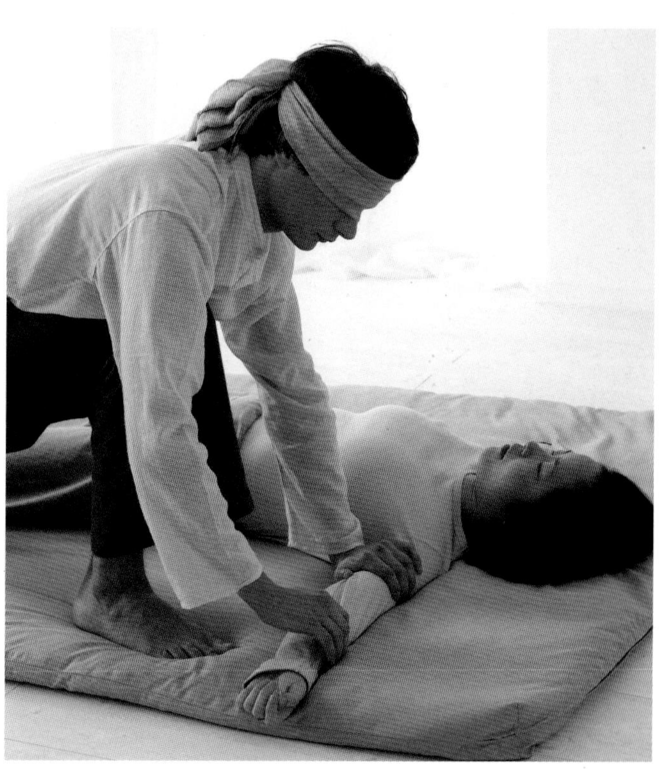

Right Covering your eyes, so that you temporarily remove your sense of sight, gives you an opportunity to explore working with touch alone. This is highly valuable, as it enables you to tune into the feeling in your hands. Palming the arm is a simple and safe place to start with the blindfold exercise, although of course you can eventually expand this practice to the whole of the massage.

The Hands

Our hands are incredibly dexterous, complex and strong structures that are constantly in motion and at work. Time spent focusing on the hands will enable you to work into all the joints and pressure points and will give a sense of completeness to the massage.

Small repetitive hand movements have become part of most people's daily lives, and can lead to repetitive strain injuries. Stimulating the acupressure points and creating space within the joints relaxes the hands and influences the flow of energy throughout the upper body. The sequence shown here is only a general guide – feel free to explore and play with what feels good for your partner.

Right This artwork shows specific acupressure points that can be worked on the hands in a Thai massage.

Getting it right

✗ Don't massage cut or bruised areas. Be careful of arthritic joints and don't massage when they are inflamed.

USING PRESSURE POINTS ON THE HANDS

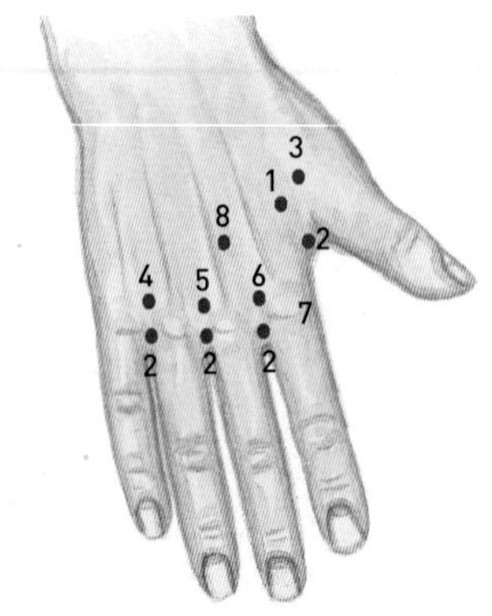

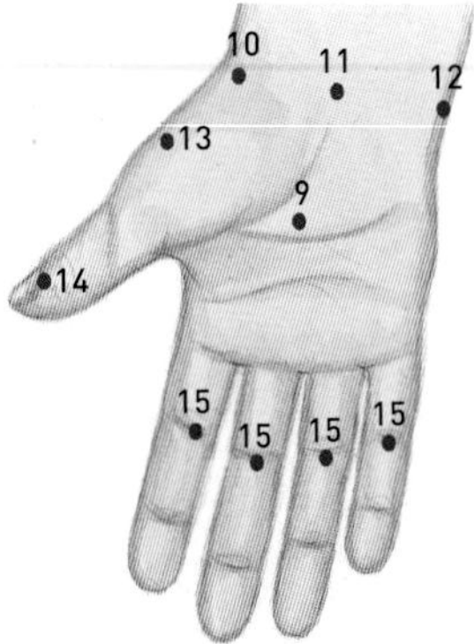

Key to the pressure points

Back of the hand:

1 hegu point, for all kinds of pain
2 and 3 headache and toothache
4 sciatica and hip pain
5 sore throat and toothache
6 tension in neck
7 shoulder pain
8 tension in neck, shoulder and arm, plus migraine and various stomach pains

Palm of the hand:

9 heatstroke and nausea
10 asthma, plus pain in chest, back, shoulder and wrist
11 wrist pain and arm paralysis
12 insomnia
13 coughs, asthma, fevers, sore throat and tendon problems
14 sore throat, fevers, fainting and respiratory problems
15 whooping cough and arthritis of the fingers

Working the Points on the Hands

Like the feet, the hands have specific acupressure points to focus on. For a general relaxing massage use the outline below, then for specific conditions you can focus on working particular acupressure points.

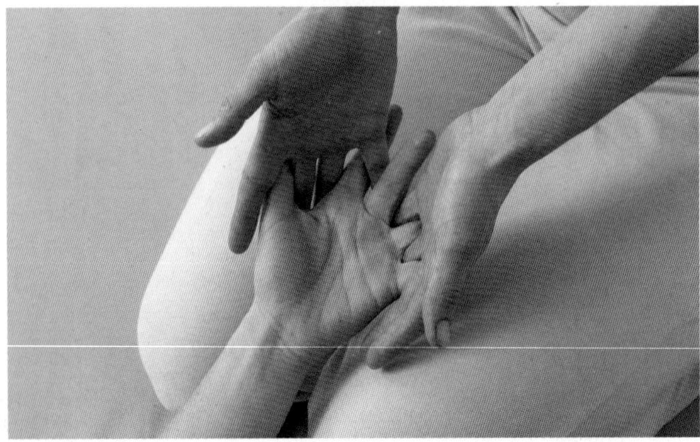

1 Palm opener Sit comfortably and let your partner's hand and wrist rest in your lap. Turn your hands palms up and slide your fingers between your partner's, leaving their middle finger free. Use the resistance of your fingers against the back of their hand to open their palm.

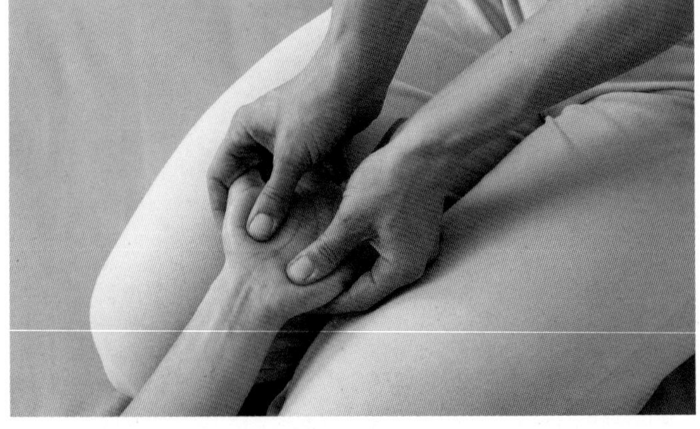

2 Stroking the palm Using your thumbs, firmly stroke from the wrist down to the centre of the palm. Use your fingers at the back of the hand as counter-pressure. Most people find this very relaxing, so work here for as long as your partner likes, exploring the whole palm with your thumbs.

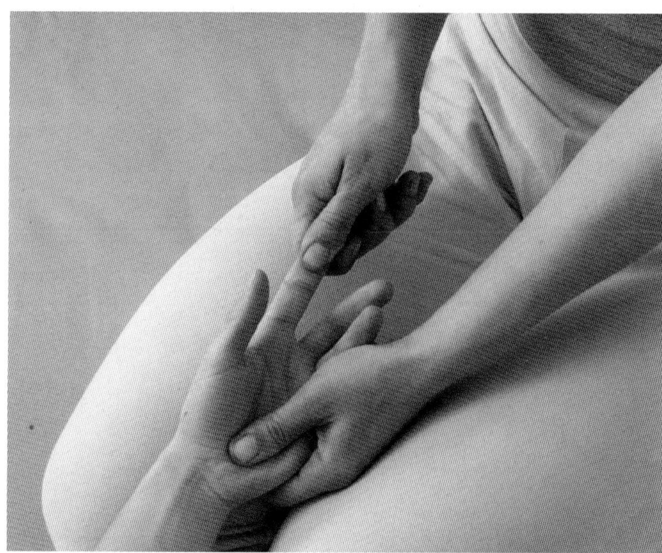

3 Finger squeeze This exercise creates space in the finger joints and relieves and enlivens stiff, tired fingers. Firmly hold the palm of your partner's hand in place and use your thumb and forefinger to rotate around all the joints of each finger, working from knuckle to tip and squeezing and lengthening each finger in turn.

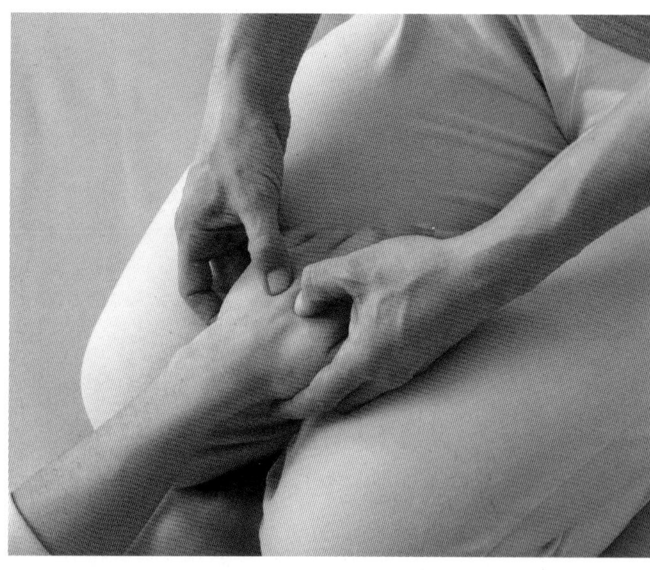

4 Opening the back of the hand Turn the hand over and work as you did the top of the feet. You can stimulate the many points on the back of your partner's hand by working in between the tendons. Use your thumbs to massage firmly from the wrist up towards the knuckles, giving a gentle pinch to the webbing between the fingers.

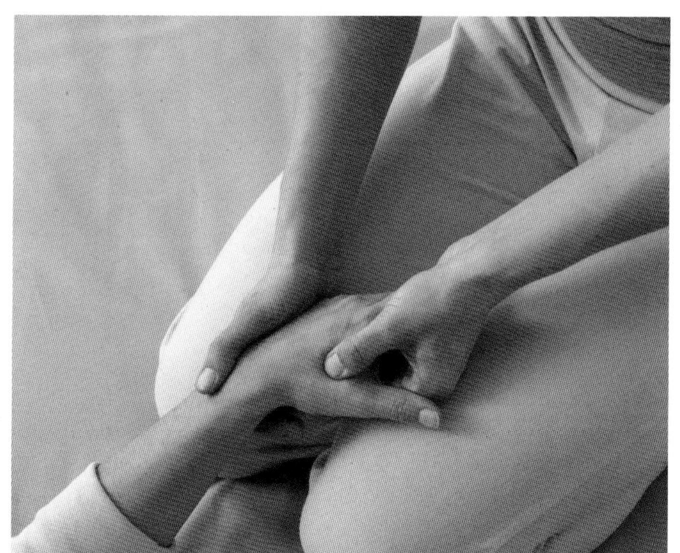

5 Hegu point To locate this point, turn your partner's hand slightly on its side. Go right up into the webbing of the hand and come away from the joint slightly. Angle towards the finger joint. Pinch firmly with thumb and forefinger for maximum effect – if it feels painful you've hit the spot. Encourage your partner to breathe. For a relaxing massage you can rub around the area, but for therapeutic use, work with very strong pressure and hold for as long as possible before releasing. The feeling should be one of a good pain, which eases as soon as you ease off the pressure. Now repeat several times.

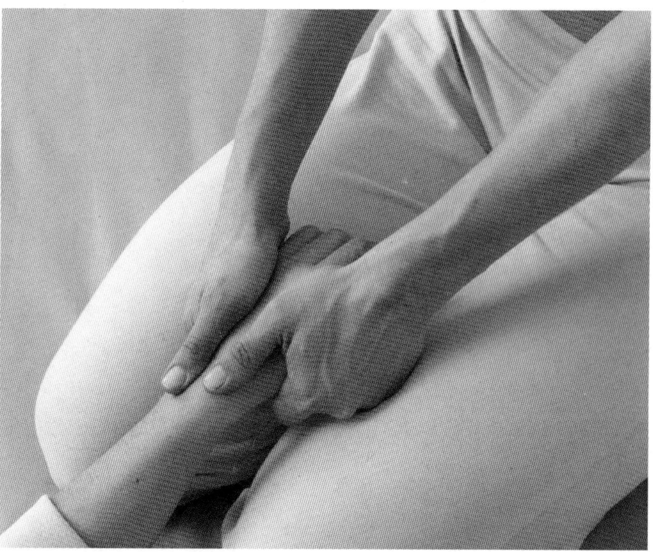

6 Kneading hands This is a very relaxing movement so explore and enjoy it. You can work the hands in a slow pulsing, squeezing movement from the wrist towards the fingertips. Use your hands alternately or simultaneously.

Caution

The hegu point is used in Chinese medicine as a natural painkiller and powerful detoxifier. Often called the Great Eliminator, it is specifically good for headaches and toothache. Never use during pregnancy, due to its strong eliminating effect.

Opening the Wrists

The wrists are extremely sensitive, much-used joints that often suffer from compression and strain. These exercises bring a wonderful feeling of freedom and release to the wrists.

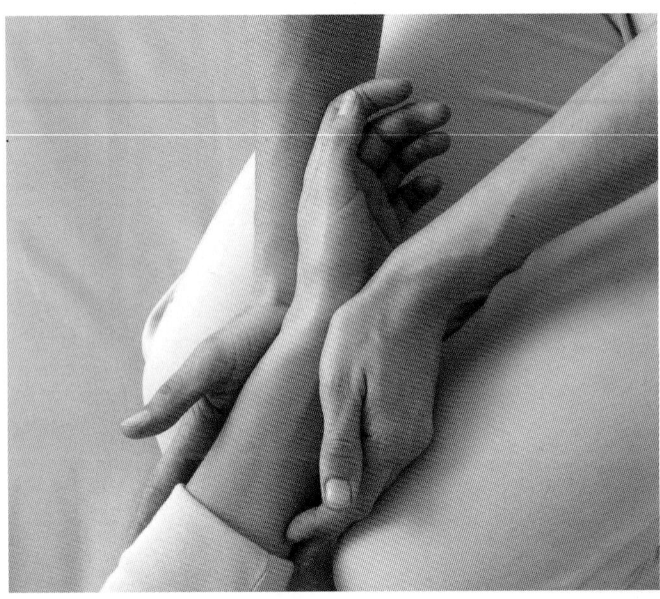

1 Wrist rub Hold your partner's wrist between the heels of your hands and let their hand relax completely. Rub your hands together, letting their fingers flop back and forth as you do so.

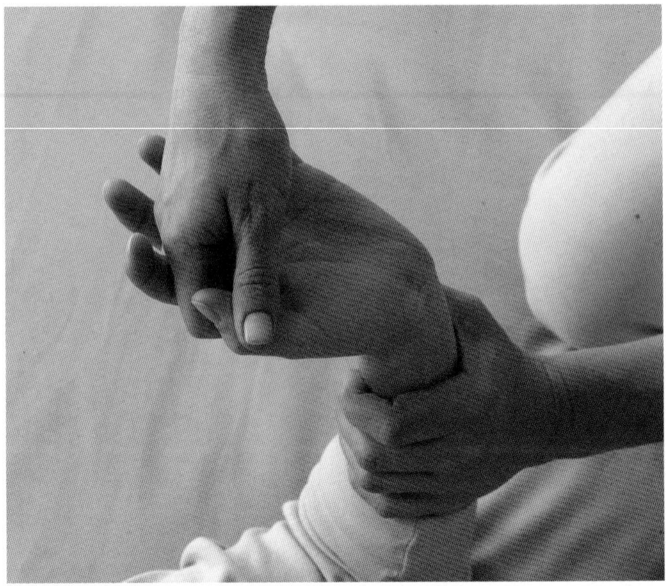

2 Opening the wrists The wrists are often restricted in their movement because the forearms are tight, so this exercise focuses on opening the wrists and the forearms simultaneously. With one hand on the forearm, press your partner's elbow down into the mat. Place the fingers of your other hand between their fingers and lengthen their fingers away, creating space throughout the front of the wrist.

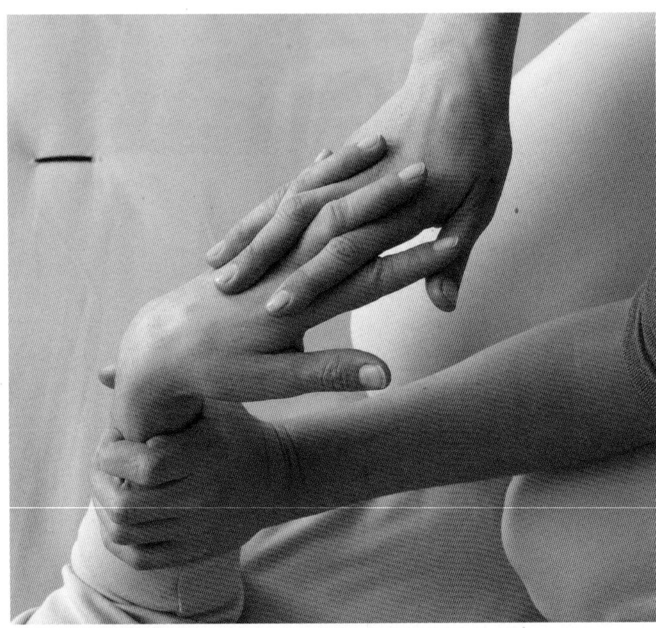

3 Maintaining a feeling of length through the palm, take the fingers over to the other side and stretch open the back of the wrist and the back of the forearm. Repeat gently back and forth three times.

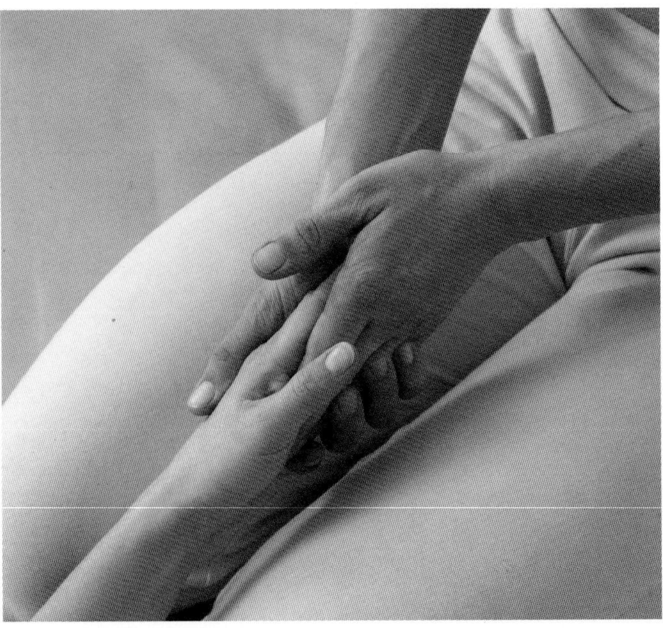

4 Hold and sweep To finish the hand massage, hold your partner's hand between yours and sweep firmly from the wrist to the fingertips. Repeat several times.

Review: Arms and Hands

Now repeat the whole arm and hand sequence on the other side of the body, using the pictures below as a reminder. As before, make sure that you are confident about working this part of the body before moving on.

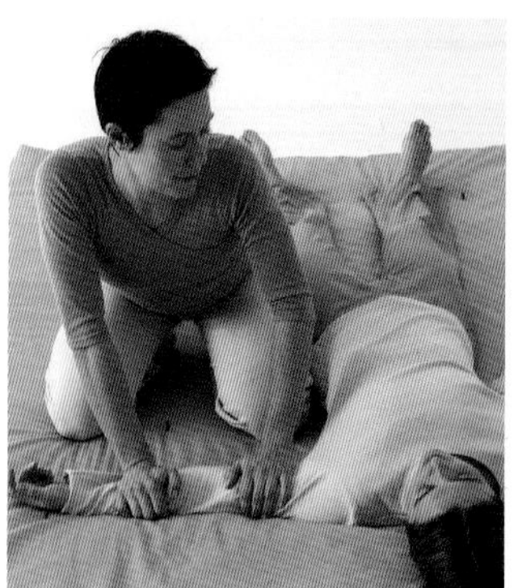

Palming the arm

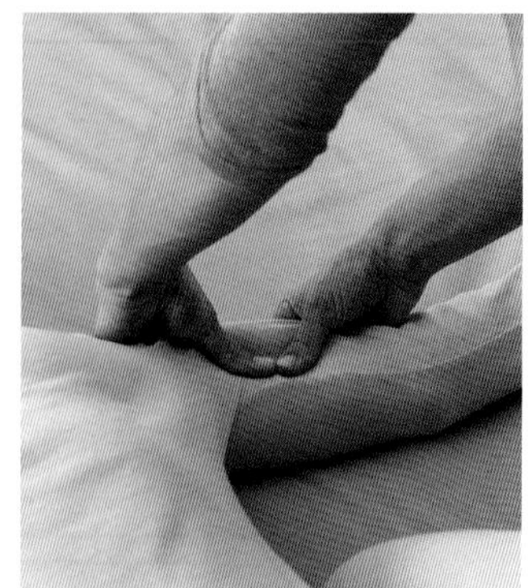

Thumbing the arm

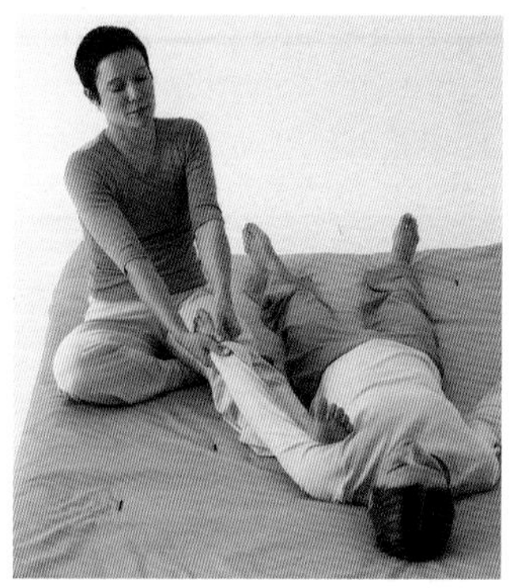

Arm stretch I

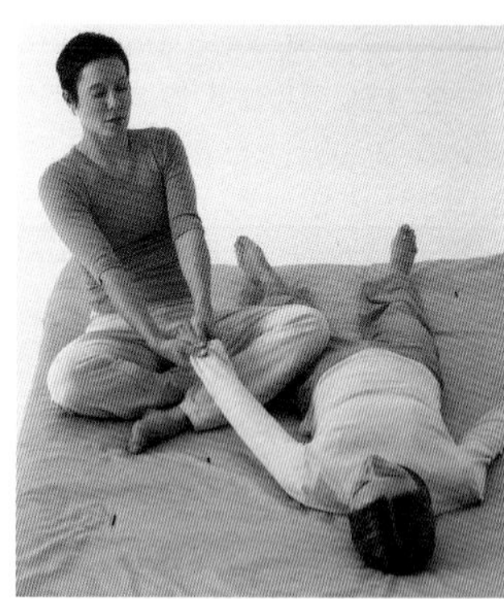

Arm stretch II

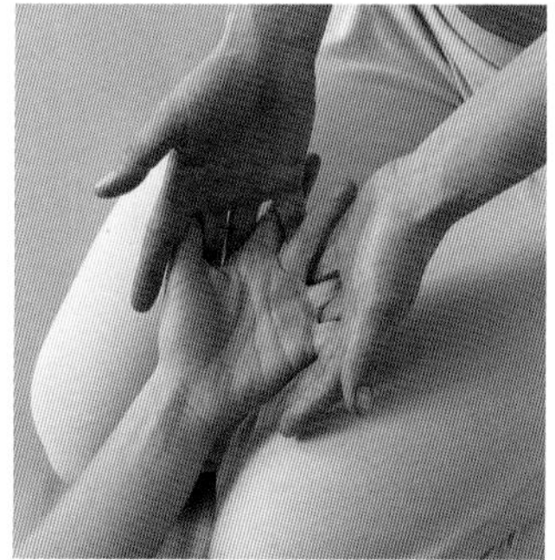

Palm opener

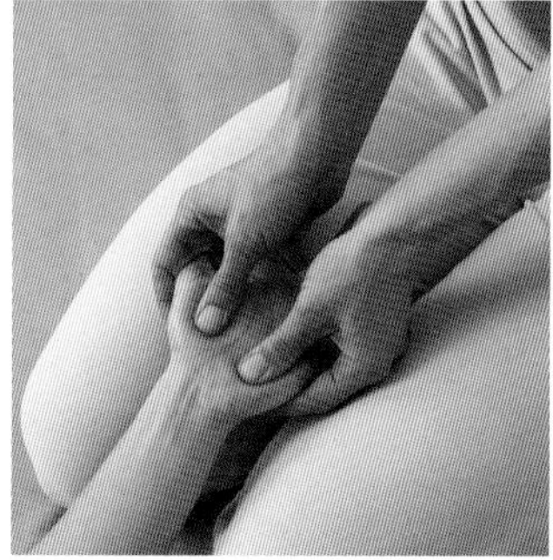

Stroking the palm

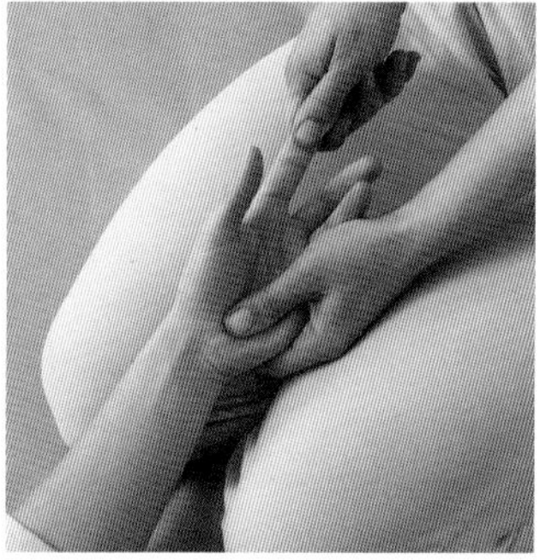

Finger squeeze

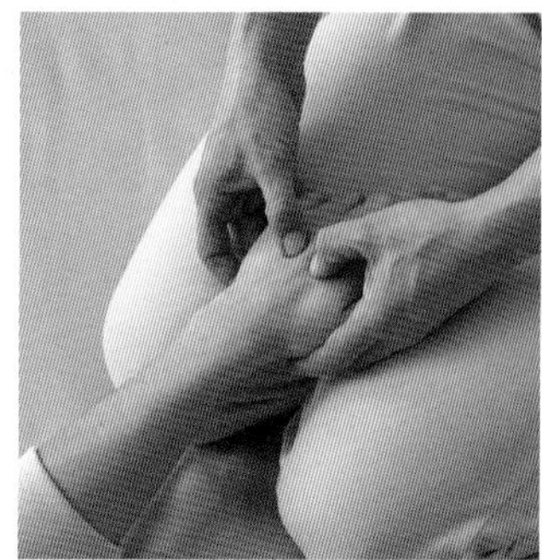

Opening the back of the hand

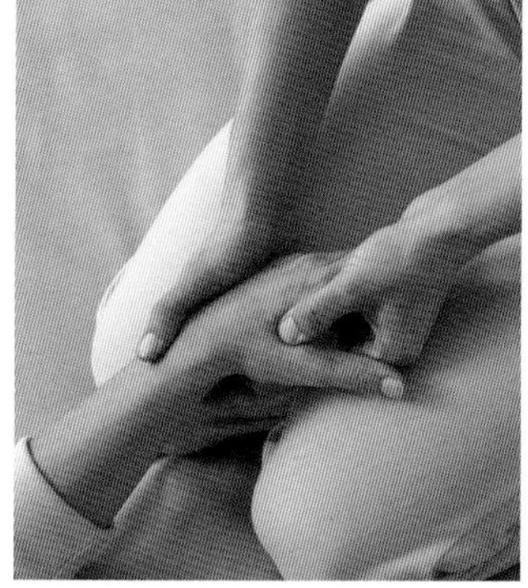

Hegu point

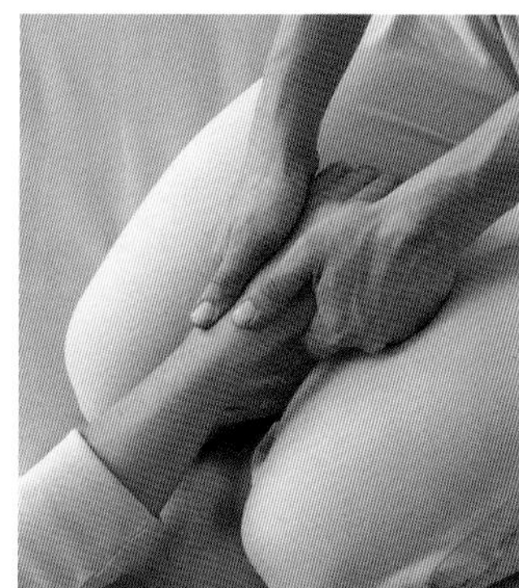

Kneading hands

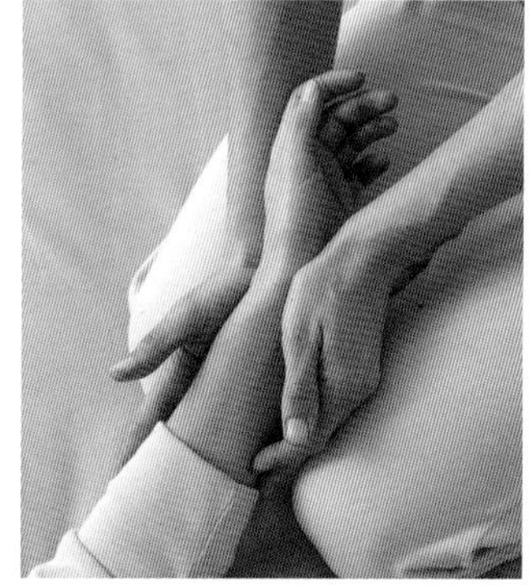

Wrist rub

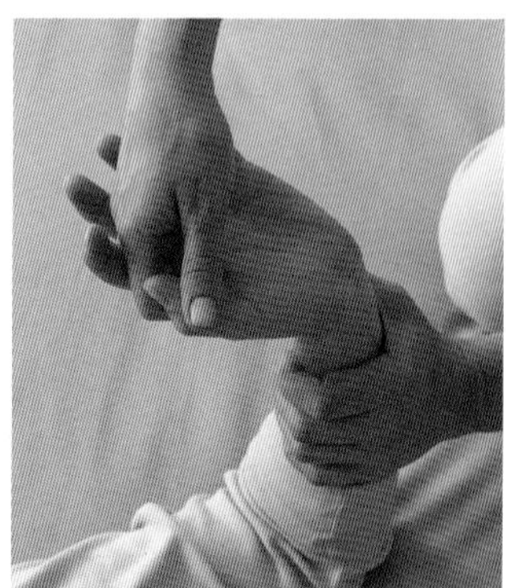

Opening the wrists

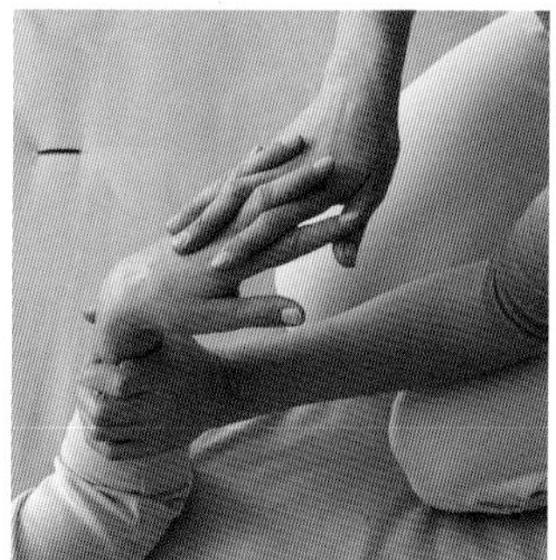

Opening the wrists

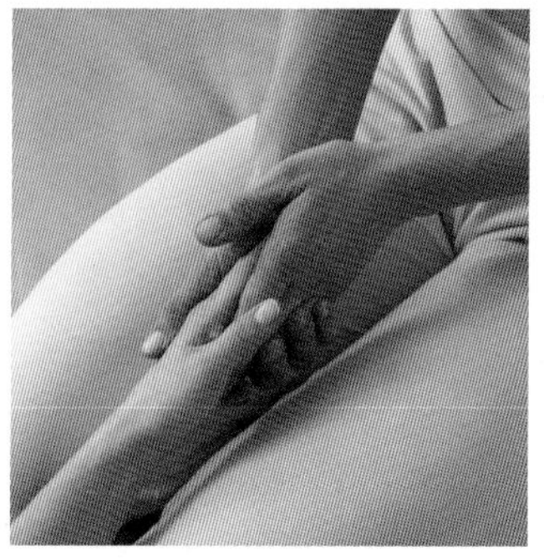

Hold and sweep

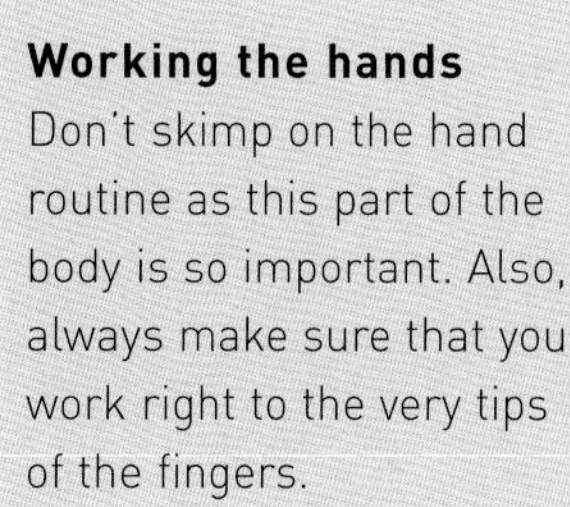

Working the hands

Don't skimp on the hand routine as this part of the body is so important. Also, always make sure that you work right to the very tips of the fingers.

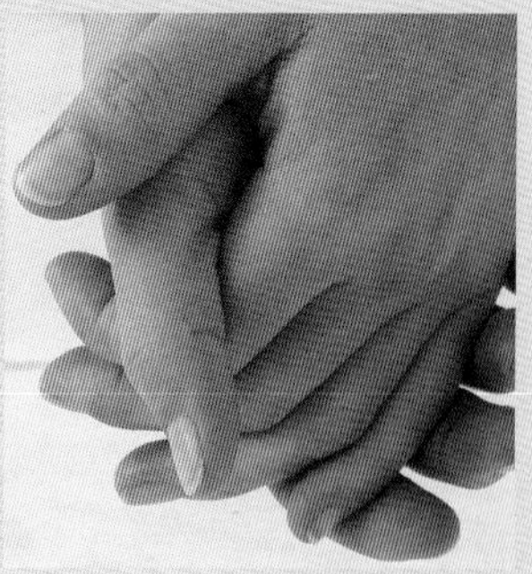

The Shoulders and Neck

You will discover that the side position is a particularly effective one for helping to free up energy that has become blocked around the shoulders and the neck.

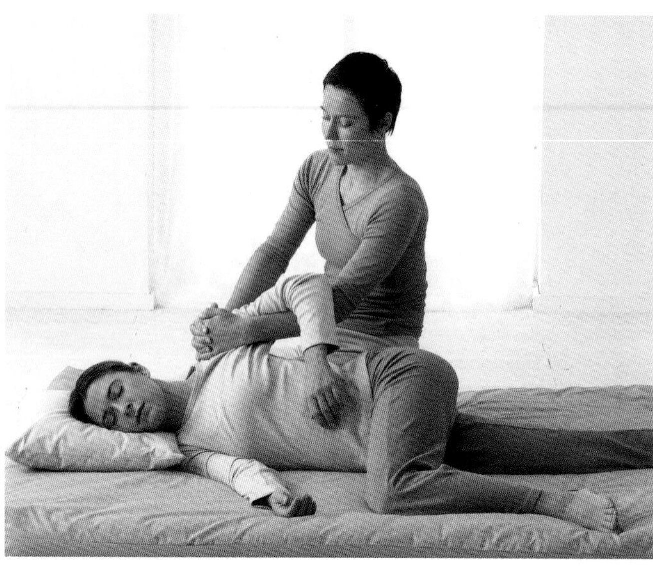

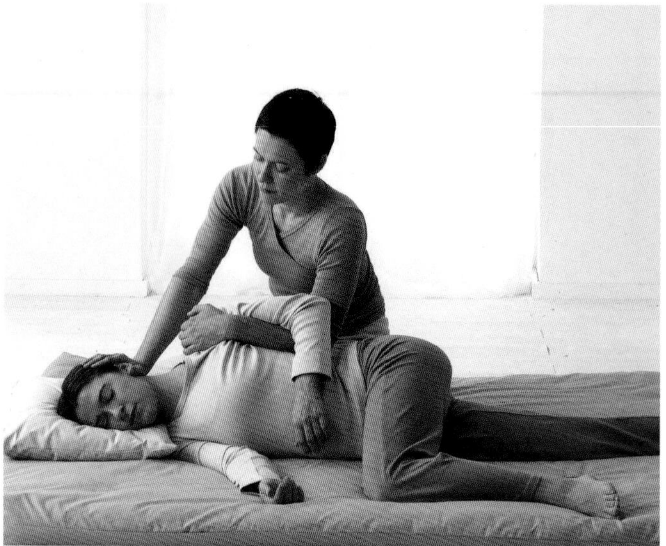

1 Shoulder circles This is an easy general movement that relaxes the neck and the whole of the shoulder joint. For very stiff people it helps to free up the chest area. Kneel behind your partner's shoulder blade and slide your body close up against their upper back. Circle your arm under theirs and clasp one hand around the front and one hand around the back of the shoulder. Make sure your partner's forearm is nice and floppy. Now slowly rotate the whole of the shoulder joint, drawing as big a circle as possible. Rotate several times in both directions.

2 Neck stretch Now that you have loosened the shoulder, this stretch will work deeper into the neck and up into the base of the skull. Keeping the front hand clasped around the top of your partner's shoulder, slide your other hand up the neck so that its heel rests against the occipital ridge at the base of the skull. Fix your hand here and lean away to create space between the shoulder and the ear. Check the pressure with your partner as it can be deceptively strong.

Shiva Pose

This mirrors the yoga pose, Natarajasana (Lord Shiva's pose). It gives a wonderful expansive feeling through the front of the body, opens up the front of the hip and belly and stimulates the sen in the front of the abdomen, as well as the spine and sen sumana.

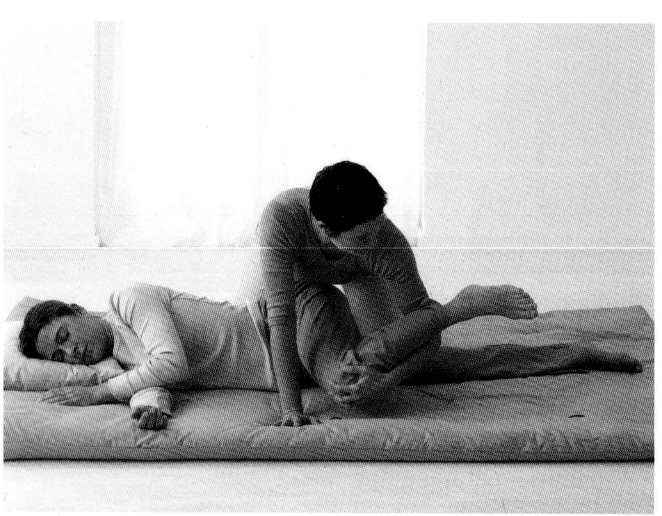

1 Kneeling behind your partner, reach forward and support their knee with your hand and their lower leg with your forearm. Keep your elbow wide, as if there is a circle emanating from your breastbone to your fingertips. This will help maintain the framework of the stretch. With your other hand, push yourself back to upright, using your partner's hip joint to support you.

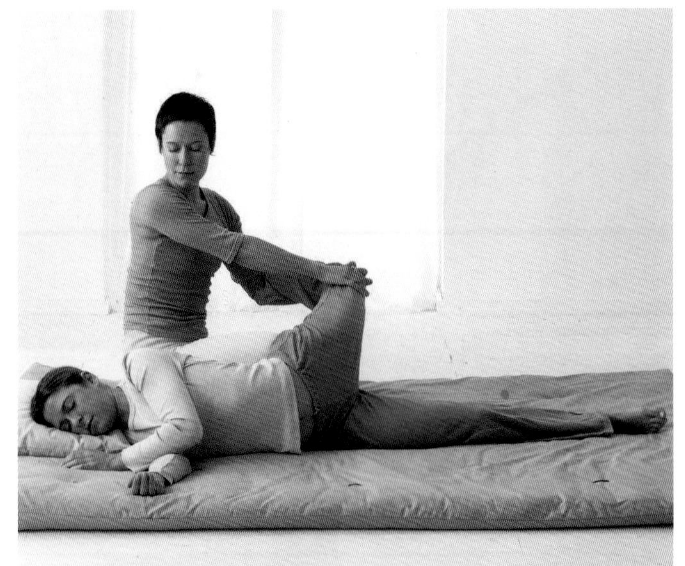

2 Raise your knee (keep the toes flat) and place into your partner's buttock. Clasp both hands around the front of their knee for support. To move into the stretch, sink your knee into the buttock and lean away with your upper body. Ease in and out of the stretch three times without undoing the pose totally. To end, keep a good support under their knee and circle the leg down to the floor.

Step 2 positioning
Note the position of the masseur's knee and foot. This is a similar position to the knee lift featured in the physical preparatory exercises.

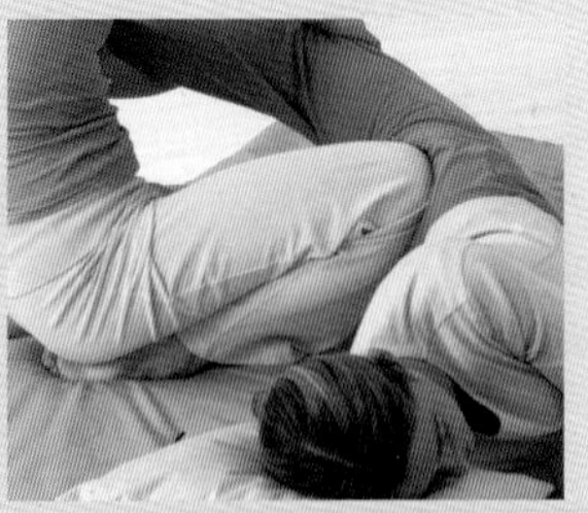

Variations to the Shiva pose

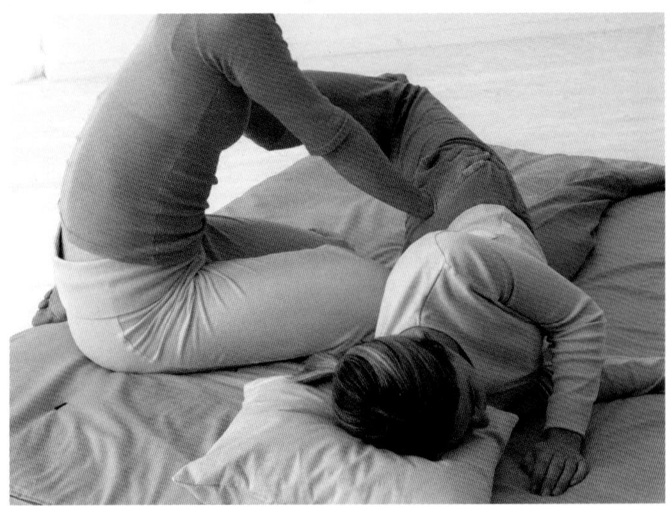

Above For a gentler stretch, use this alternative method. Kneel down and place your hand on your partner's buttock. Sink your hips down to one side of your feet. Keep your arm straight and lean into your hand, bringing the movement out through their thigh and knee. Continue the circle with their leg by leaning away with your other arm. Work to the point of resistance, then ease off. Repeat three times before releasing the whole posture.

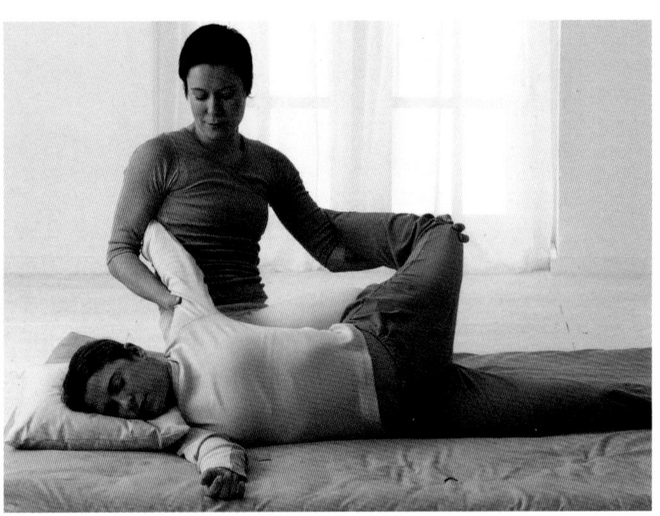

Above There are a large number of different variations of this pose within the Thai massage tradition. The one shown here adds a shoulder stretch, in order to open up the chest and the armpit.

Getting it right

✗ Don't do this exercise if your partner suffers from disc problems in their lower back or from lower back pain. Also, avoid it if your partner is much bigger and heavier than you.

✓ Make sure you are working with the breath, exhaling as you move deeper into the stretch.

✓ Ask whether the stretch is too strong – you can't see your partner's face to judge their reaction.

✓ You need to support your partner's body throughout so that they can stay very relaxed in the thigh and buttocks. Remind them to let the weight of their leg drop completely into your arm.

✓ Always keep your partner's knee in alignment with their hip joint. To maintain the correct angle, imagine that you are drawing a circle with their leg so that if the foot carried on round it would eventually reach the top of the head.

The Back of the Body

A COMPLETE BODY ROUTINE

The back of the body is like a protective shell and is where we tend to habitually hold tension, often over many years. The massage sequence given over the following pages aims to soften this shell and re-integrate the energy previously held as tension, letting it flow freely through the body from the feet to the head.

The exercises directly influence the structure of the spine, which provides fundamental support for the whole skeleton. It works with deep layers of tension held around the spine, which can restrict the flow of energy and blood to the spinal nerves, with implications for the whole nervous system. Most people feel very relaxed lying on their belly, so this sequence provides a chance to consolidate the stronger work of the side position.

Below Thai-style palming done in this position is a very traditional way of working the back. Its beautiful contained shape shows how one body can support the other.

THAI MASSAGE AND BACK PAIN

Back pain is something that many of us suffer from to some degree during our lives. Many cases are not too serious and are the result of tight or aching muscles. However, back pain may be caused by injury, and one common spinal injury is a slipped or herniated disc. You may have experienced this for yourself or be massaging someone who has, so it can be useful to have a little understanding of what it involves.

The spine is a column of 26 vertebrae interspersed with discs, which are gel-like shock absorbers. The spine is healthy and flexible only if the discs remain healthy. Movement keeps the inside of each disc nourished with a good flow of blood, but if the spine is not used to moving in all directions, a disc can become weak. If it is then put under too much stress, it may become herniated: fluid leaks out of the disc membrane. When this happens at the back of the spinal column the

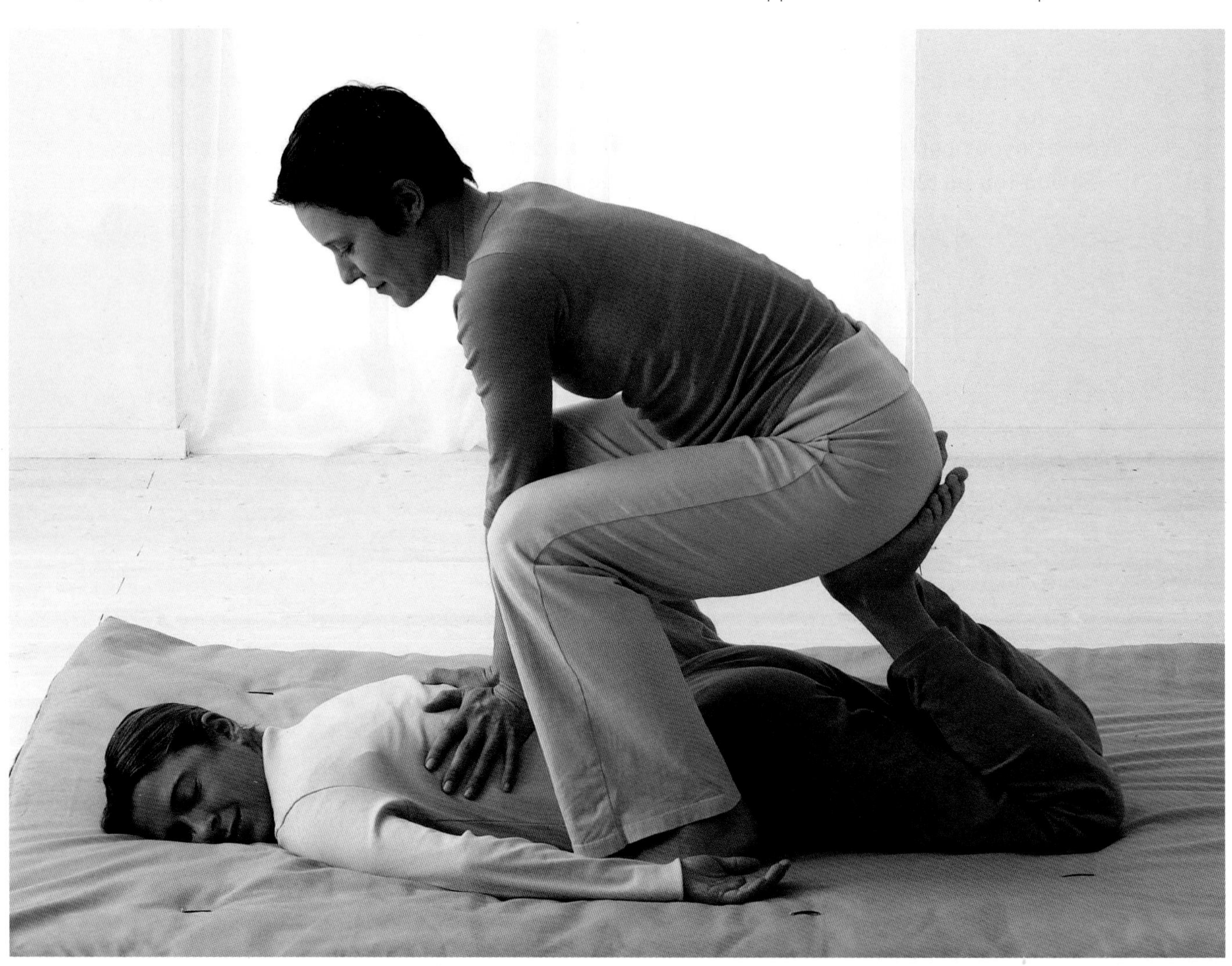

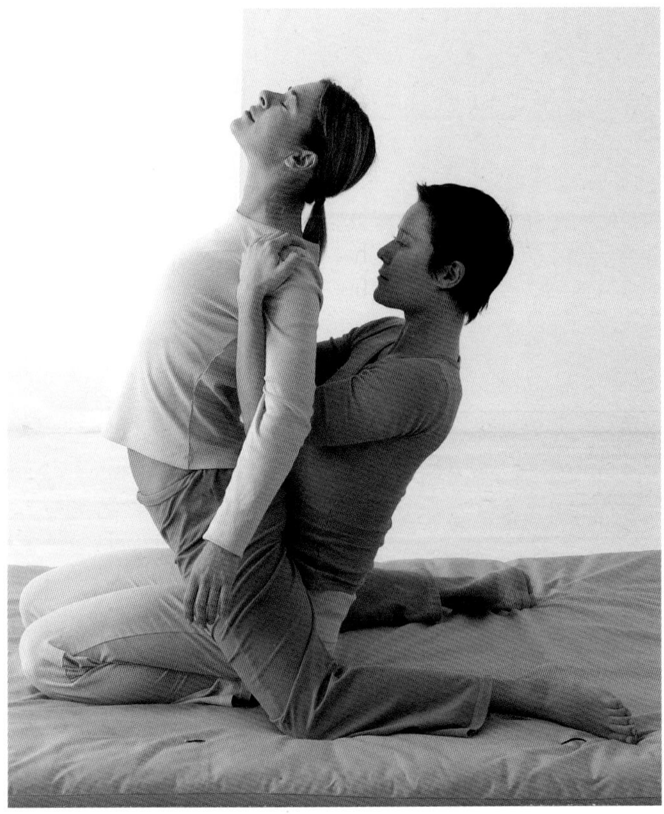

Getting it right

✗ Do not use stretches on those suffering from spinal injuries or disc problems. If you are in any doubt about the state of your partner's health following an injury or back problem, then you must consult an experienced physiotherapist or osteopath.

✗ Remember not to work directly on the bone itself.

✓ Work with the breath. It can be useful to remind your partner to focus on their breath. Work with a slow and smooth rhythm as you apply and release pressure. Sink with your body weight, don't push with your strength.

✓ Check the strength of the stretches and pressure with your partner as you will not be able to take cues from their facial expressions.

Left The King of Cobras is a beautiful pose, suited only to advanced practitioners and recipients, that shows the potential of a healthy back, allowing an opening all the way through the spinal column.

fluid presses on the spinal nerves, causing pain. It can also occur at the front of the spine. As there are no nerves here no pain is experienced, but the integrity of the body is still affected.

We need exercises that help prevent these weak areas from developing. We need to keep the joints in the spinal column well nourished with good blood flow and strong, healthy energy flow. This increased flow can come about only through movement, and Thai massage, with its emphasis on dynamic and passive movement, is very beneficial for maintaining a healthy spine.

SLIPPED DISCS

Avoid working on your partner's spine if they are suffering from, or have recently suffered from, a slipped (herniated) disc. The condition may take up to three months to heal, and during this time it is very important to avoid any movements that might aggravate the situation. However, you can help to alleviate the discomfort and tension around the affected area by gently working the energy lines of the back. Work with your partner's permission and constant feedback.

MAKING YOUR PARTNER COMFORTABLE

Ensure that your partner is as comfortable as possible so that they are able to relax fully. Some people are unused to lying flat on their front with their arms down by their side, in which case you may need to provide a little extra support. A pillow or folded blanket under the chest or hips can help create more space through the upper spine so that the neck feels free. Support under the front of the ankles can alleviate any pressure or discomfort in the knees. If your partner suffers from a very weak or painful lower back then you may need to raise the feet slightly higher, again using some padding under the front of their feet.

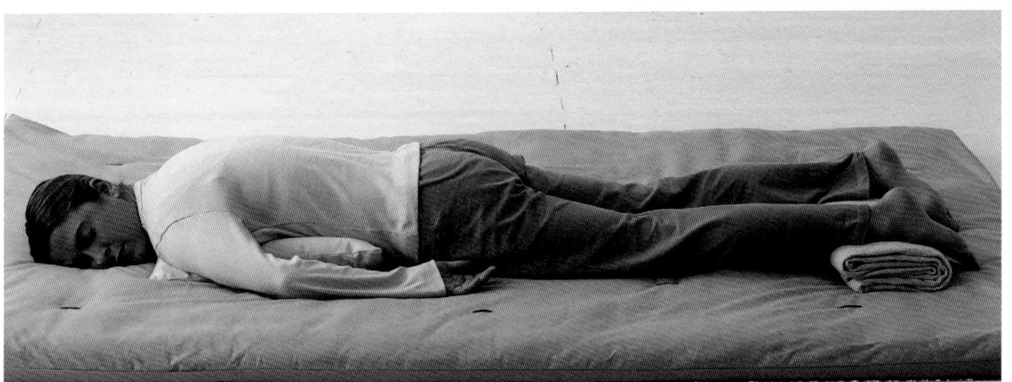

Left You may need to add extra support – with pillows or folded blankets for example – to ensure that your partner is totally comfortable and relaxed.

The Sequence for the Back of the Body

There are many different aspects to working the back of the body. As this is a long sequence, it is advised that you practise it section by section until you feel more confident about putting all of the aspects together. The initial section of the sequence focuses on additional work for the feet and ankles, before providing some gentle warm-up exercises for the legs and hips. The sequence then moves on to exercises that cover ways of working the energy lines of the back, as well as stretches that provide a deeper level of opening.

Integrating the Back of the Body

This exercise, like the ones that follow, acknowledges the all-important energetic and physiological connection between the feet, the legs and the back.

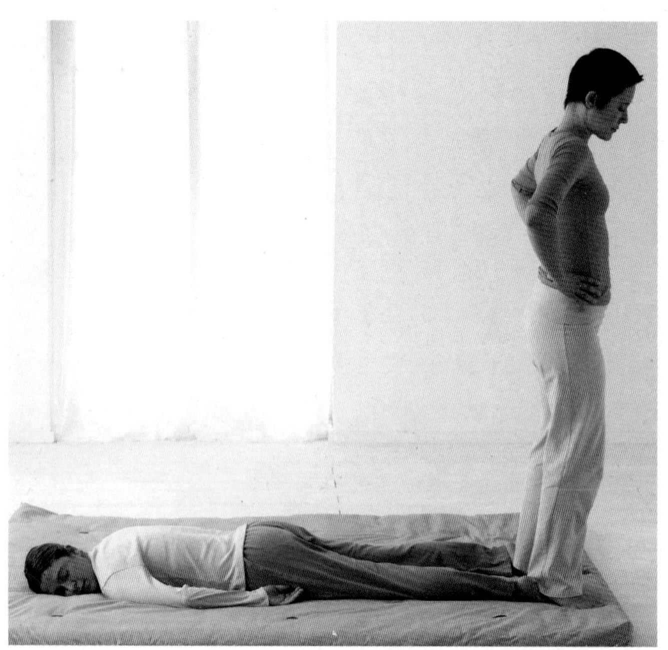

1 Walking on the feet This is very easy and very satisfying for your partner, but do not attempt it unless their heels fall comfortably out to the side with their ankles touching the mat. Facing away from your partner is easier – use a chair for support, if necessary. Stand with the front of your feet on the mat and place your heels on your partner's insteps. Shift your weight from side to side, as if you were walking on the spot. Check the pressure with your partner (most people love the sensation).

Step 1 foot position
Make sure that your heels are well away from the balls of your partner's feet – to avoid putting direct pressure on the joints.

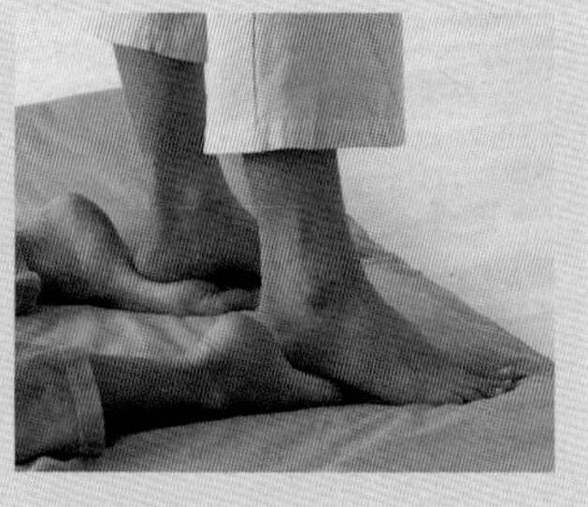

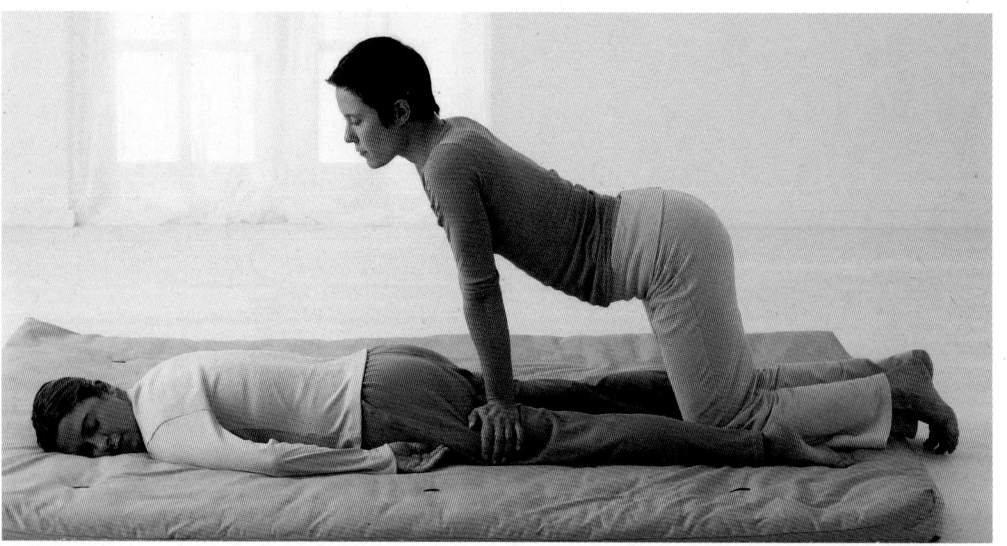

2 Palming the backs of the legs Palm both of the legs simultaneously. Work from the Achilles tendon directly up the legs until you feel the buttock bone. Ease off the pressure as you pass over the knees. This additional palming for the backs of the legs will help to relax both the hips and the lower back.

Feet to Sacrum

This exercise helps to open the lower back and works to lengthen through the front of the hips and into the thighs, as well as opening the ankle joints. Three variations are shown here for varying degrees of flexibility.

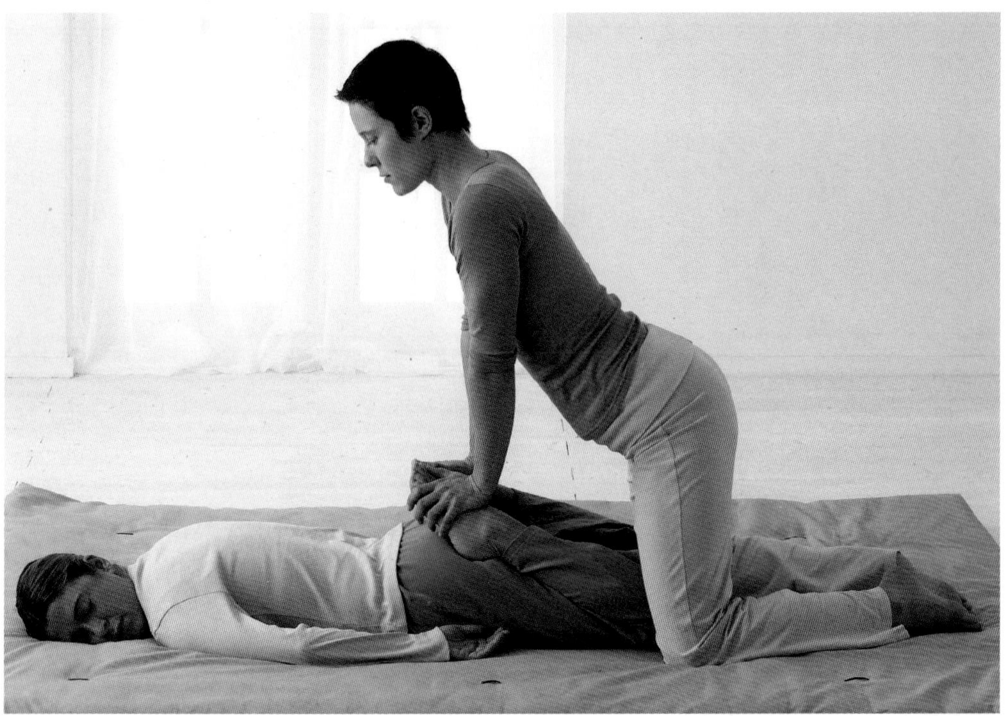

Pose 1 This is the main version, suitable for a wide range of people. Position yourself at your partner's feet. Take both their feet up towards their buttocks, and lengthen through the front of their toes. Keep your posture wide and your arms straight. Sink your body weight on to their feet so that their heels press in towards their buttocks.

Variation for less flexible people

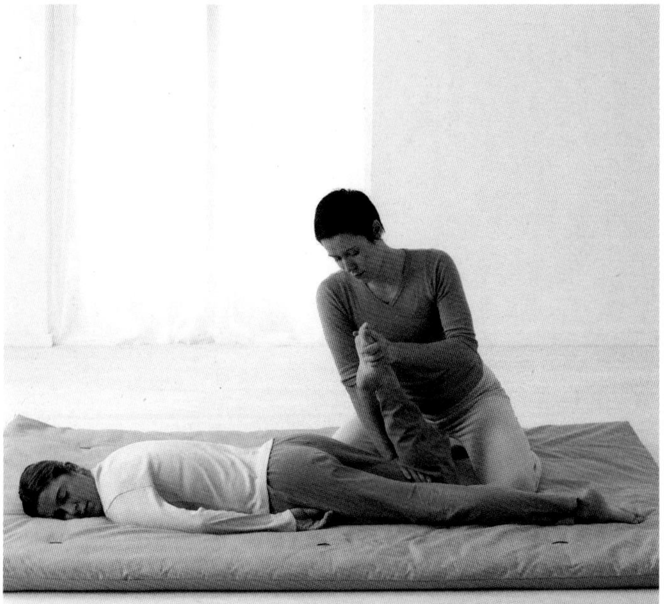

Pose 2 This version is for stiffer people who experience restriction through the fronts of the thighs or discomfort in the lower back. Kneel at the outside of the leg, facing sideways on to your partner. Place your upper hand behind the knee and take the front of the foot up and towards the buttock as far as it will go. Encourage your partner to remain relaxed and heavy in the front of the hips.

Variation for protecting the back

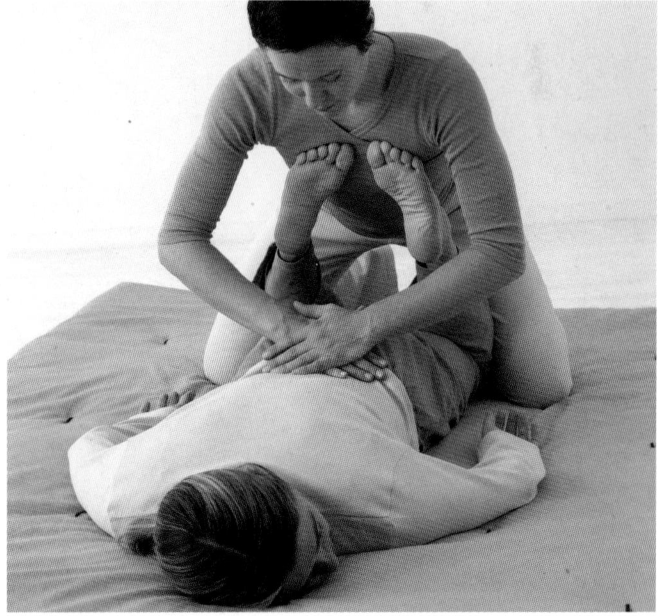

Pose 3 This pose lengthens the sacrum as you bring the feet in towards the buttocks, so it is ideal for those whose lower back needs protection and stability. Wide-kneel at your partner's feet. Lift up their feet to rest against your chest. Cup your hands over their sacrum, with your fingers pointing in and your elbows wide. As you lean forward with the feet, scoop the sacrum back towards you with your hands.

The Locust

In this pose, lengthen through the sacrum to create a deep opening into the front of the hip and thigh. The Locust can be a strong position, so ensure that you work smoothly with the breath.

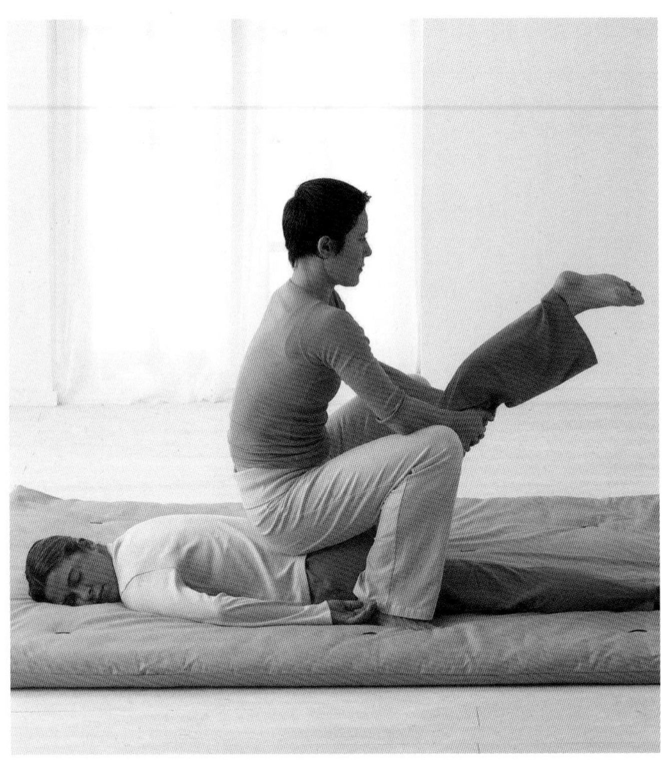

Left Squat lightly over your partner's hips, keeping most of your weight in your legs. Work one leg at a time. Cup your hands under their knee and firmly interlace your fingers, so that you have a good grip. Fix your tailbone against your partner's sacrum, then lift the knee off the ground and rest your elbows on your thighs. This is your lever and your fix in the pose.

To achieve the stretch, work on the exhalation. Make a scooping action with your hips to create length through the base of your partner's spine and lean back, lifting their knee up and away. Ease in and out two or three times, but without completely undoing the pose. Repeat the exercise with the other leg.

Getting it right

✗ Don't try this pose if your partner has a weakness in the lower back, or if they found feet to sacrum challenging. Do not attempt it if your partner is much bigger or heavier than you.

✓ As the pose can be quite strong, make sure you maintain a good level of communication with your partner.

Take a Break

This is a wonderfully relaxing pose for both you and your partner, as you can really enjoy using your body weight. The rolling action can be repeated for as long as feels good for your partner.

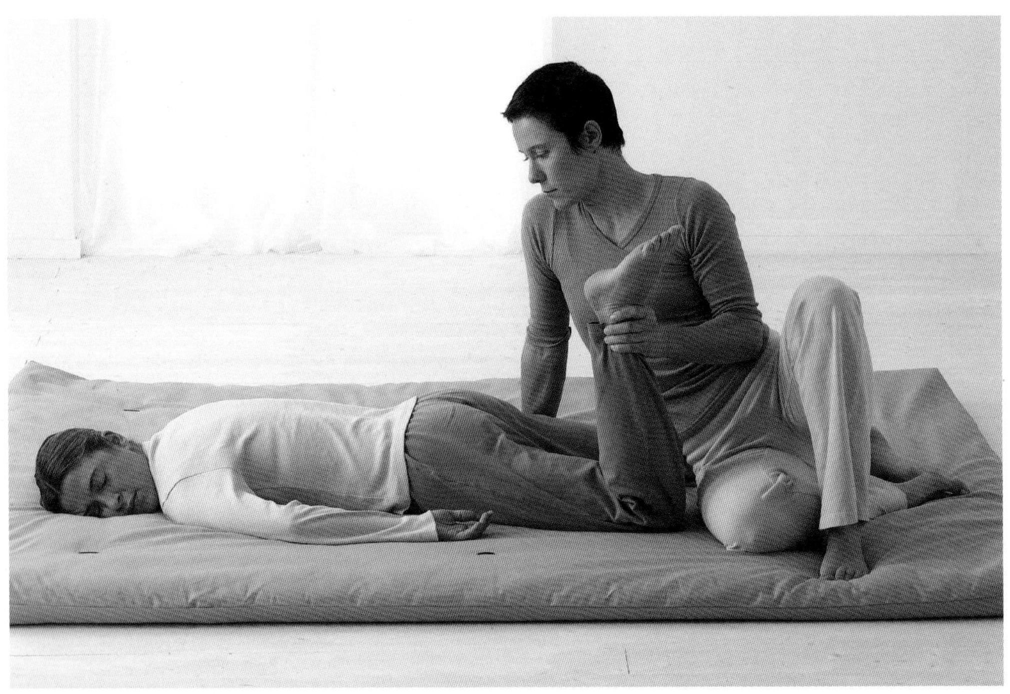

1 This is a very snug pose, so you have to get close in to your partner. Bend their knee up and, with your lower hand, hold firmly around the ankle joint. Support yourself properly by placing your other hand on the floor.

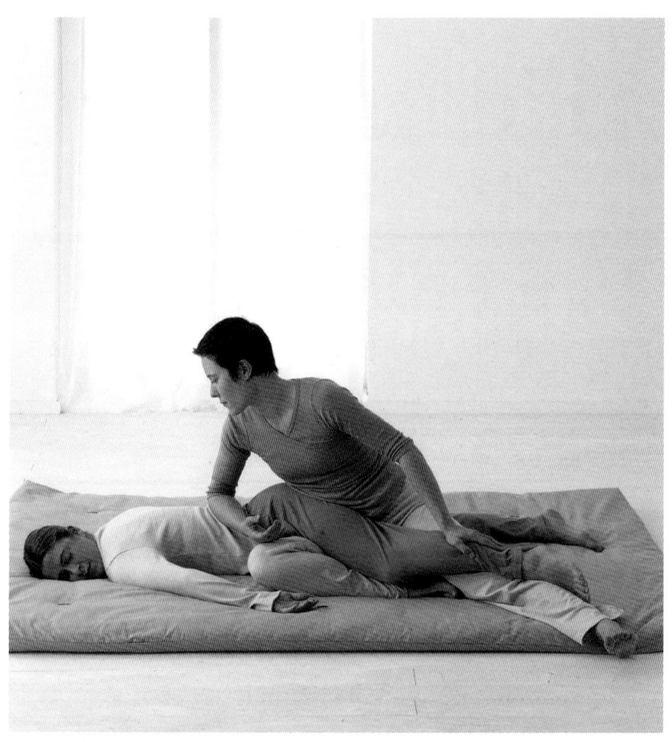

2 Catch hold under your partner's knee and lift their leg high so that you can slide your thigh all the way up under the front of their hip. Extend your lower leg to provide support for their calf. Fix your lower hand on their calf.

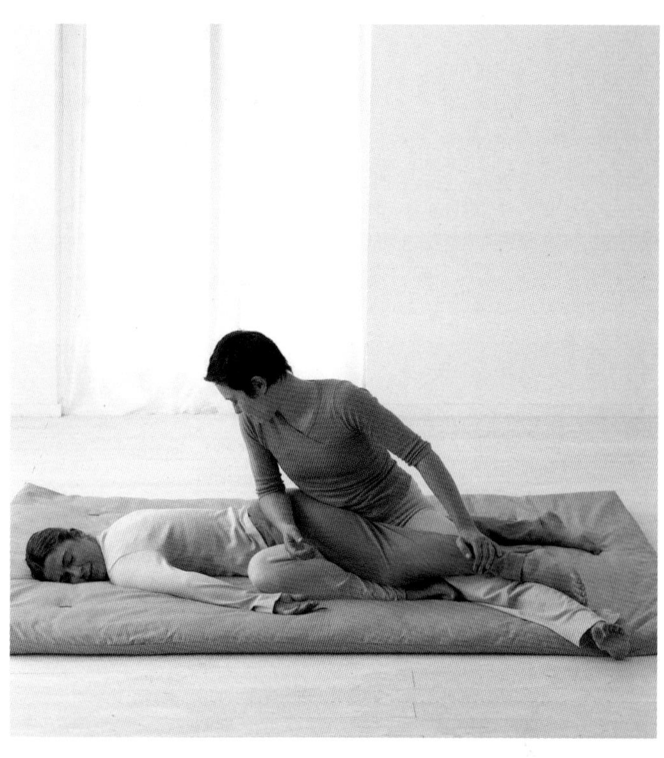

3 With your upper arm, roll over the thigh, buttock and lower back of your partner, using the fleshy part of your forearm. As you roll, keep your other hand securely on their lower leg, as shown.

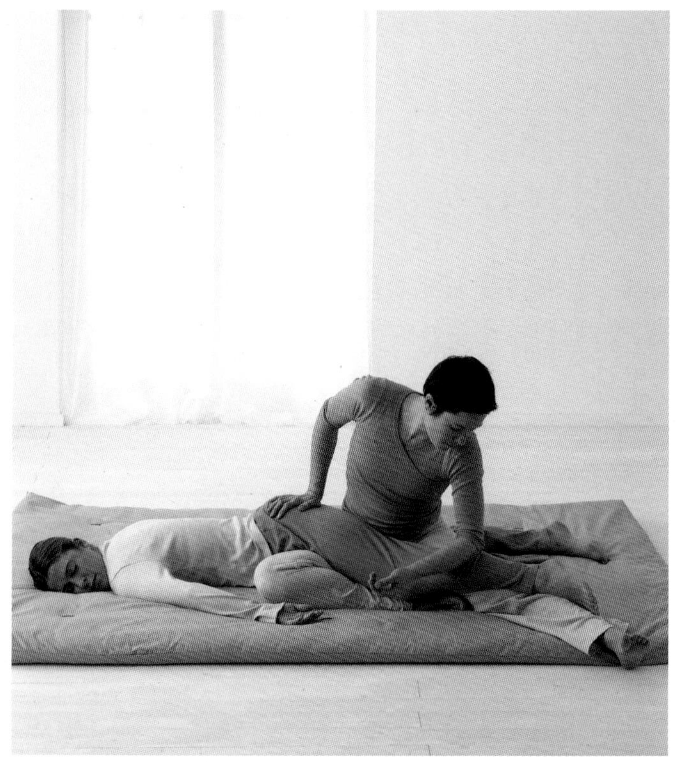

4 Now fix your upper hand on the hip and, using your lower forearm, roll away across the calf, working only on the fleshy part of the leg.

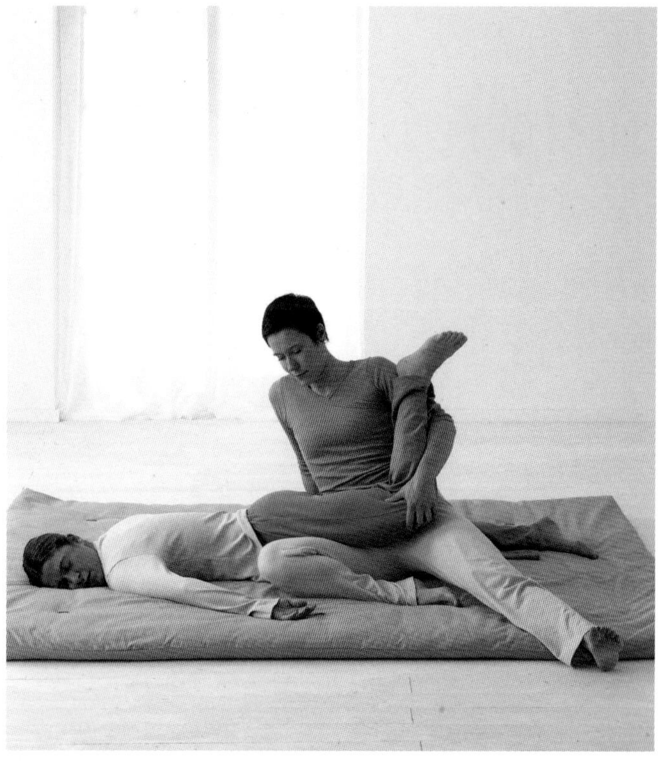

5 Your partner should be extremely relaxed by now, so ease your way out, causing the least disturbance possible. Support your partner's knee as you gently lift their thigh in order to slide your body out carefully. Repeat the exercise with the other leg.

Working the Energy Lines of the Back

Working the back lines is an important part of the massage as it affects the whole body. Sen sumana runs through the spinal column and is regarded as the location of the body's main chakras, or energy centres.

Two energy lines run up the back. Line 1 has two aspects: sen ittha, running up the left side of the body, and sen pingkhala, which runs up the right. To work line 1, begin just above the sacrum and apply pressure into the shallow dip either side of the spinal column. Line 2, sen kalathari, begins just above the hips, about a thumb's width out from line 1. You may notice a muscular ridge running either side of the spine. This is the pathway for line 2: work up and down this ridge.

YOUR POSTURE

To tune into your partner properly, you must establish a comfortable, stable working posture. Half-kneel astride your partner, with your hips in line with their back. Change legs as often as you need to. Depending on the length of your partner's back, you may need to adjust your pose several times in order to keep your centre of gravity directly over the area that you are working.

THE BACK LINES

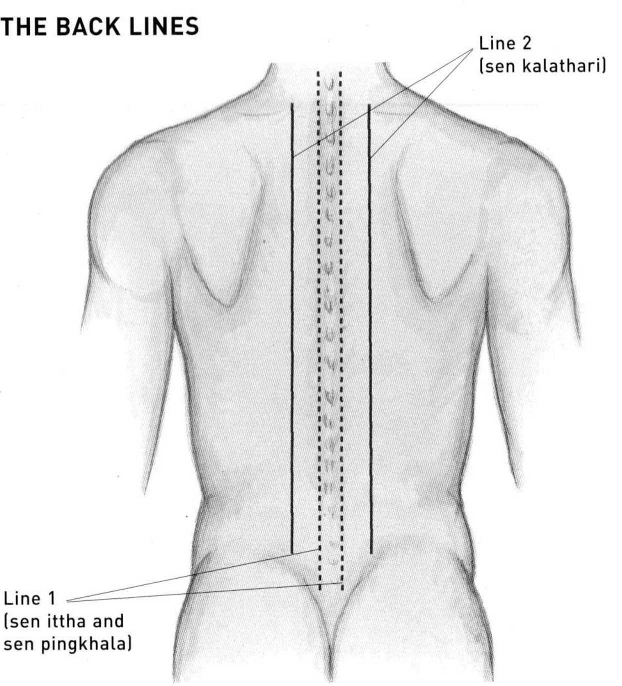

Above This picture shows the paths of the two sen, or energy lines, that are worked on the back.

Palming and Thumbing the Back Lines

Use exactly the same kind of slow and rhythmic rocking movement as for the leg and arm lines, but instead of working alternately, apply the pressure with both of your hands simultaneously.

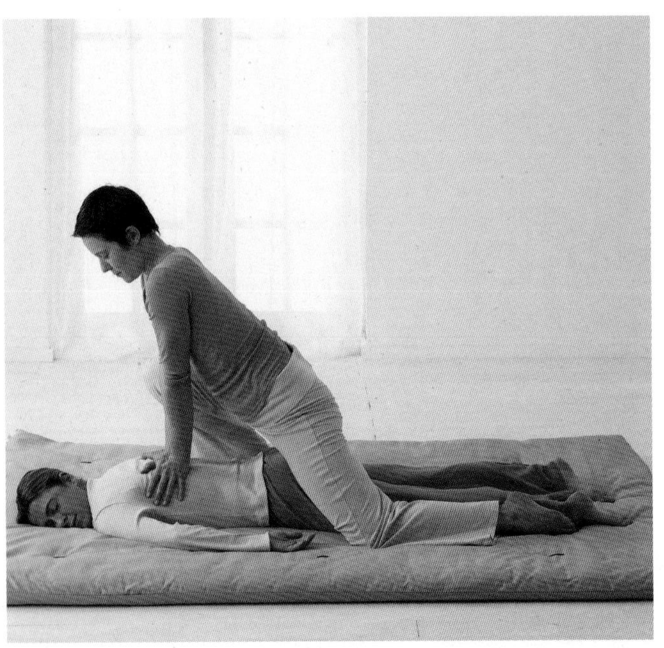

1 Palming the back lines A broad, general pressure on the sen deepens and slows the breath and prepares the body. To begin, place your hands lightly on your partner's back to get a feel for their breathing rhythm. As they inhale, let their ribcage expand under your hands and, as they exhale, sink (don't press or push) your body weight down through your arms and hands, helping to expel their exhalation. Reposition your hands and work with the breath up and down line 1. Repeat for line 2.

Line 1 hand position
Palm with the pressure coming down through the heel of your hand. Your fingers should be relaxed around the ribcage.

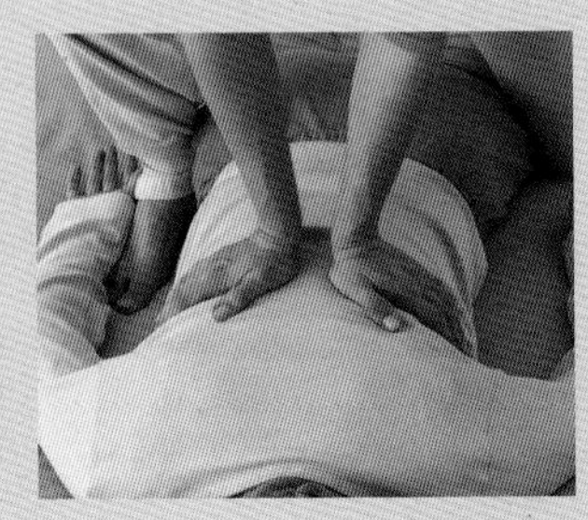

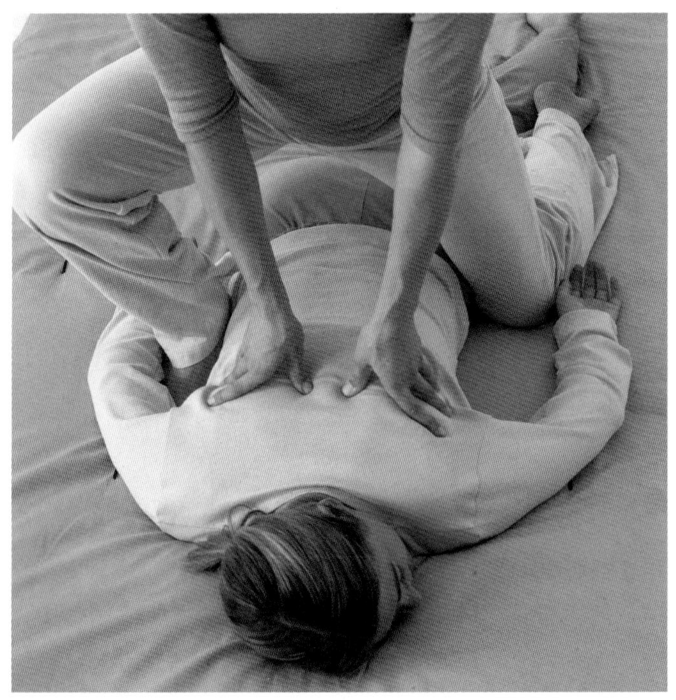

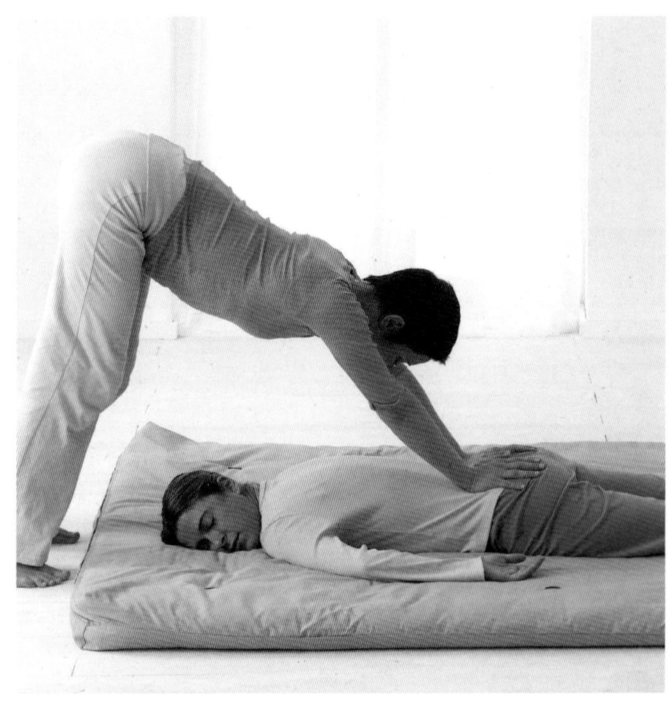

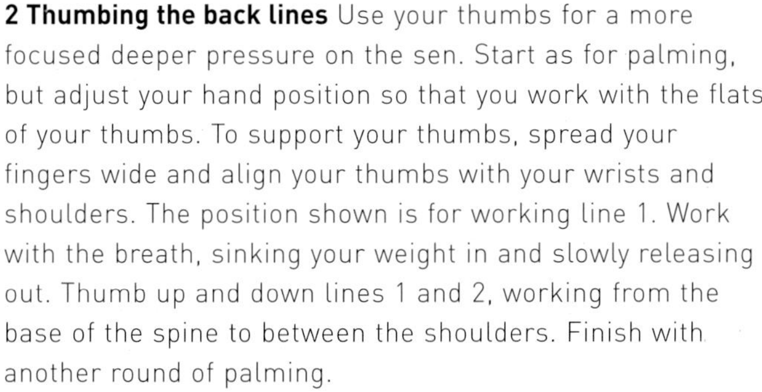

2 Thumbing the back lines Use your thumbs for a more focused deeper pressure on the sen. Start as for palming, but adjust your hand position so that you work with the flats of your thumbs. To support your thumbs, spread your fingers wide and align your thumbs with your wrists and shoulders. The position shown is for working line 1. Work with the breath, sinking your weight in and slowly releasing out. Thumb up and down lines 1 and 2, working from the base of the spine to between the shoulders. Finish with another round of palming.

3 Sacrum lengthener Get into a kneeling position above your partner's head and slide the heels of your hands down to their hipbones. This is your fix on the pose. As your partner exhales, lift up your hips. Enjoy a few breaths, feeling the opening of your own body as your partner enjoys the openness in theirs. This delicious stretch creates length all the way through the spine. It is particularly soothing for tired and tight lower backs.

Accessing the upper back

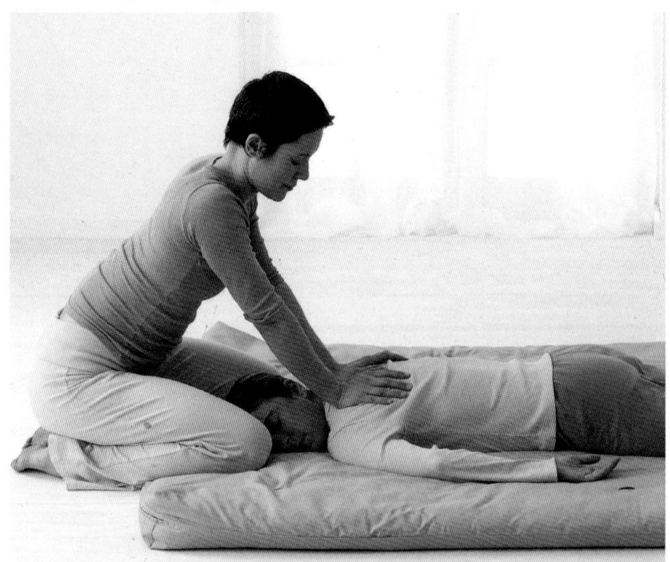

Above In order to work lines 1 and 2 effectively right up into the upper back, you will find that it is often easier and much more comfortable for you if you change your position. Wide-kneel above your partner's head and work your hands alternately, like a cat pawing in a relaxed way.

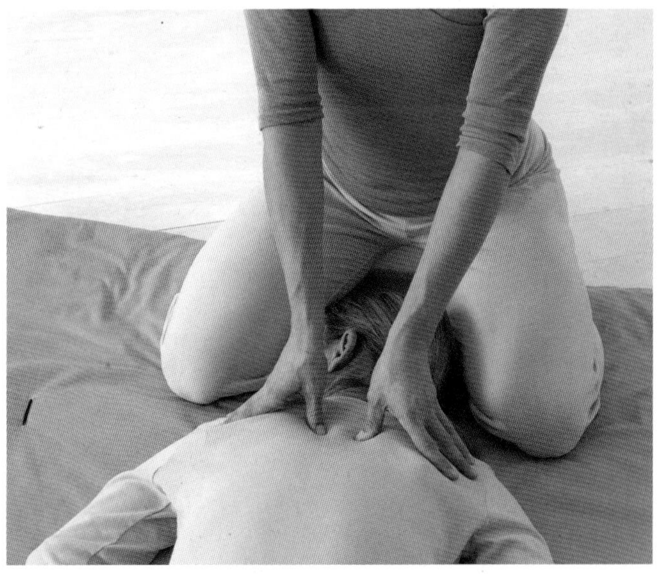

Above To thumb your partner's back lines much more easily, tuck your toes under, in order to raise your centre of gravity. Work with both of your thumbs either simultaneously or alternately – whatever feels best for you.

Dynamic Back Stretches

After you have warmed up the body thoroughly by working the two back lines and simulating the flow of energy up and down your partner's spine, you can now move on to some more dynamic stretches for the back of the body. You'll see that the stretching exercises that follow involve some active lifting of your partner. Remember to move into the stretches sensitively and with awareness, using your body weight and breath, rather than your strength – this will make the lifting much easier.

The Cobra

This energizing back bend stimulates the upper spine, chest and shoulders, while also encouraging deeper breathing. As the focus is on opening the upper back, the lower back should feel no discomfort.

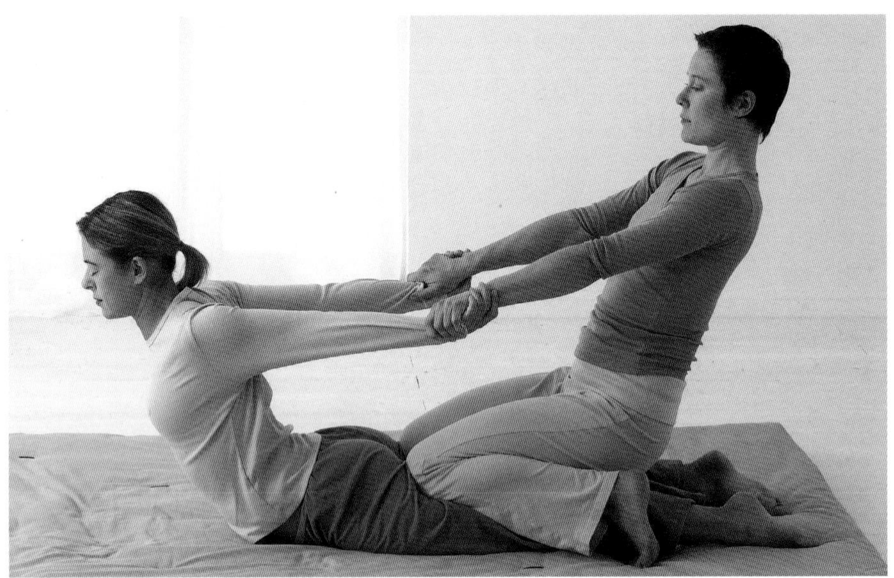

Left Make sure that your partner's toes are pointing inwards and their ankles outwards. Kneel gently on their thighs, keeping your feet outside their legs. Leave a space between your knees and your partner's buttocks so that they have enough room to come up fully into the pose. Ask them to place their forehead on the floor and to take hold around your wrists as you hold theirs.

Gently lean back, lifting their upper body off the ground. You can work on either the inhalation or the exhalation. The former gives a greater lift and opening through the front of the body; the latter gives more control and lengthens the spine more effectively. Explore which feels best for you and your partner. Work in and out of the posture three times, resting completely on the ground between stretches.

Variation to the pose

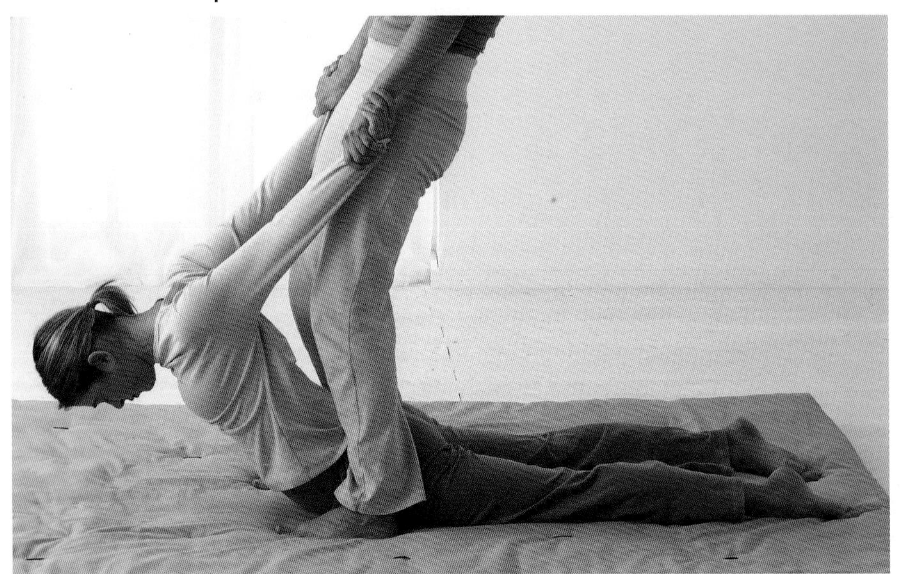

Left The shoulder lift This is a gentle alternative to the cobra for stiff or heavy people. Fix your feet very snugly against your partner's hips. Bend your knees, keeping your back straight. Hold on to each other's wrists. As you exhale, stand up using the power in your legs. Encourage your partner to let their arms and head relax. Repeat three times.

Cross-legged Forward Bend

This is a lovely counter-pose for the cobra position. Remember that you can alter the degree to which your partner's legs are crossed in order to stretch both of their hips to whatever level feels comfortable to them.

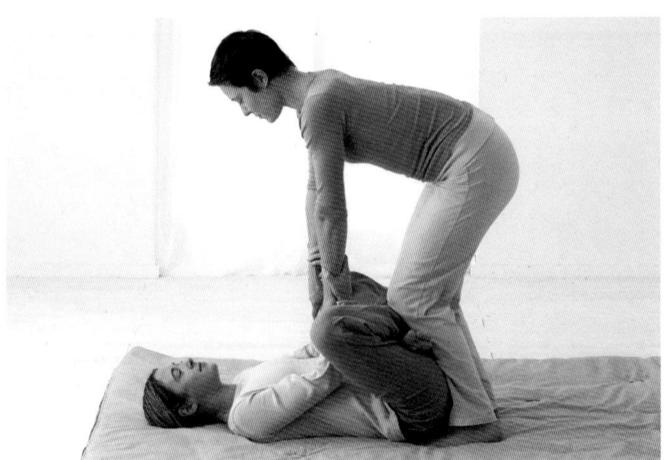

1 Ask your partner to roll on to their back and bring their knees up to their chest as if they were sitting cross-legged. Stand with your knees together and your feet wide, as close up against your partner's shins as possible. Make sure that their feet are crossed below your knees to fix the pose. Bend your knees and clasp around each other's wrists.

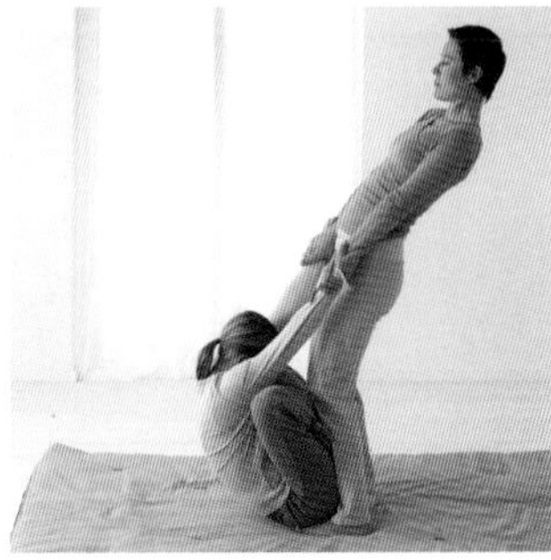

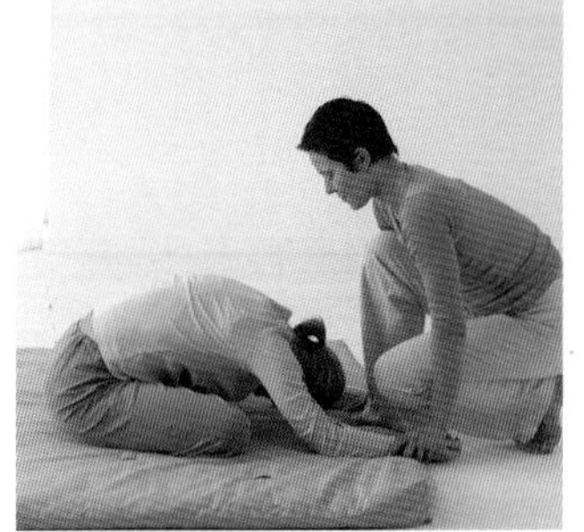

2 (above left) On the exhalation, straighten your legs and, leaning away, lift your partner's upper body off the mat. Keep your shoulders relaxed. Sink your knees inward slightly for a deeper stretch. Release your partner back down to the mat.

3 (above right) Repeat three times, but on the third stretch, step away with your feet and extend your partner's arms to rest on the mat in front of them. You can give them extra support here by placing a bolster or cushion underneath their upper body.

Percussion

The vibration of these percussive techniques penetrates deep inside the body. They are very invigorating for the energy system and have a grounding effect on the body. Keep your shoulders and wrists relaxed, and remember to avoid contact with the spine.

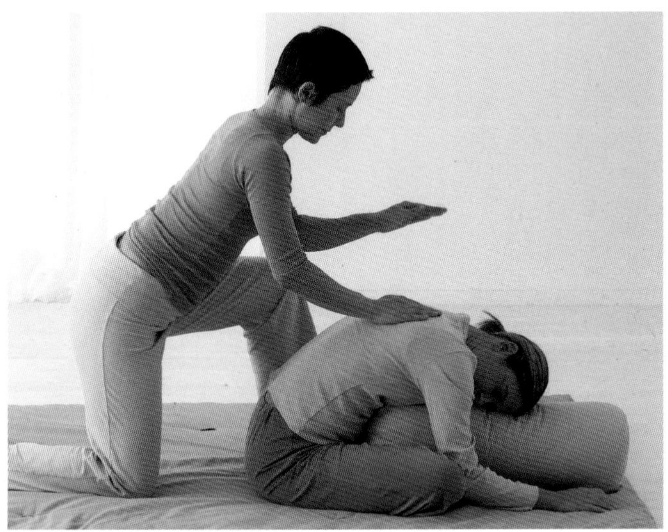

1 Cupping Make a shallow cup with each palm, keeping your thumbs tucked in and your wrists soft. Alternately cup up and down either side of the spine, experimenting to find a rhythm and speed that suits your partner.

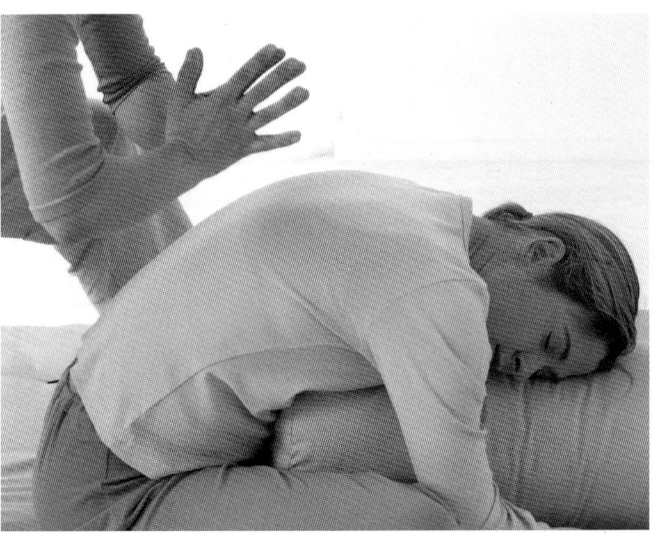

2 Prayer hands "Glue" the heels of your hands together and imagine that the pads of your fingers are stuck lightly together. Keep your elbows wide and make a chopping action with your hands. Contact the body with the sides of your little fingers. You will know when you have it just right, as your fingers will make a very satisfying clacking sound.

Technique improver

Occasionally you may work with someone who is suffering from severe pain or acute sensitivity in their back and who is unable to receive any of the dynamic work or acupressure of traditional Thai massage. However, they may still benefit enormously from some hands-on therapy and there are alternative ways of working the energy lines of the back that are very soothing and effective – namely, using herbs and oils.

Traditional Thai medicine has several different aspects, of which physical massage is just one. Herbs are also used therapeutically, and in Thailand it is common to see herbal steam baths offered alongside Thai massage treatments. These baths are a wonderful way to complement the relaxing and detoxifying effects of a Thai massage.

Most of us do not have ready access to steam bath facilities. However, you can easily introduce herbal therapy in the form of compresses, for use during the massage. These compresses are very effective at helping to ease congestion and tension. Traditionally, each practitioner would make up a blend of herbs appropriate to an individual patient's condition, but a simple compress of something warming and stimulating such as ginger can be just as beneficial.

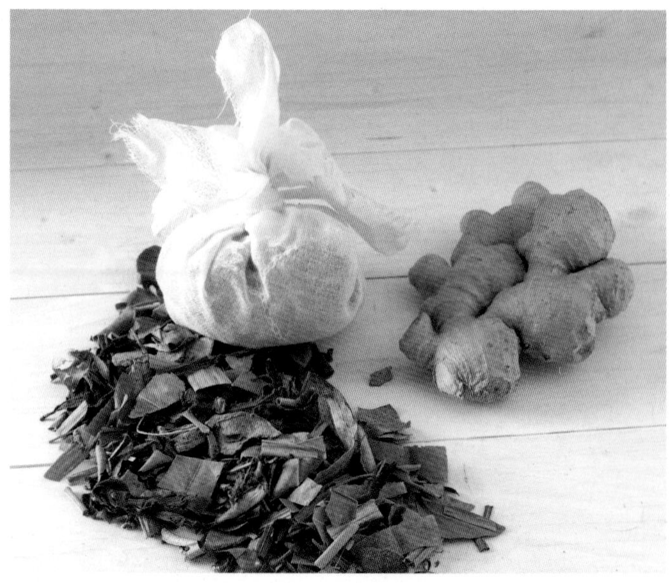

Above Preparing a ginger compress To make a simple compress, roughly chop plenty of fresh ginger into a pan and then add boiling water and let it simmer so that its warming properties are released. Wrap the ginger in a piece of muslin (cheesecloth) and then, checking that it is not too hot, apply the compress directly to the energy lines, using a padding movement, in the same smooth rhythmic way as when palming the lines.

Right Using oil Although not a standard part of traditional Thai practice, working with oil is a very soothing alternative to applying direct acupressure to the energy lines. No special oil is required: you can use grapeseed, sweet almond or even sunflower oil. Try to use organic oils if you can, so that no impurities are absorbed into the skin.

Make sure that your partner is warm enough. Use the same body posture as when thumbing the energy lines but instead of applying downward pressure, simply glide your thumbs up and down the path of the energy lines, checking the pressure with your partner.

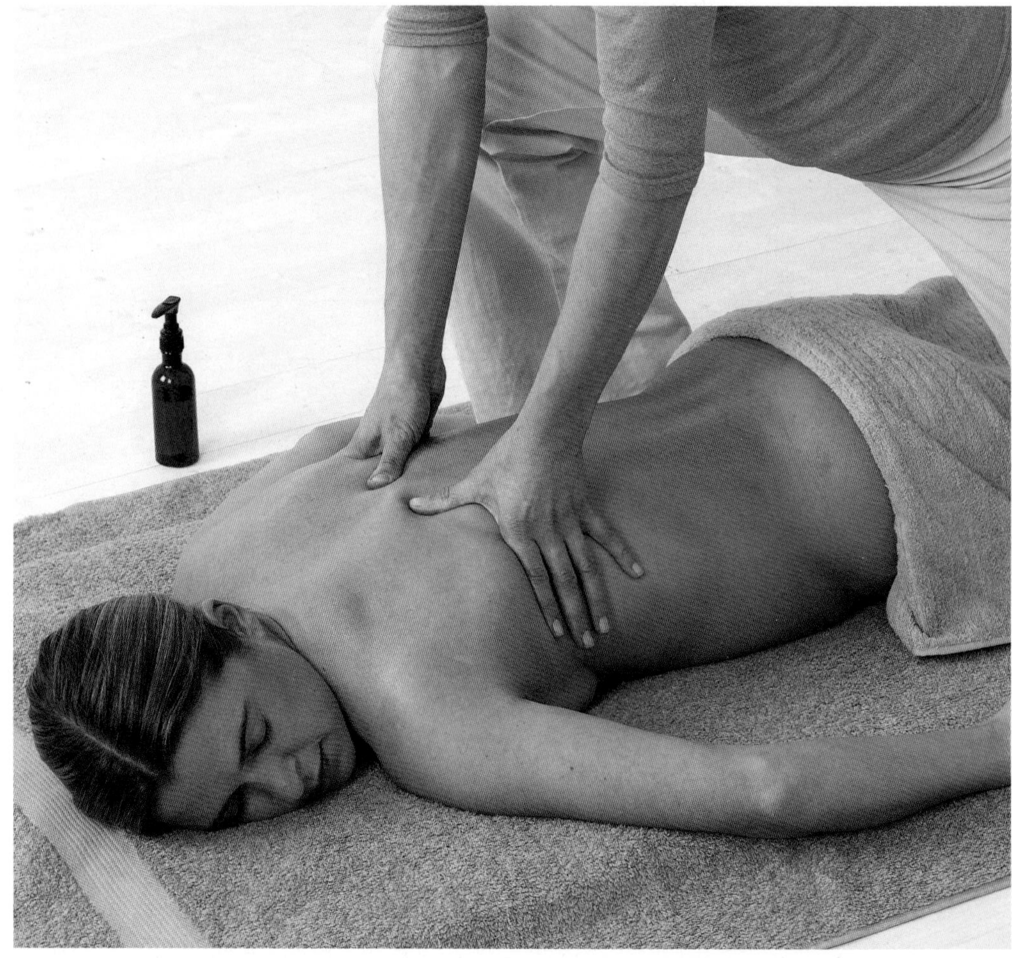

Review: the Back of the Body

Use the pictures below as a reminder of the main flow of the sequence. As before, take time to feel comfortable with massaging this part of the body before moving on to the next, and work to your partner's specific needs.

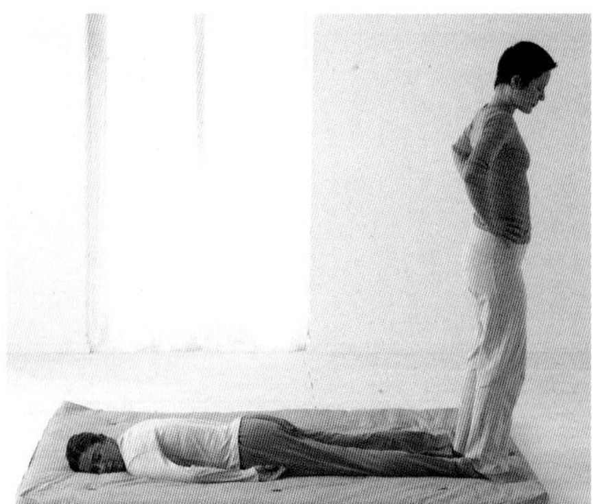

Walking on the feet

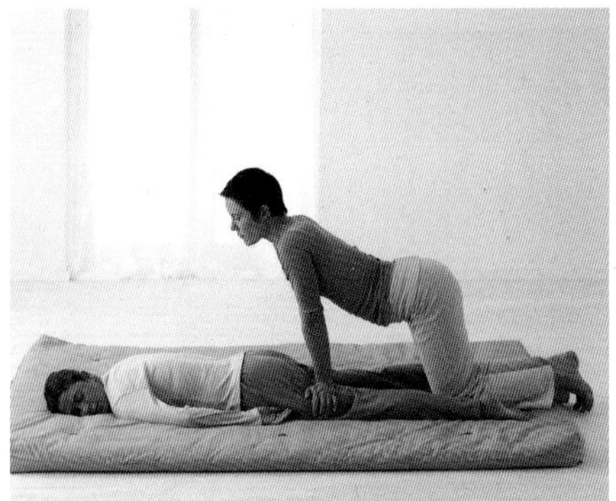

Palming the backs of the legs

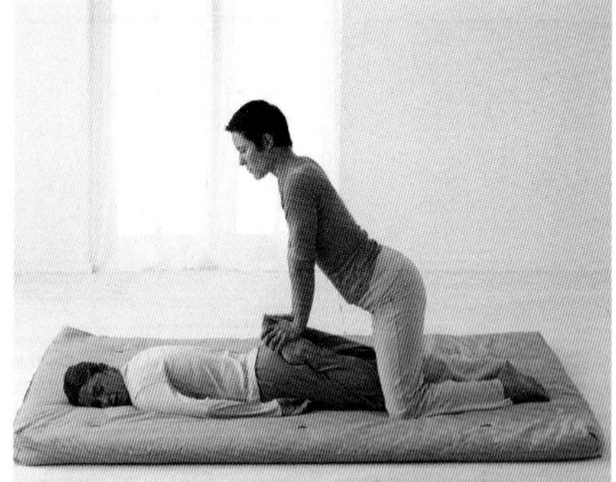

Feet to sacrum

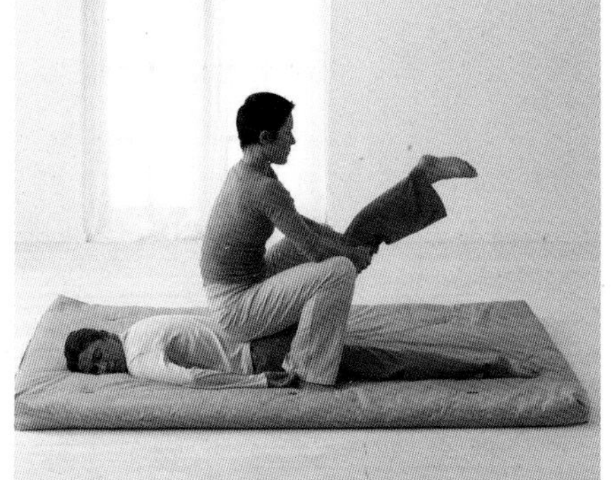

The locust

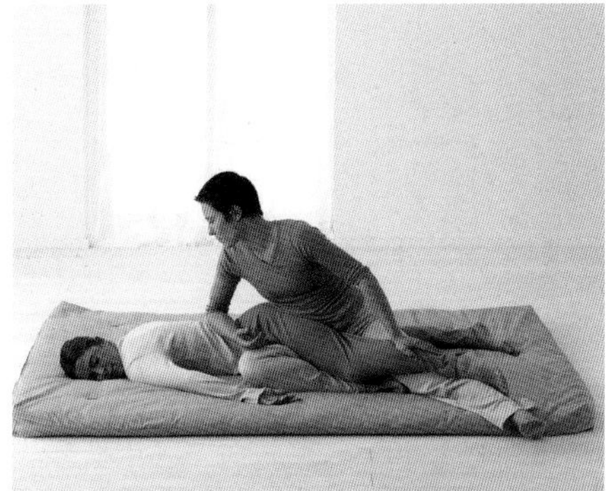

Take a break

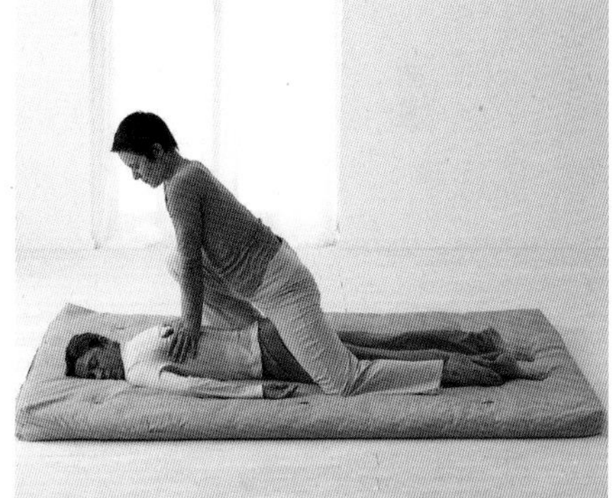

Working the back lines

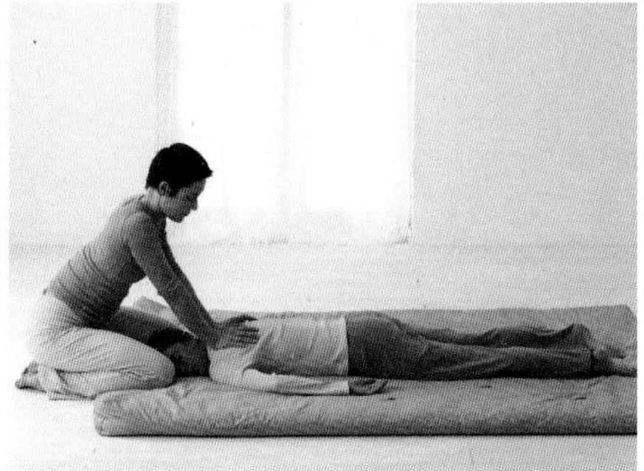

Palming and thumbing

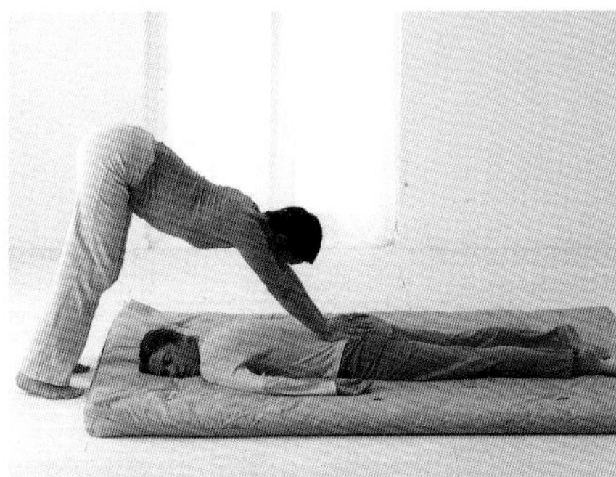

Sacrum lengthener

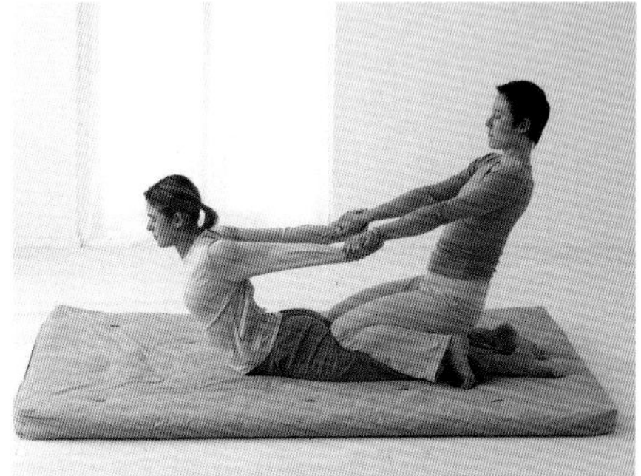

The cobra

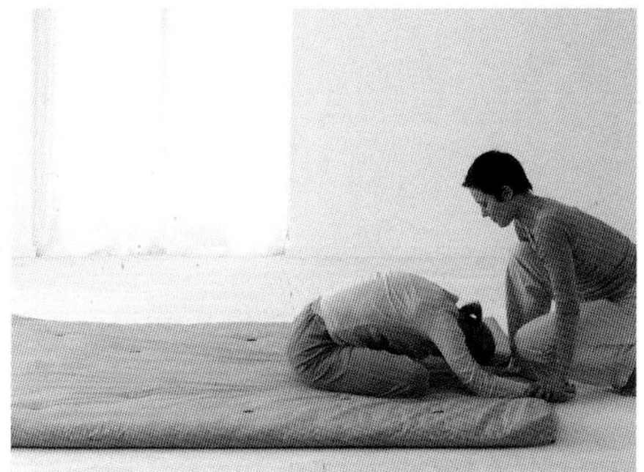

Cross-legged forward bend

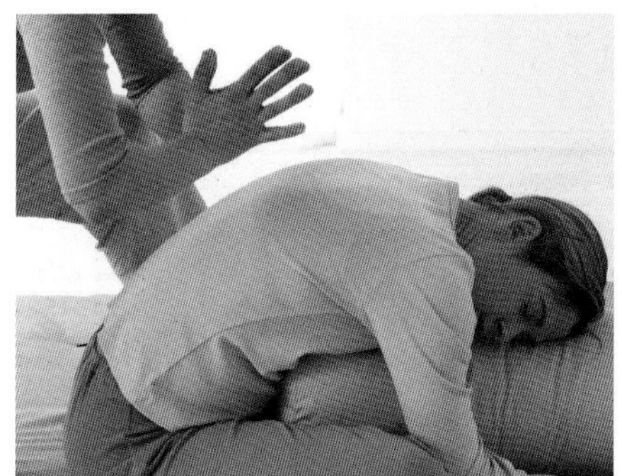

Percussion

Caution

Remember when carrying out percussive techniques that you should keep your hand contact soft and never strike your partner's spine directly.

Seated Sequence for the Upper Body

For the exercises that follow, featuring the head, neck and upper body, your partner will be in a seated position. This makes these exercises very versatile, as it means they can be done anywhere, unrestricted by lack of space or equipment. Most of the exercises could be given with your partner sitting on a stool or low chair.

Modern lifestyles can leave us feeling depleted, tired and weighed down, particularly in the upper chest, shoulders and neck. The stimulating sequence that follows eases the upper body and helps clear the mind. The work here focuses on releasing what is often long-term tension held in the upper body.

SITTING WITH EASE AND LIGHTNESS

To ensure that your partner gains maximum benefit from this sequence, take time to check that they are relaxed and supported in their sitting position, so that the whole of their spine, right up into their head and neck, feels light and free. Maintaining a healthy posture is beneficial not only for the physical body but also for the energetic body, which is central to Thai massage.

Below It can help to raise the hips slightly higher than the knees, using a folded blanket or block. If necessary, place extra support under the knees to prevent any strain in the joints.

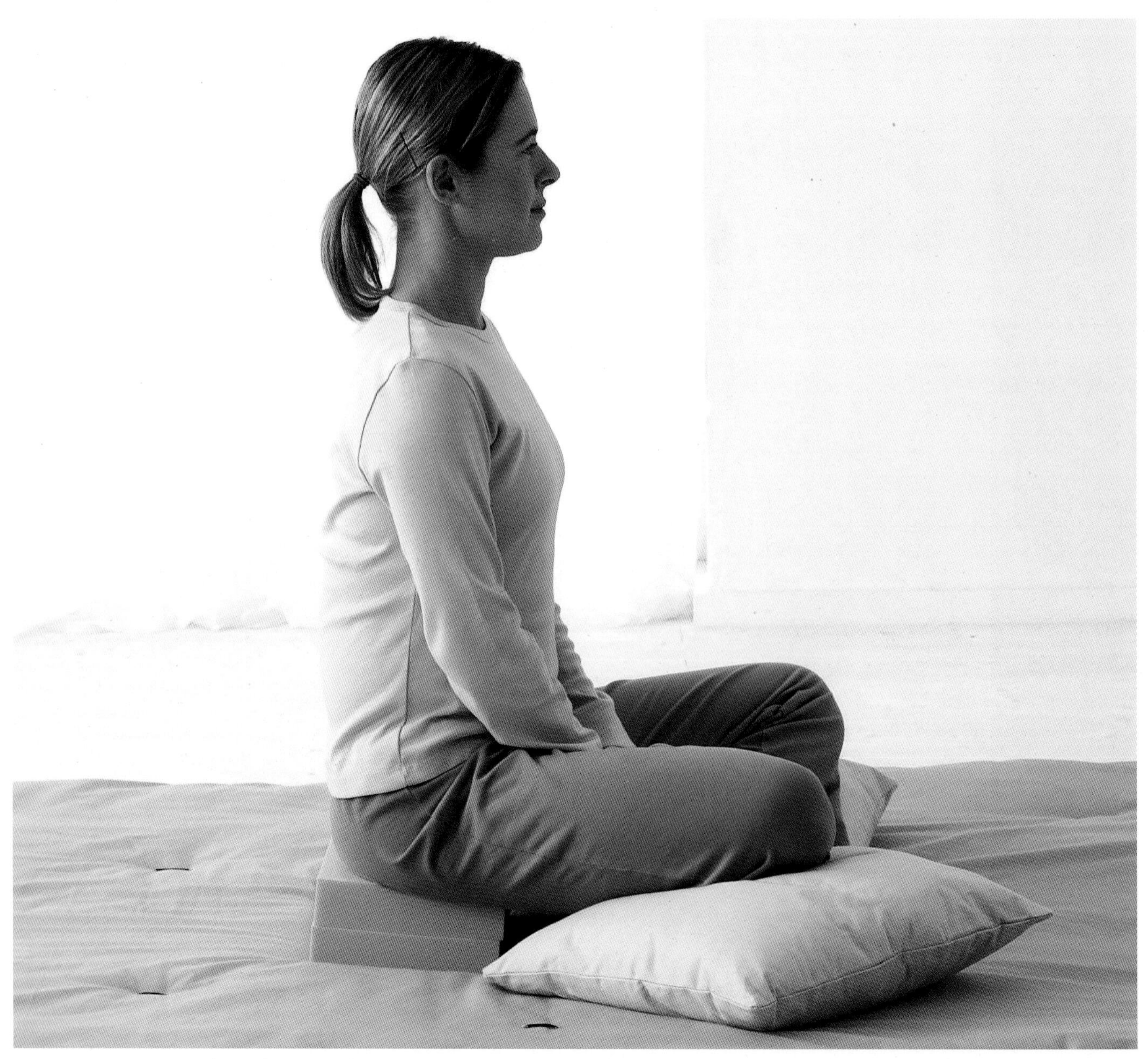

Warming up the Shoulders

Working this area helps to release habitual tension in the shoulders and neck and stimulate deeper breathing. It creates a feeling of space between the shoulders and ears, encouraging greater freedom of movement in the neck.

ENERGY POINTS IN THE SHOULDERS

The exercises shown below work along three important acupressure points located on the top of the shoulders. These are very effective for releasing tension in and around the base of the neck and upper back. They are described in the order given below for learning purposes only, but once you are familiar with their location it may feel more natural to start at the base of the neck and work outwards.

Getting it right

✓ Ask if your partner has suffered from any neck injuries, including whiplash, and if so proceed with due sensitivity and caution.

✓ Be aware of how much tension people can hold in their upper body. Some people find deep pressure very beneficial while others are extremely sensitive.

✓ Work with the breath. Encourage your partner to focus on their exhalation, so that they actively release the tension in the shoulders.

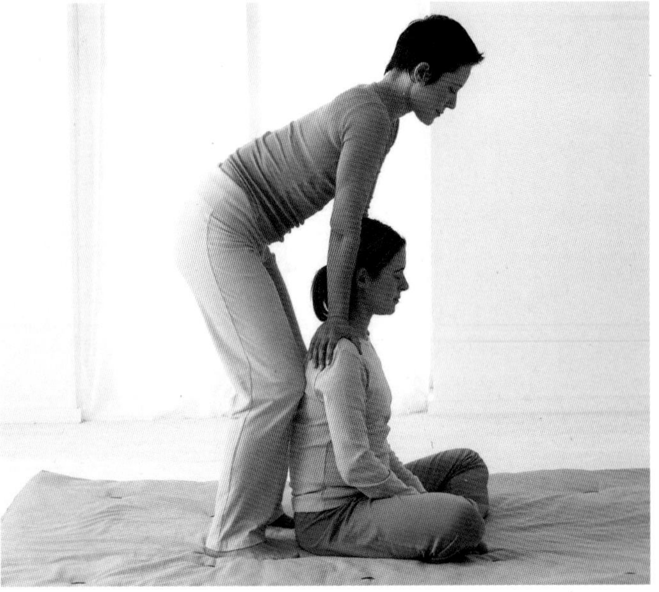

1 Palming the shoulders This general pressure loosens and warms up the shoulders. Come close in to your partner's body so they feel supported from behind. Make sure you are stable and your feet are relaxed. Turn your wrists forward, with your fingers pointing back towards you, and place your palms on the fleshy part of the shoulders, as shown. Use your body weight to sink into the shoulders. Slowly apply as much pressure as your partner enjoys.

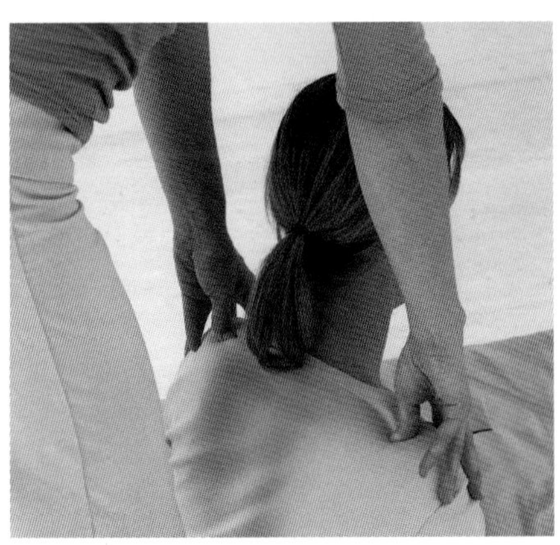

2 Thumbing the shoulder points Work into these points with the pads, rather than the tips, of your thumbs. Stabilize your hand position by spreading your fingers wide. Locate point A by sliding each thumb away from the neck and coming to rest in the small dip at the "V" where your partner's collarbone and shoulder blade meet.

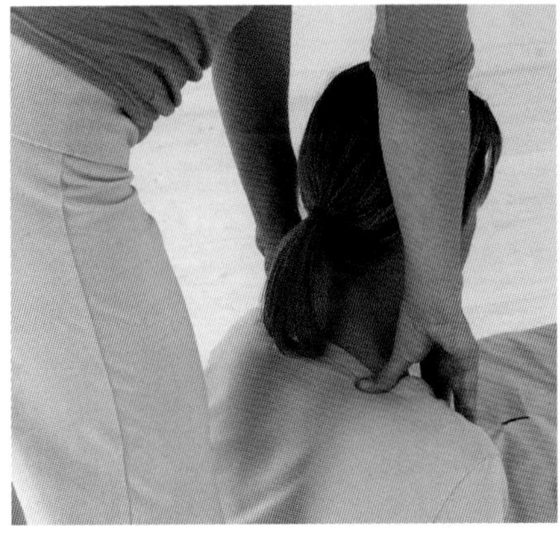

3 Where the shoulder meets the neck, drop back slightly off the top of the muscular ridge of the shoulder to find point C.

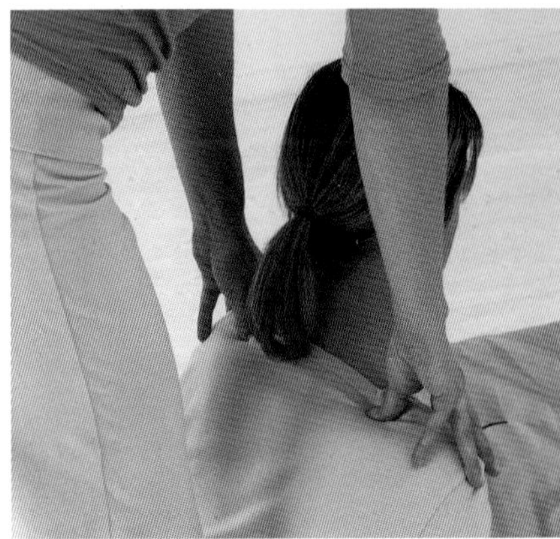

4 Midway between points A and C is point B. It often has a slightly different quality to it, and may naturally feel quite dense.

The Head and Neck

This part of the sequence concentrates on smaller, more sensitive movements for the neck and head. The energy flow can readily become blocked here and this can result in feeling "stuck in the head" and slightly disconnected from the sensations and inner cues of the body.

THE OCCIPUTAL RIDGE

The area at the base of the skull, where the spinal column feeds up into the head, is known as the occipital ridge and can be described as being like a physical junction between the body and the mind. Keeping a free flow of energy here maintains a healthy supply of blood to the brain and scalp. It also helps to preserve an integrated sense of the body, where the body and the mind are held in equal regard and where neither the sensations of the body nor the chattering of the mind dominate the other.

Right This artwork shows some of the acupressure points that you can work around the base of the skull. They can be located by letting the head drop back slightly until the thumb falls into a natural dip up against the bone.

USING PRESSURE POINTS IN THE NECK AREA

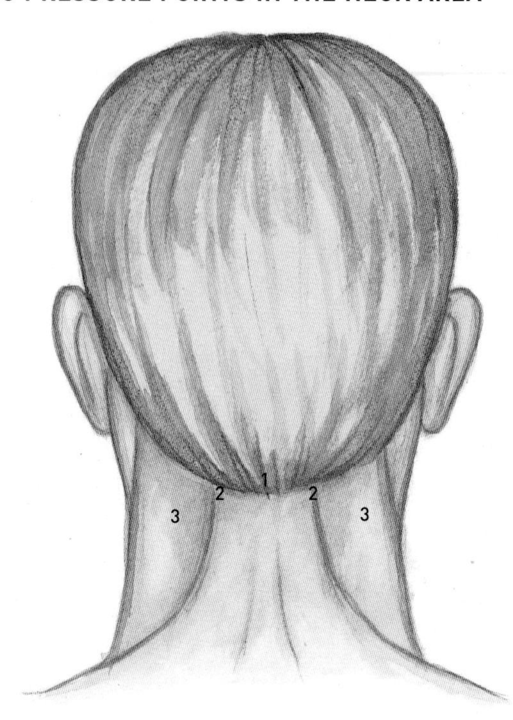

Working the Occiput

By working the acupressure points along the occiputal ridge and easing tension from the neck, you help to keep the energy flowing freely and the body and mind in balance.

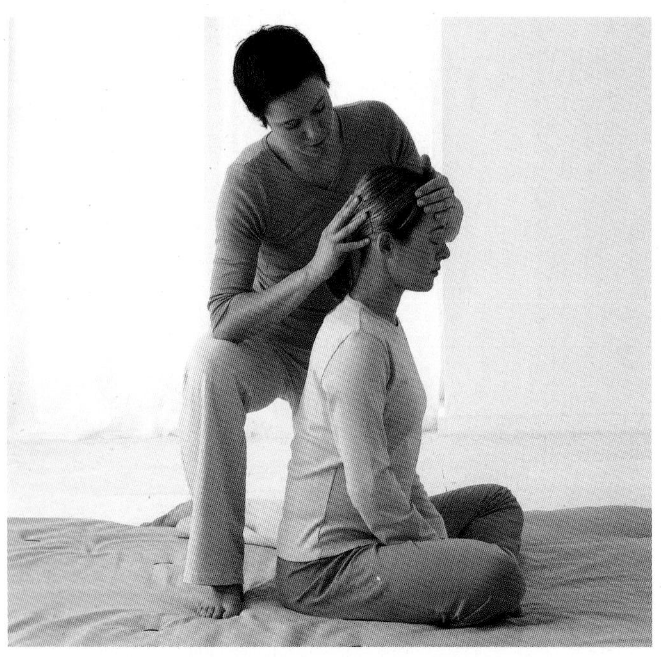

1 Half-kneel behind your partner – making sure that you are in a stable and comfortable position – and lightly support their forehead with your hand. Use the thumb of your other hand to work on the points. Keep your fingers spread wide for support against the back of the skull. Work with an inward and upward motion, using slow, firm pressure.

Remember that these points can be sensitive but you can work them more deeply if your partner consciously works with their breath as you apply the pressure. As with all the other exercises it is important for masseur and receiver to communicate well with each other throughout.

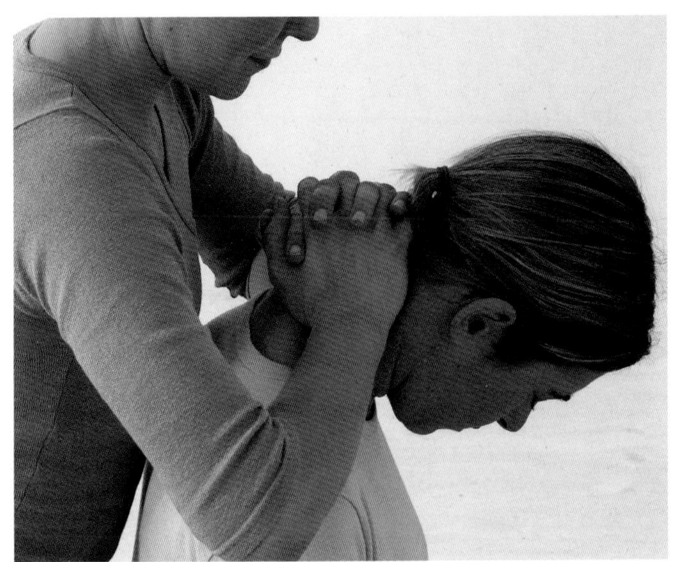

2 Palming the neck As with the butterfly squeeze (single leg sequence), interlace your fingers and, using the heels of your hands, gently squeeze up and down the back of the neck. Work from the shoulders up to the base of the skull. Be aware of how strong the pressure in your hands can be.

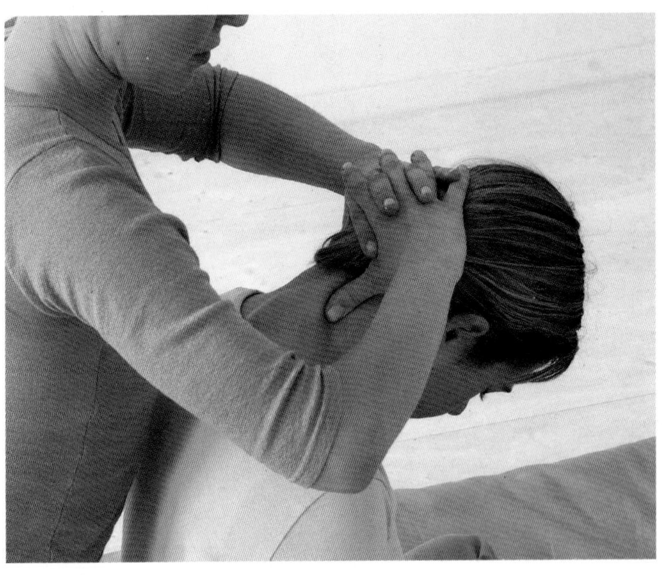

3 Thumbing the points on the neck Undo your clasp slightly and take your elbows wide, turning your thumbs face down. Use the pads of your thumbs to work up and down the muscular ridge on either side of the spine.

Head Massage

This is a simple but wonderfully releasing part of the sequence. Working into the roots of the hair stimulates blood flow to the scalp, resulting in healthy hair, and helps to relieve headaches and sluggishness, leaving your partner more alert and rejuvenated. The following techniques are simply suggestions – be playful and use your intuition.

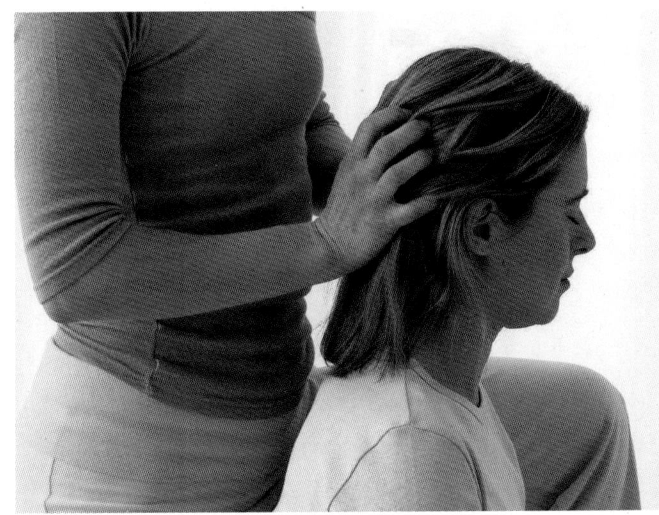

1 Shampooing Work right into the hair and rub the scalp vigorously with the tips of your fingers.

Getting it right

☒ Never work on wet hair, as it can damage the hair and also feels very uncomfortable.

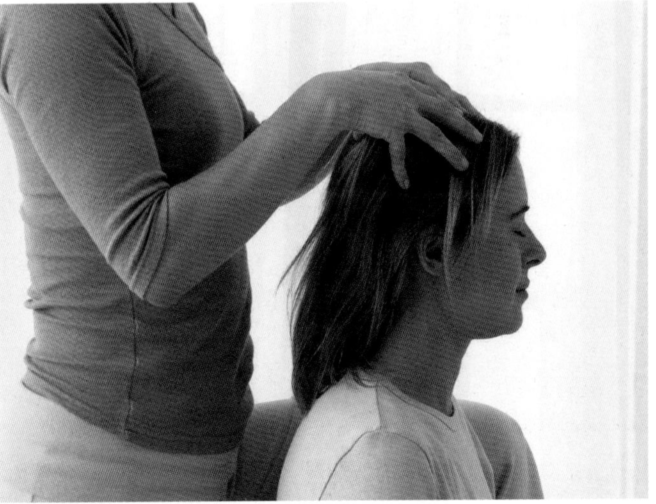

2 Plucking This technique is a little more specific. Place the pads of your fingers firmly against the skull and then briskly pluck your hands away. Repeat, covering the whole of the scalp.

People tend to either love or hate these kinds of techniques, so always check with your partner that they enjoy having their scalp massaged before you begin.

Expanding the Upper Body

At this stage we move on to working with the whole of your partner's upper body. The sequence of exercises and techniques that follows involves some wonderful stretches that are aimed at integrating the flow of energy throughout the upper body. They should open up this whole area and help to release any held tensions. As a result, your partner should be left feeling fully relaxed and yet refreshed.

Stretch Sequence

This sequence features just some of the more expansive and opening exercises that can help to release energy which has become held deep inside the shoulder joints, the ribs, and the upper back.

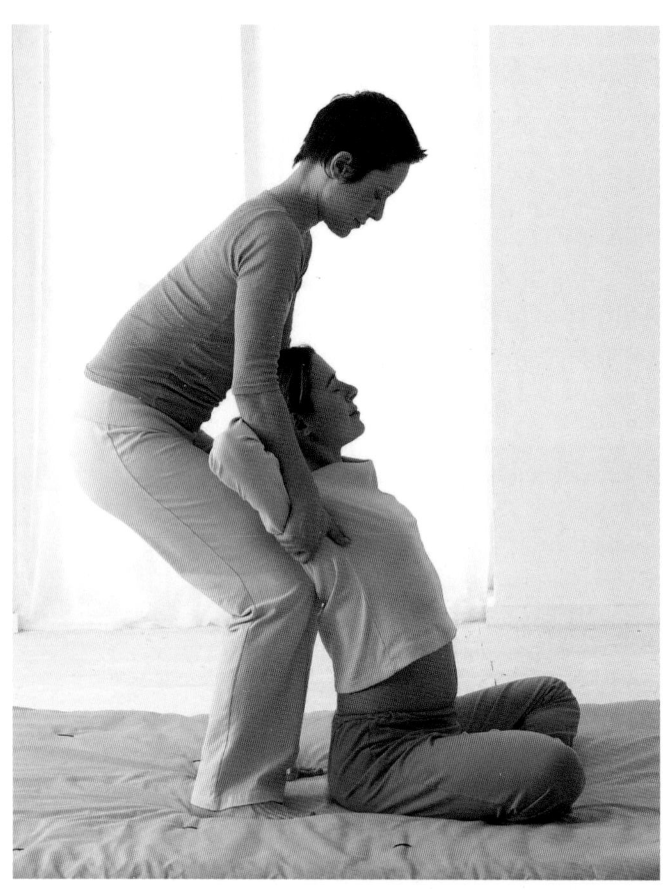

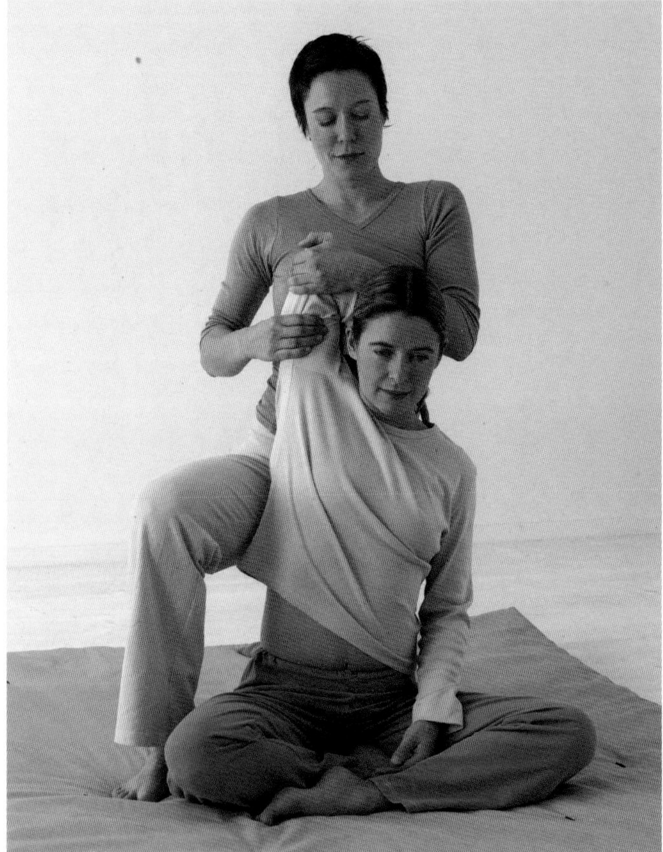

1 Hello world Stand close in behind your partner, but make sure that you leave a small gap between your knees and their back. Ask them to interlace their hands behind their head. Reach over and clasp around their upper arms, close to the armpits.

Let your partner lean back on to your knees. On the exhalation, lift their arms up and out. Encourage your partner to drop their weight into their hips as they open up through the front of their body. Repeat the stretch three times, making sure that you do not undo the position completely in between.

2 Opening the armpit Half-kneel behind your partner. Take their arm and lift the hand up to the ceiling to create space all the way through the side of the body. Drop their upper arm behind their head and, using your inside hand, support their elbow against your body. With your outside hand squeeze up and down the upper arm, from the armpit to the elbow, using the flats of your fingers. Change arms and repeat on the other side.

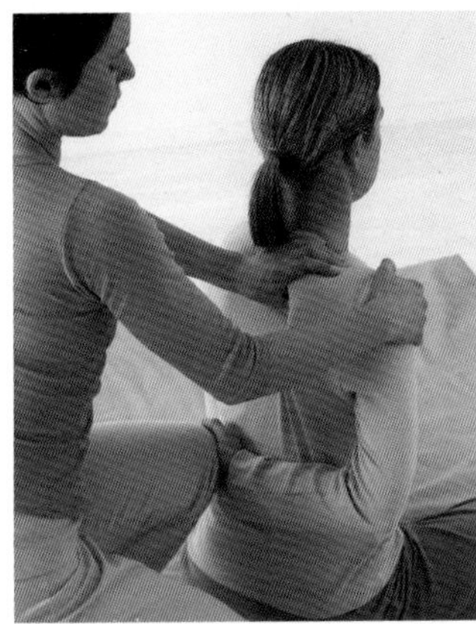

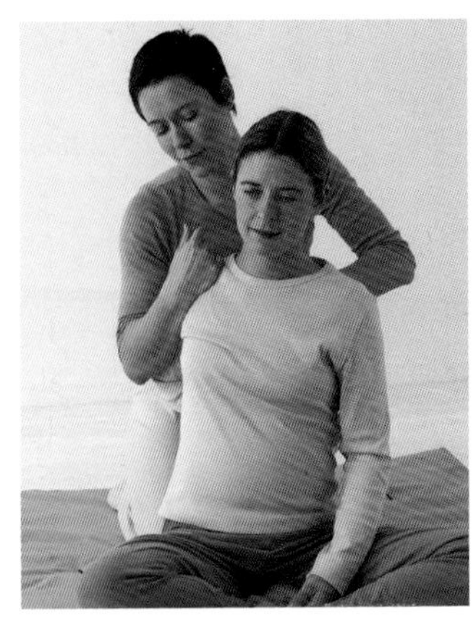

3 Finding your wings (above) This exercise opens up the hidden places behind the shoulder blade (scapula), and introduces a slight twist through the upper body. Take your partner's hand behind them and bring it across to the other side of their spine. Put your knee into their palm to fix their hand in place. This position helps to create space behind the shoulder blade.

4 (above right) Support the front of the shoulder joint with your outside hand. Place the thumb of your inside hand behind the shoulder blade and lean back. Release, reposition your thumb and continue working all around the shoulder blade. Repeat on the other side.

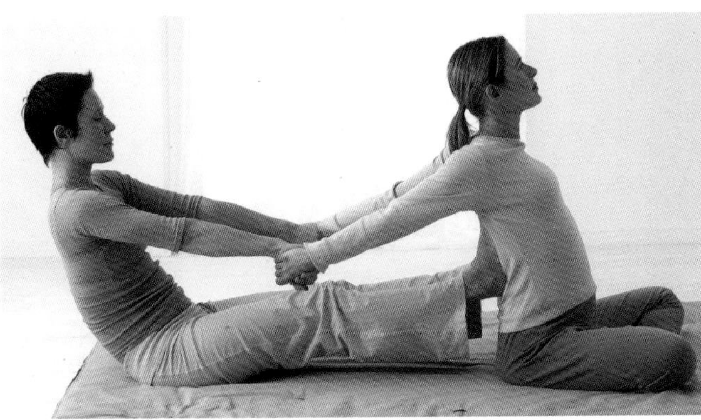

6 Back walk This is a lovely release for the back and provides a gentle stretch for the front. Sit far enough behind your partner so that you can almost stretch your legs out straight. Place your feet in their back, just either side of the spine, below the shoulder blades. Take hold of your partner's hands, clasping around their thumbs.

As you straighten your legs, encourage your partner to let their weight fall back on to your feet, opening fully through their chest. Push them gently back to sitting, reposition your feet slightly and repeat. Work up and down the back but don't take the feet too low, or your partner may feel discomfort in their lower back.

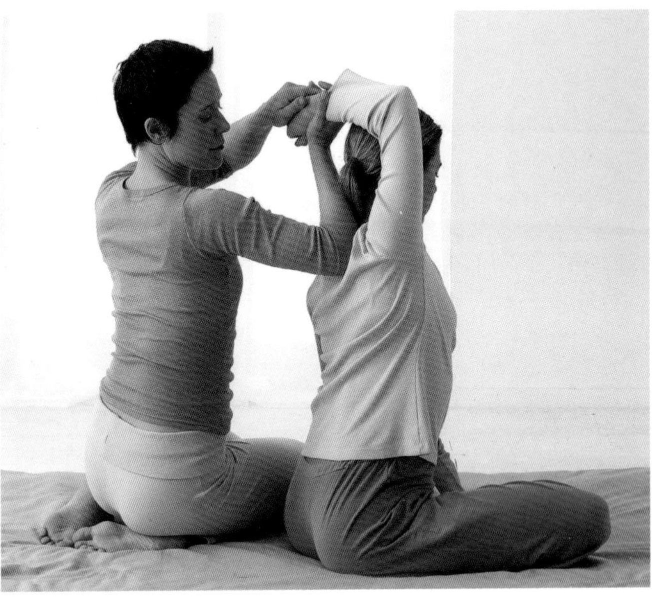

5 Spanish dancer This is a stronger opening for the shoulder and armpit, working into the little pocket of tension at the top corner of the shoulder blade. Kneel beside and slightly behind your partner, facing away slightly. Take their hand and circle it up and behind their head, maintaining its natural direction. Use your inside arm as the lever: hold their wrist and place your elbow in the small space between the spine and the corner of the shoulder blade.

As you sink your hips towards your partner, lean in with your elbow and away with your hands. Sink in and out of this stretch several times, repositioning your elbow very slightly each time.

Advanced stretch

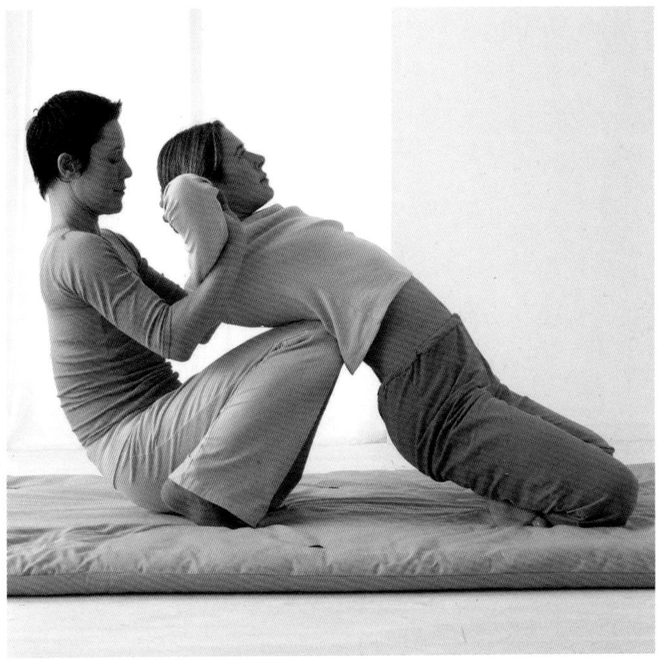

Above This pose, for advanced participants only, shows just how flexible and free your partner can feel in their spine towards the end of the massage.

Completing the Seated Sequence

The gentle sitting twist and forward bends that are shown below are aimed at consolidating the whole sequence of exercises that have been done with your partner in the seated position. These two exercises are excellent counter-poses for the back bends and chest-openers that have gone before. They integrate the energy, working through the whole length of your partner's spine. This should bring a feeling of completeness to the body and therefore prepare it properly for final relaxation.

Gentle Sitting Twist

This is a good all-round twist that is accessible for most body types.

Right Ask your partner to clasp their hands behind their head. Stand behind them, slightly to one side, and gently fix their thigh with your instep. Clasp their upper arms, close to the armpits. On an exhalation, encourage your partner to sink into their hips and allow their upper body to undo into a twist. Ease out of the twist on the inhalation and deepen into it on the exhalation. Do not force, but work gently with their breathing rhythm. Repeat on the other side.

Getting it right

✗ Avoid twists if your partner has any spinal problems.

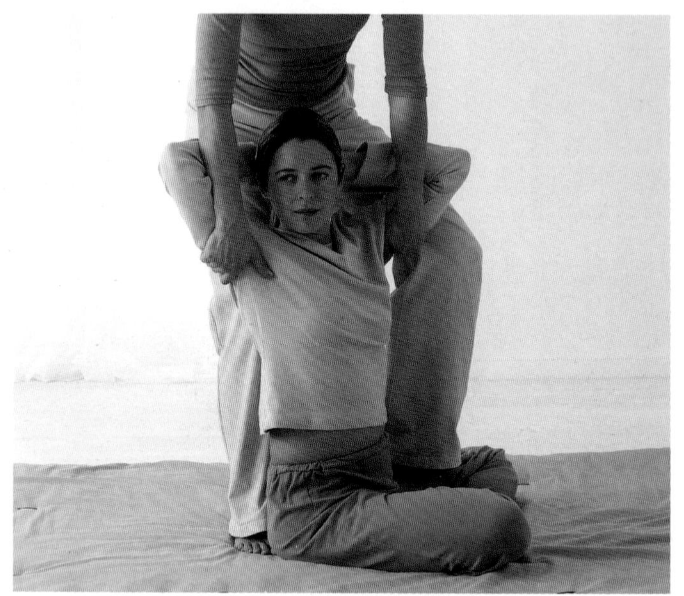

Forward Bends

These assisted forward bends help to bring your partner's focus inwards, preparing them for deep relaxation. The three variations provide options for different levels of flexibility. Find the one that gives your partner the deepest sense of release.

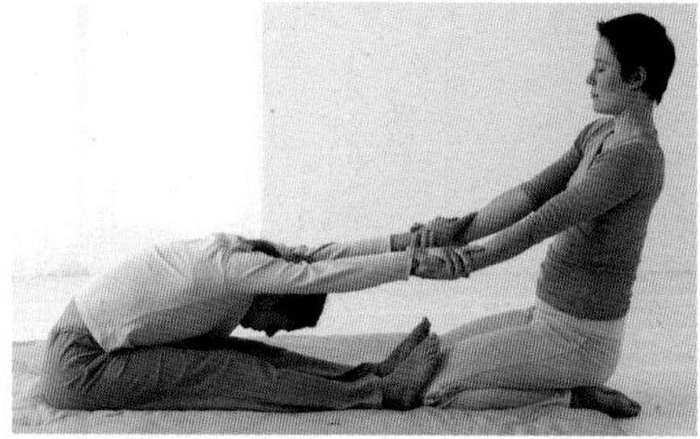

1 For average flexibility Rest your knees against your partner's insteps, as shown, and hold on to each other's wrists. As they inhale, lift slightly through the front of their spine. As they exhale, lean away, lengthening your partner's torso towards their feet. Repeat in and out several times.

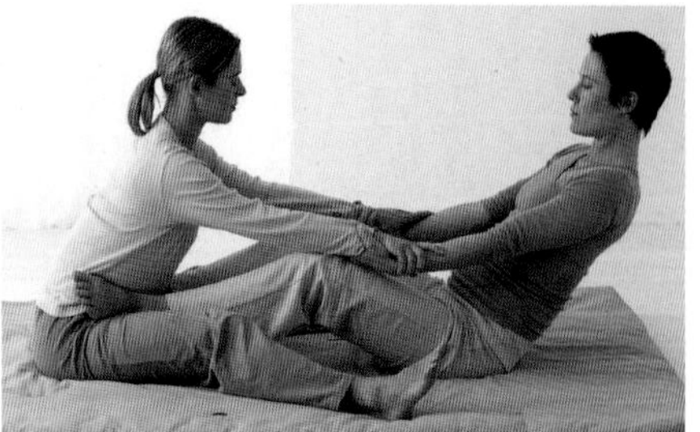

2 For stiffer people With this variation, your partner needs to sit with wide legs and bent knees, so that their pelvis and the base of their spine feel free. Fix your insteps into the front of their hips. As your partner exhales, lean your upper body away and push into their hips with your feet.

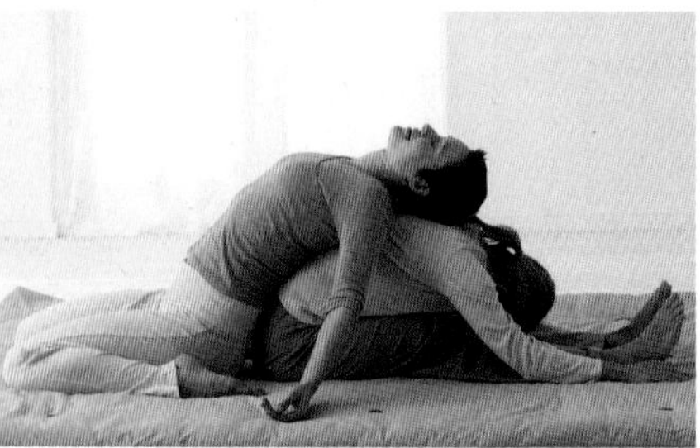

3 Back-to-back This suits those who find version 1 comfortable. Both parties achieve release here: one in the back of the body, the other in the front. Kneel down sacrum to sacrum, with your feet either side of their hips. Relax totally. Slowly release your body weight along their back, feeling their spine lengthen.

Advanced position – the flying pose

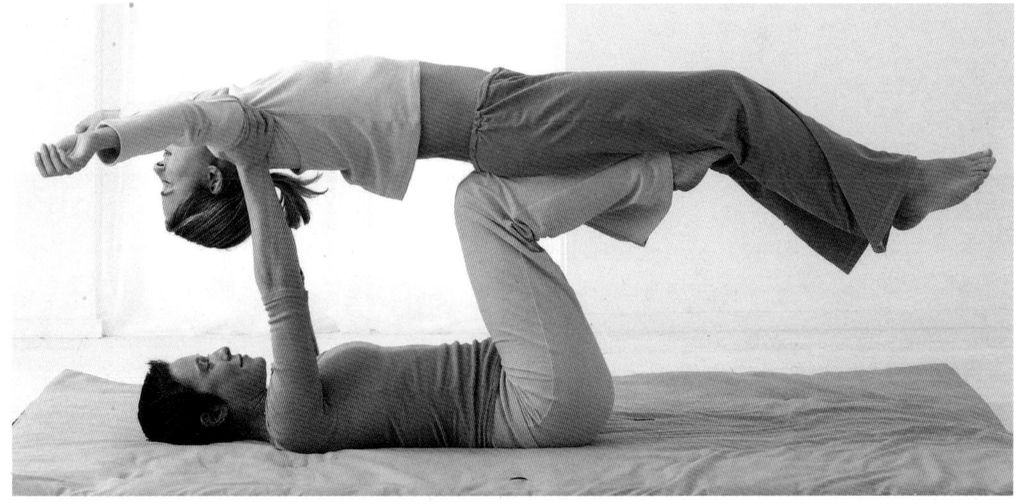

Left The flying pose is one of several advanced positions that facilitate a feeling of complete surrender at the end of a massage. Like all advanced positions, it should be done by experienced participants only, under expert guidance.

Review: Seated Sequence

Use the pictures below as a reminder of the main flow of the sequence performed in the seated position. Remember to keep checking that your posture feels comfortable and to maintain good communication with your partner.

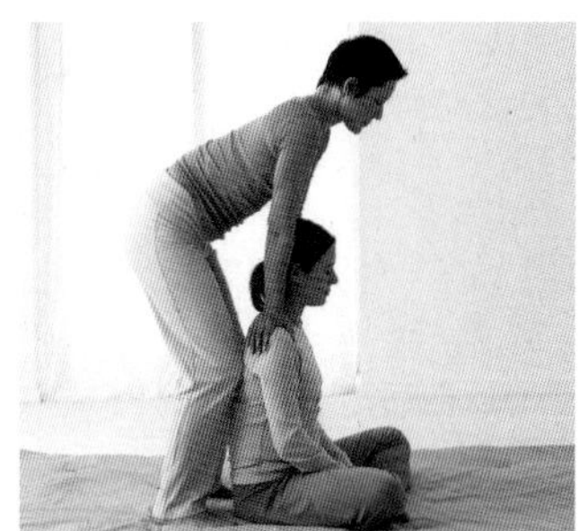

Palming the shoulders

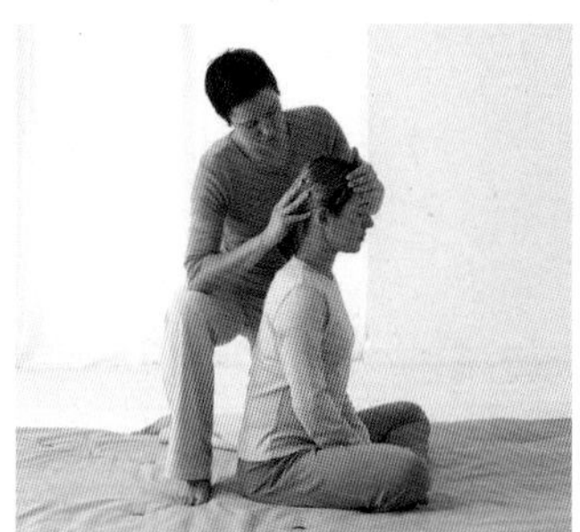

Working the occiput

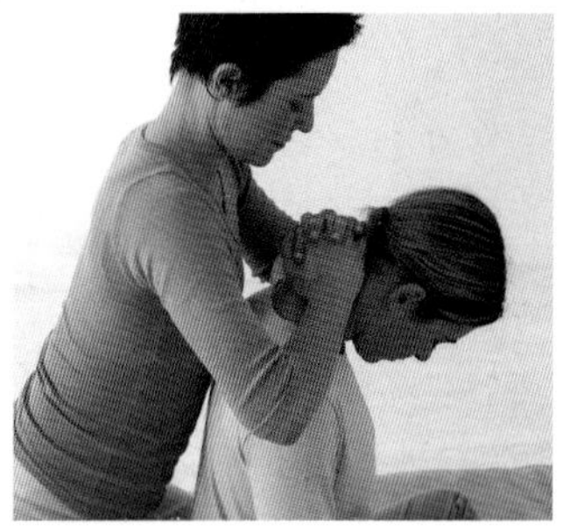

Palming the neck

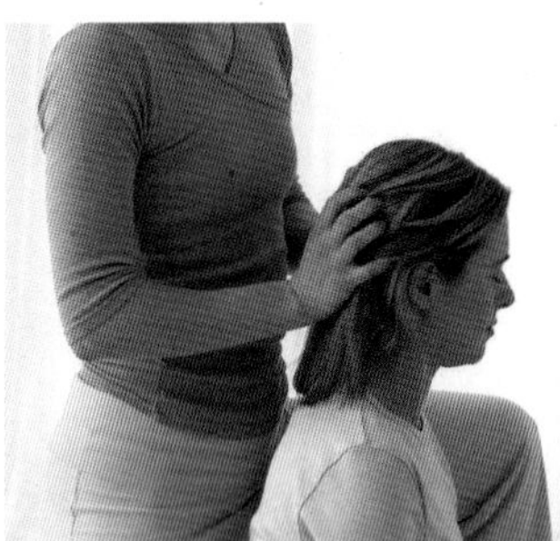

Head massage

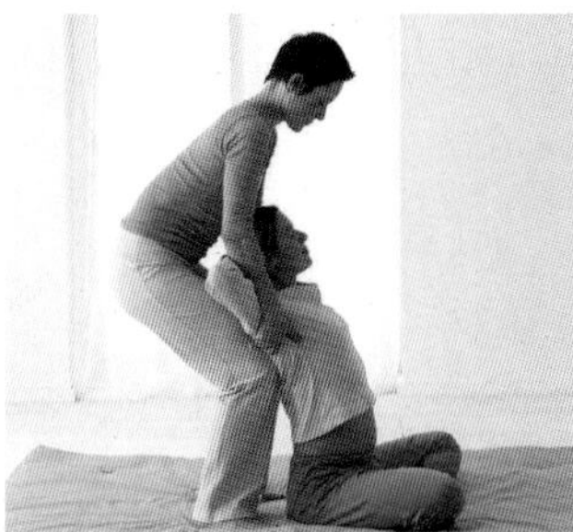

Hello world

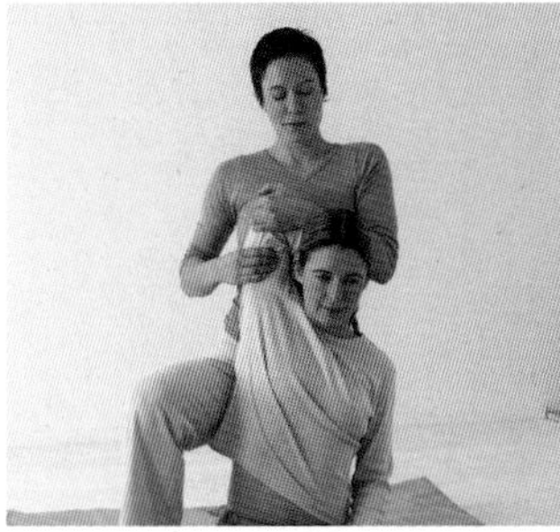

Opening the armpit

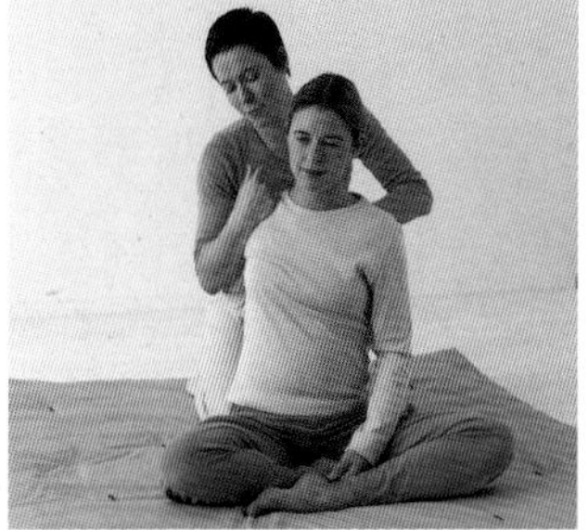

Finding your wings

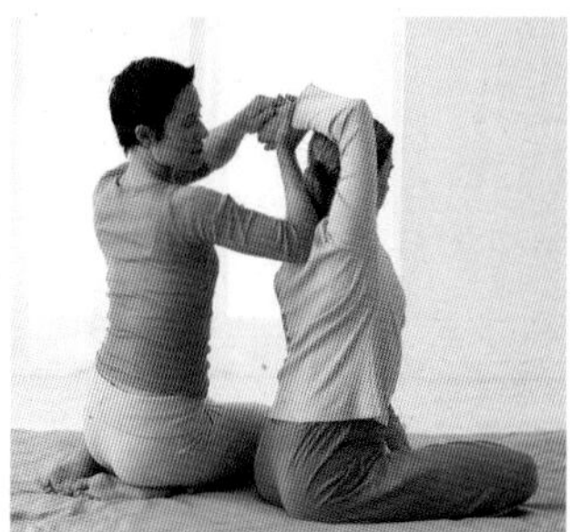

Spanish dancer

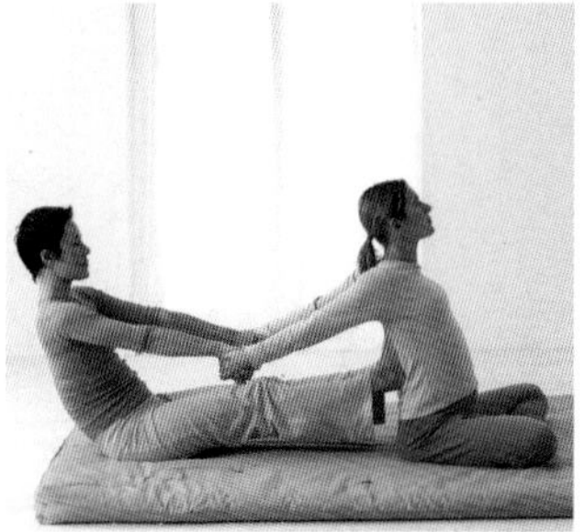

Back walk

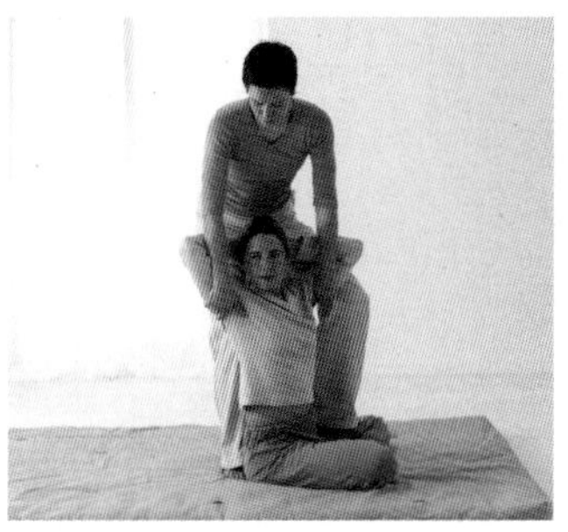

Gentle sitting twist

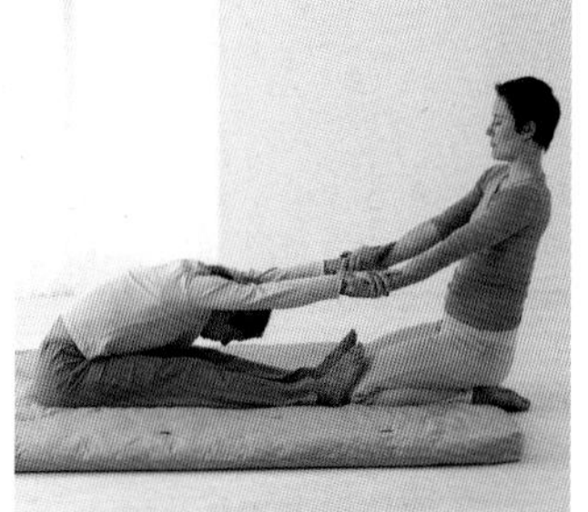

Forward bend

Caution

Once again, you must find out if your partner has any old or current injuries in their neck, shoulders or lower back before proceeding.

The Face

A face massage is a welcome and relaxing treat at any time. Given at the end of a full-body Thai massage, it is an opportunity for your partner to come to a point of stillness and quiet within their body and to release any tension that they may still be holding on to.

The face massage plays a similar role to that of relaxation after a yoga session. It is a time for the body to assimilate and consolidate the dynamic work that has preceded it. Make sure you leave a good ten minutes for the head and face massage; economizing here can leave your partner feeling unsettled, and the massage incomplete. Use this part of the treatment as an opportunity to let your instincts guide you and your creative juices flow.

Make sure that your partner is warm enough, since their temperature will naturally drop as they relax more deeply. Some people with lower back problems may need a little support under their knees at this point - you can use a bolster or a rolled-up blanket. Your partner may also want the support of a cushion or pillow under their head to help keep the back of their neck relaxed. Make sure that you are comfortable too – there is no point in ending the massage with an aching back. Place some support under your hips to help keep your upper spine free from tension.

Getting it right

✓ If your partner suffers from low blood pressure, then you may want to make the face massage more stimulating than relaxing. Also, remind your partner to get up slowly to avoid feeling dizzy.

✓ If you decide to use a little oil for the face massage, ensure that your partner doesn't have any allergies and that they like the smell.

✓ Make sure that your hands are clean, warm and dry. If you know they get a little sticky, use some talcum powder.

Using oils

Traditionally, oil is not used in Thai massage. However, massaging the face is a wonderful opportunity to introduce some essential oils to help relax or invigorate your partner. The oil is meant to enhance the quality of the face massage rather than dominate it, so use only a small amount. Apply the oil after you have done any acupressure point work, otherwise your hands will be slippery. Do not use essential oils neat on the skin. Always add them to a base oil such as sweet almond or grapeseed. Use organic oils wherever possible. For professional advice, however, consult a qualified aromatherapist.

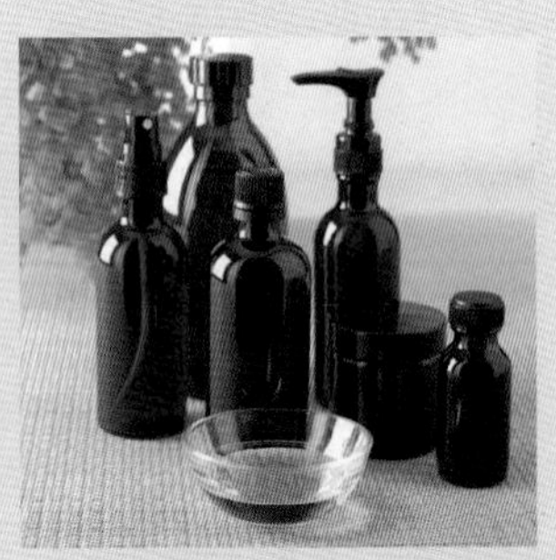

A few suggestions

- Calming/relaxing: lavender, chamomile, neroli, jasmine
- For stress: sandalwood, lavender, neroli, rose
- Grounding/supporting: lavender, frankincense, sandalwood, cedarwood
- Uplifting/refreshing: lemongrass, lemon, orange
- Comforting: rose, lavender, sandalwood
- Balancing: sandalwood, geranium

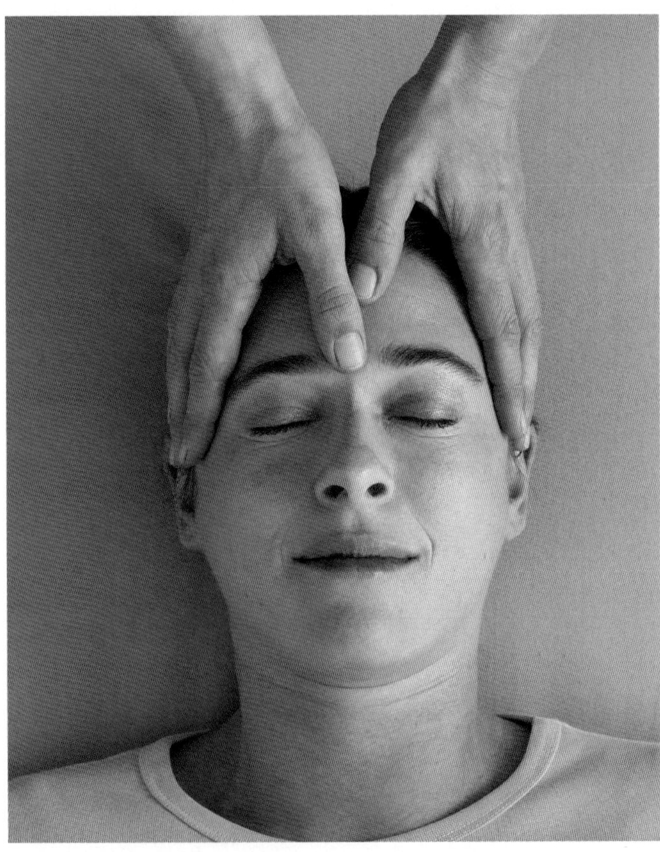

Above Simple, smooth, flowing movements are all you need for an effective and relaxing face massage.

Relaxing the Head and Neck

Start the face massage by encouraging your partner to bring their focus inwards and relax completely. Suggest that they close their eyes and listen to their breathing, letting their thoughts drift away and their body weight sink into the mat underneath them.

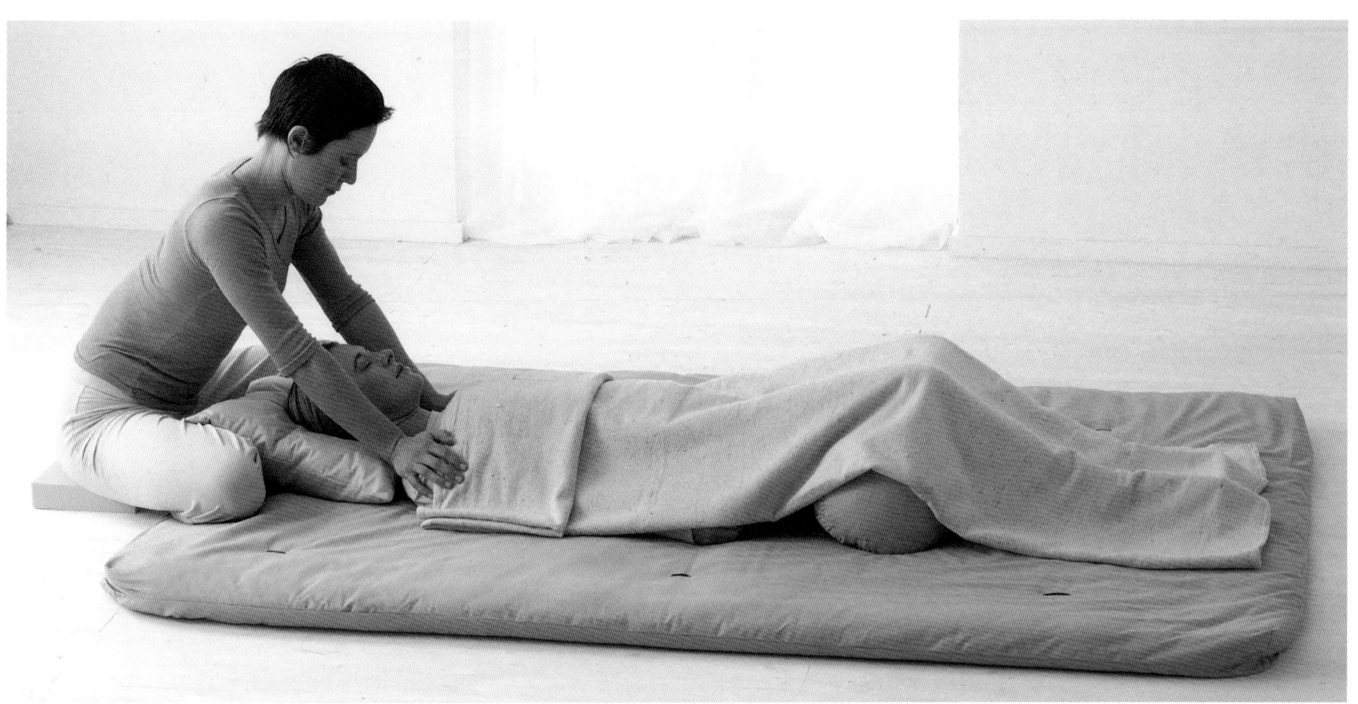

1 Relaxing the shoulders Sit down, on some support if necessary, positioned close to your partner just behind their head. Now alternately palm the shoulders, easing them away from the ears.

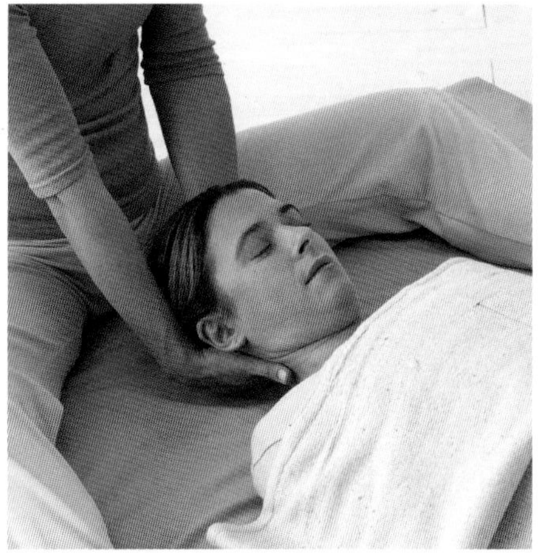

2 Neck lengthener Slide both your hands under the back of your partner's skull. Fix your palms against their occipital ridge. Now lean away, gently lengthening the back of the neck.

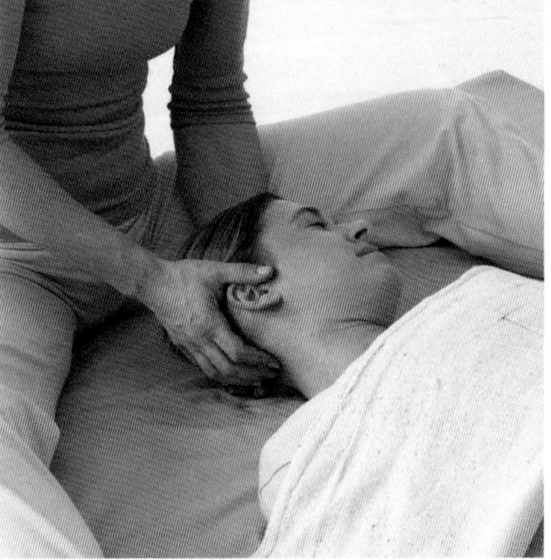

3 Cranial hold Simply supporting the weight of your partner's head in your hands can feel extremely comforting and facilitate a deep release throughout their body. To get your hands in the correct position, turn your partner's head slightly from side to side and place the flat tips of your fingers against the bony ridge of the skull. Now let your fingers and hands relax completely.

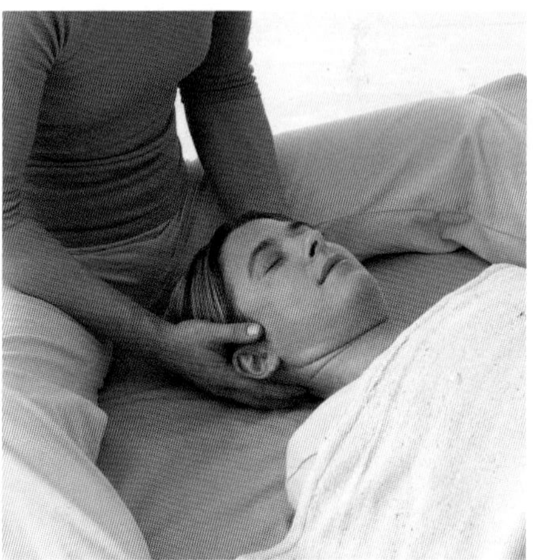

4 Keep the backs of your hands on the mat for support, as any feeling of effort or tension in your hands is quickly transferred to your partner's head. The less you do, the more effective this will be. Enjoy listening with your hands to the subtle movements and sensations in your partner's skull.

Working on the Face

As a rule, begin with repeated slow, broad, general strokes, then move on to the more focused work for the acupressure points. Work in either of two ways. For a deeply relaxing massage use slow, smooth, meditative sweeping movements. For a more stimulating massage, apply pressure with invigorating circles. The way you work depends on your partner's likes and dislikes and may also depend on what they have to do immediately after their massage. For example, if they have to drive a car or go back to a work environment, then it may be better to give them a more stimulating face massage.

Key to the pressure points

1 the third eye or ajna chakra

2 headache, insomnia, problems of the lower sinuses and dizziness

3 headache and facial paralysis

4 headache and facial paralysis

5 headache

6 facial paralysis and hypothermia

7 the temple – an important therapy point for headaches.

8 the tear ducts – therapy point for insomnia (use only gentle thumb pressure)

9–11 these small depressions next to the edge of the ear are good for treating deafness, ear pain and toothache

12 lower sinuses and facial paralysis

13 fainting, shock, sunstroke and respiratory failure

14 facial paralysis

15 migraine

USING PRESSURE POINTS ON THE FACE

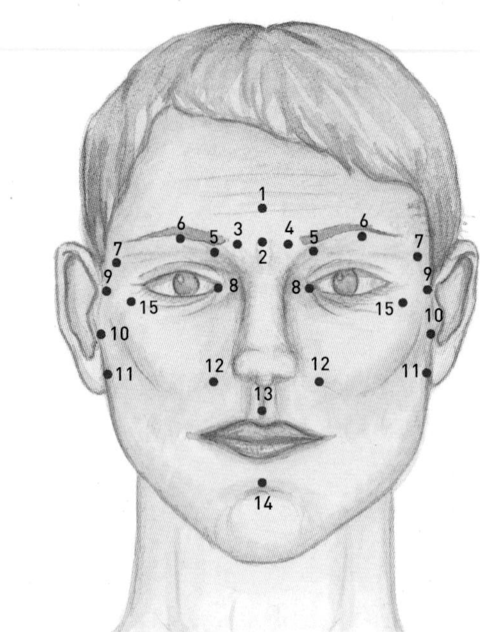

Above Thai massage stimulates a range of acupressure points. This shows a broad selection of useful ones.

Easy Massage Routine

The steps given below are just a suggestion of what you might want to try. Facial massage is an area where you can really enjoy exploring and experimenting with your own techniques.

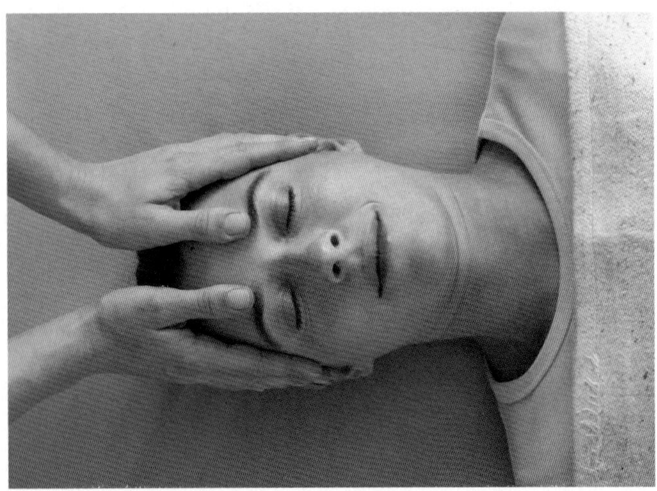

1 Brow sweep Place your fingers on your partner's temples, in order to stabilize your hands. Now use the flats of your thumbs to slide away from the centre of your partner's forehead towards their temples.

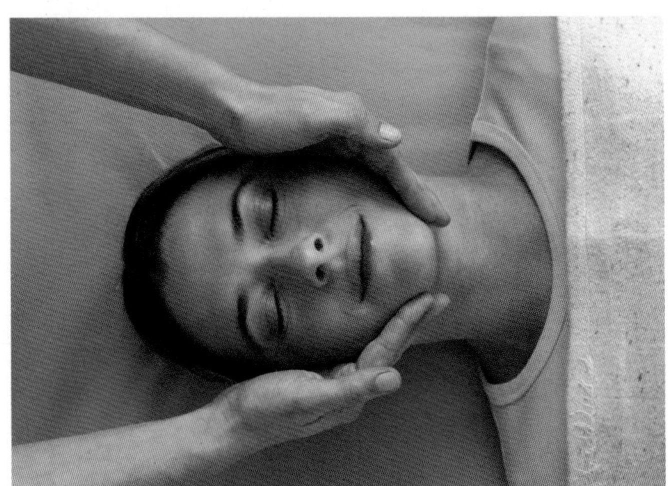

2 Jaw sweep Cup your hands around the cheeks and sweep up from the chin to the temples.

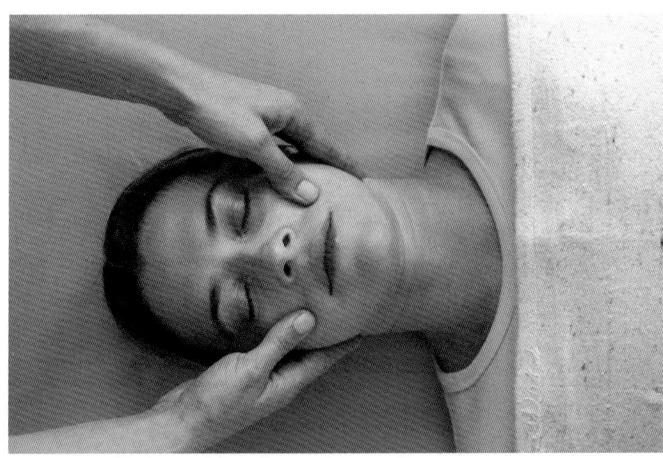

3 Cheekbone sweep Using your thumbs, sweep from the corners of the nostrils around the contours of the cheekbones and out towards the ears.

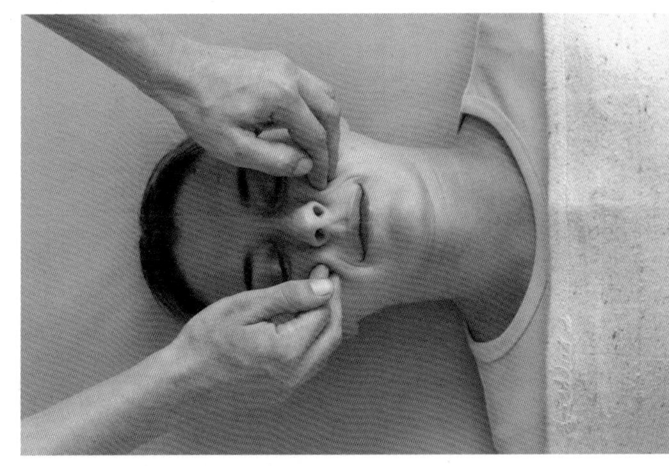

4 Sinus circles With the fingers together, circle around underneath the cheekbones.

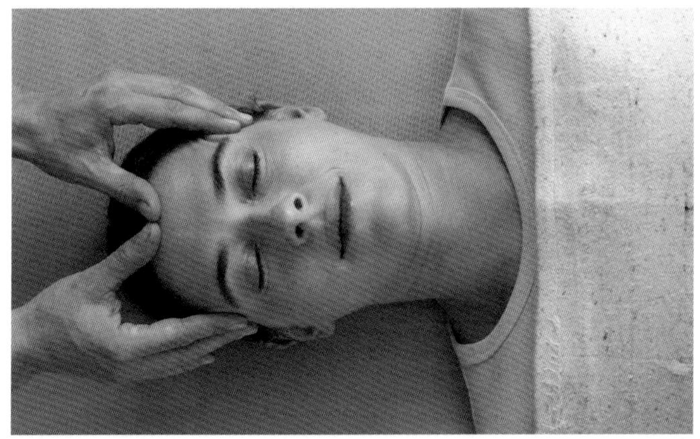

5 Temple circles With the thumbs supported on the forehead, circle gently with the flats of your fingers to ease tension from the temple area.

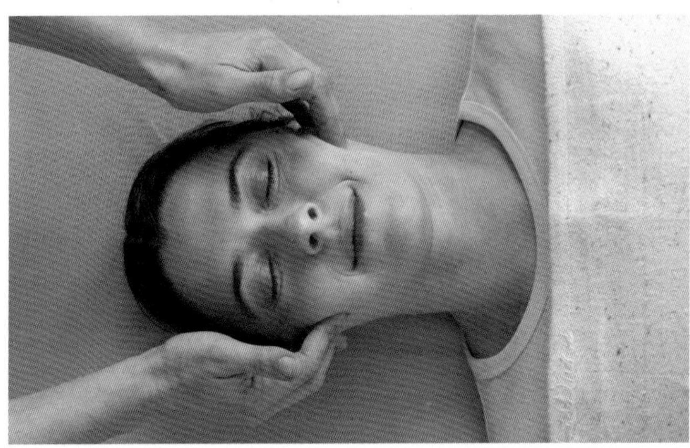

6 Jaw circles The jaw holds a surprising amount of tension. Check that your partner's jaw is relaxed and circle firmly all around this joint.

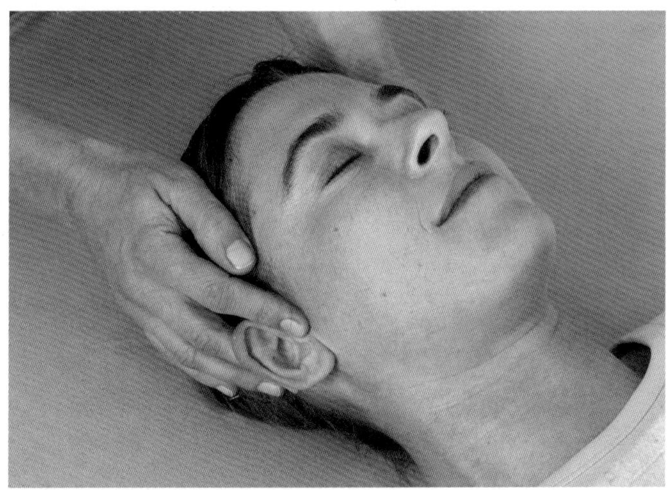

7 Ear circles Slide your fingers up either side of each ear and rub firmly around the front and back of the ear itself. There are several wonderfully releasing points around the ears and you can stimulate the whole area with firm, circular rubbing movements.

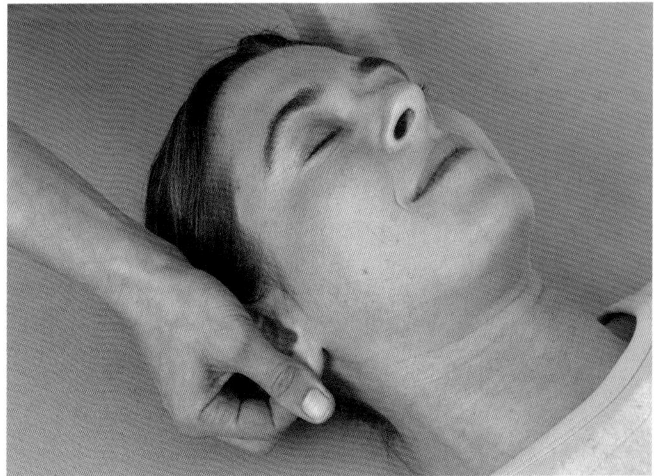

8 Stroking the earlobes The ears contain a multitude of acupressure points. Stroking and squeezing the earlobes, as well as pressing around the inside of the ear, is both soothing and stimulating.

Finishing the Full-body Massage

As the facial massage routine comes to a close, so too does the complete Thai body massage. These closing exercises can bring your partner to a place of complete rest. Never underestimate the power of stillness, of simply holding and listening. The very simple holds used to finish the facial massage will give your partner's physical and energetic body a chance to rest and rejuvenate. Enjoy this opportunity to listen, without any expectation of your own or your partner's body.

The Final Holds

Make sure that you are comfortable and your shoulders and hands are free of tension. Observe your breathing rhythm and use it to check how relaxed you are in your own body.

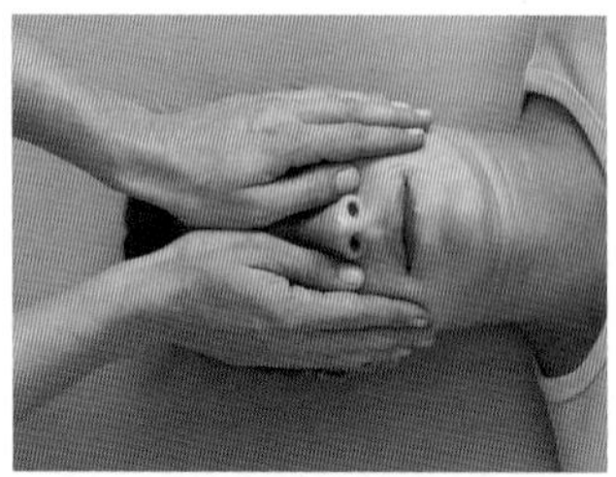

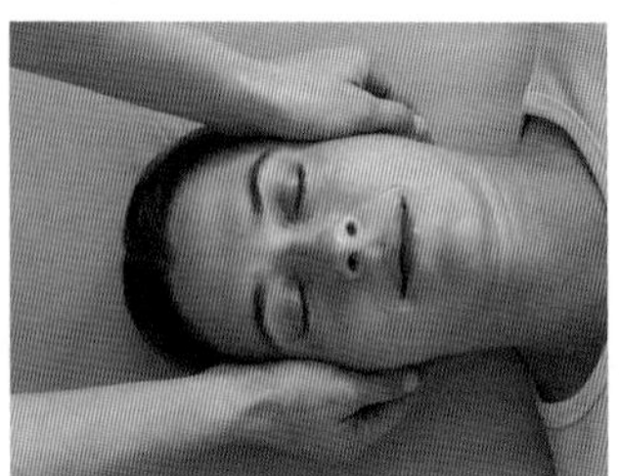

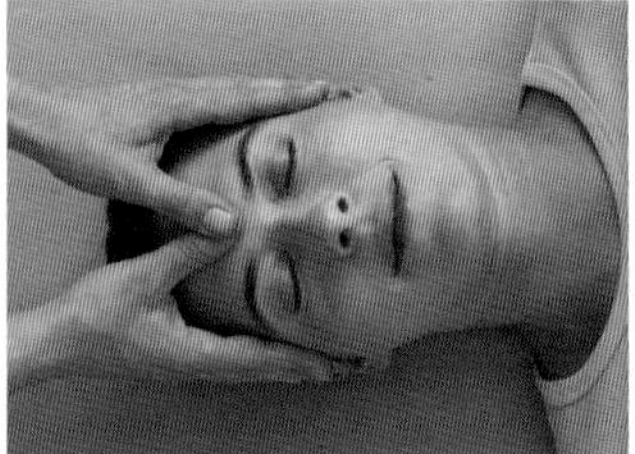

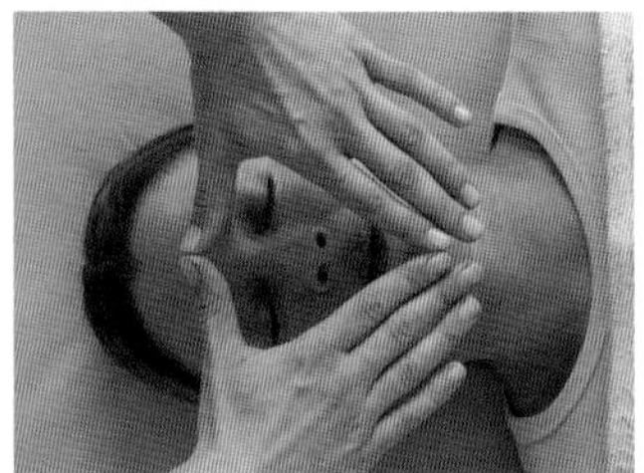

1 Eye hold (above left) Cup your hands gently over your partner's eye sockets, letting the heel of each hand rest on the brow and the fingers rest on the cheekbones.

2 Ear hold (above right) Cup your hands around your partner's ears. Shutting out external sounds helps to bring their focus inwards.

3 Third eye hold (above left) Place thumb over thumb on the ajna chakra (third eye point). This creates a focal point for the energy flow throughout the body. It helps your partner to become aware of the potential of infinite space within them.

4 Bodhi mudra (above right) A *mudra* is a yogic posture, in this case a hand gesture, that influences the body to function in a certain way. Using this mudra here enhances energy flow to the face and third eye.

Finishing Prayer

Just as you began the complete body massage with a prayer, with an intention of working with healing touch, it is important to complete it in a similar way, honouring the experience you have shared with your partner.

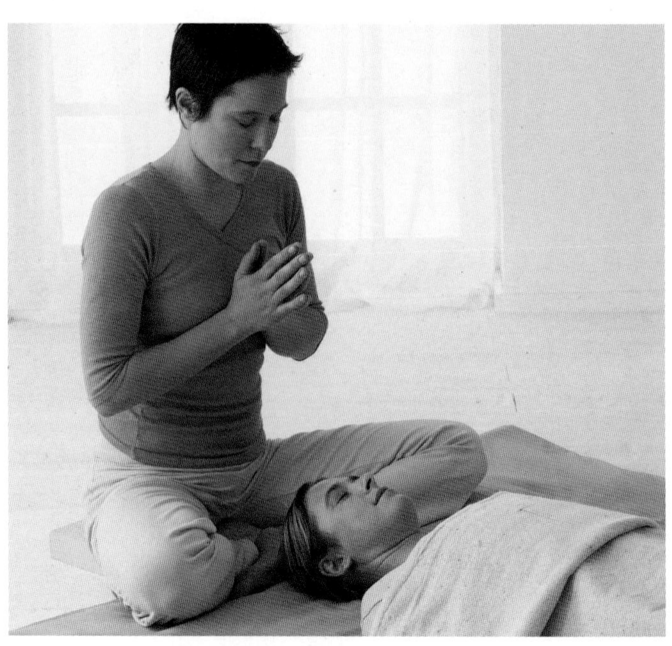

Right Taking care of your partner after a massage After you have completed the treatment, leave your partner to rest quietly for a few moments without interruption. It is often the undisturbed moments, after the hands-on aspect of a massage has finished, that deeper healing occurs. In addition it can be a good idea to offer them a glass of water, as Thai massage can be strongly detoxifying.

Review: the Face and Closing Holds

Use the pictures below as a reminder of the main flow of the facial massage sequence. As mentioned, the precise sequence for the facial massage is not crucial, but you may prefer to follow the order given until you feel confident enough to experiment.

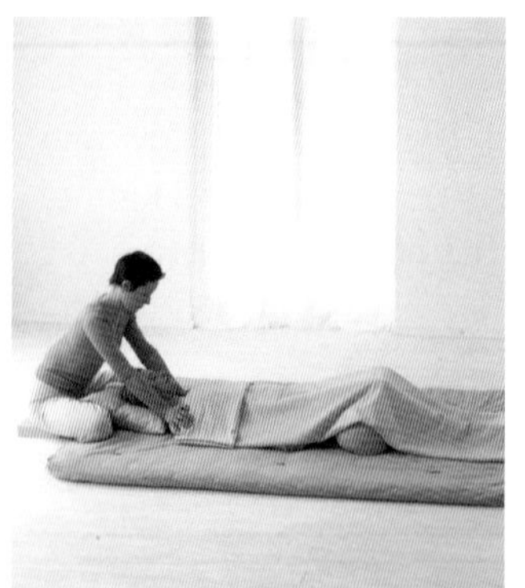
Relaxing the shoulders

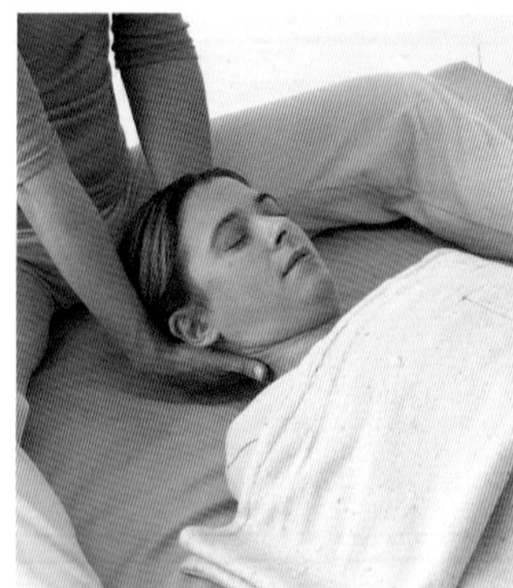
Neck lengthener

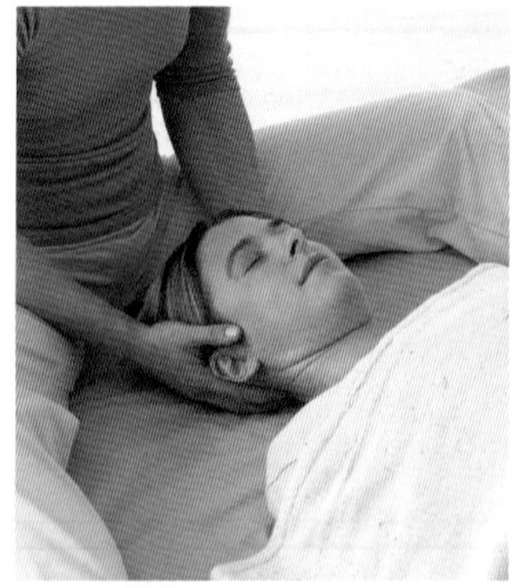
Cranial hold

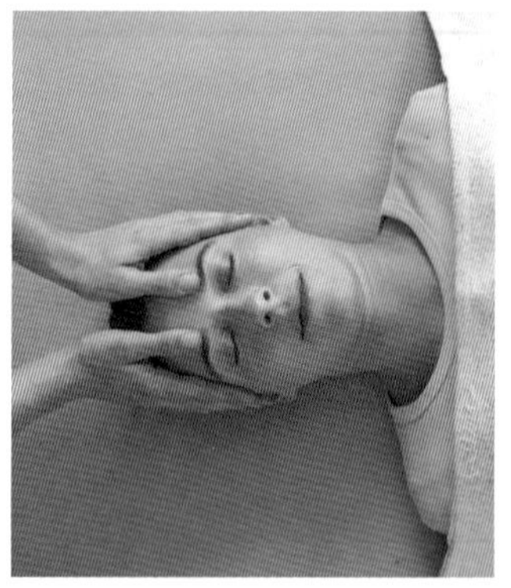
Brow sweep

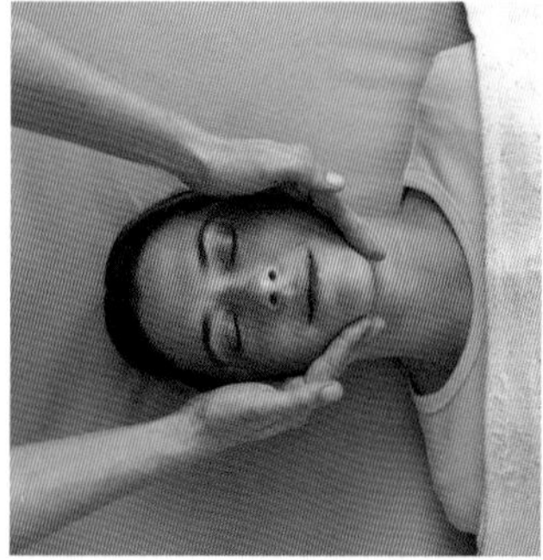
Jaw sweep

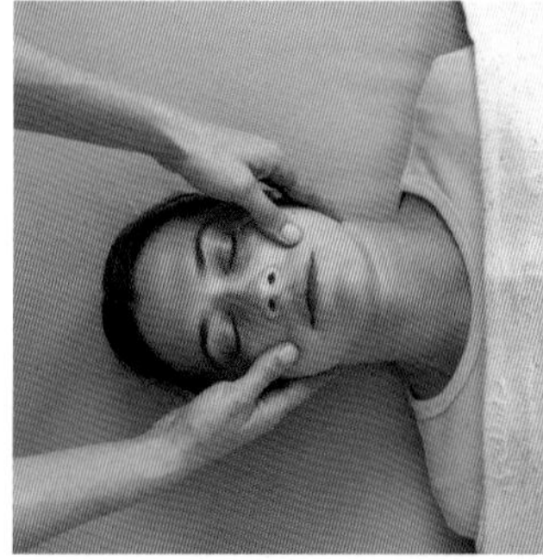
Cheekbone sweep

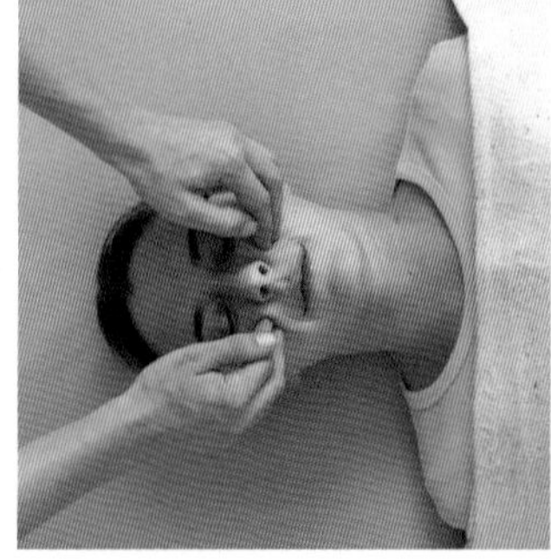
Sinus circles

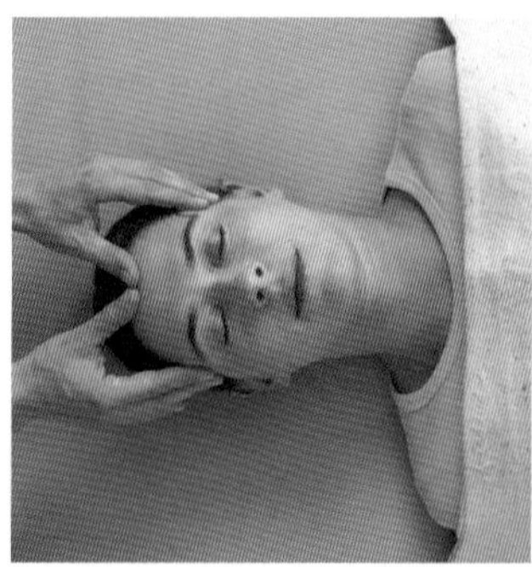
Temple circles

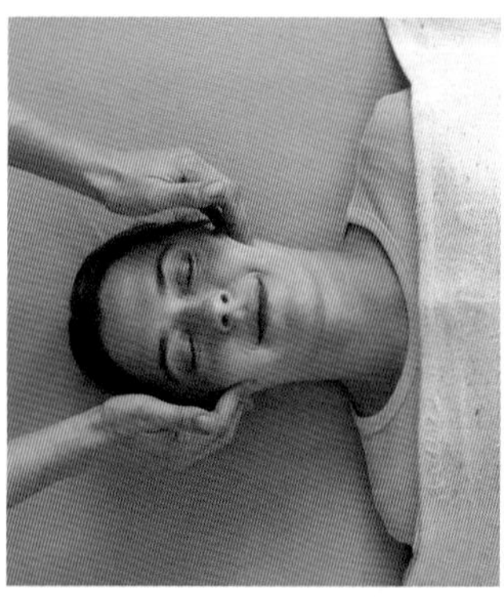
Jaw circles

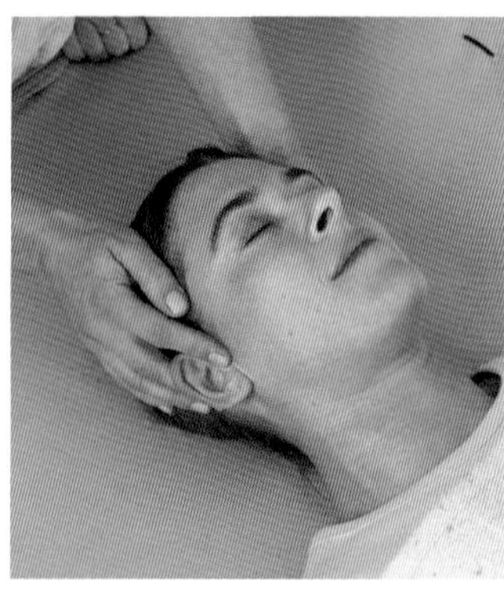
Ear circles

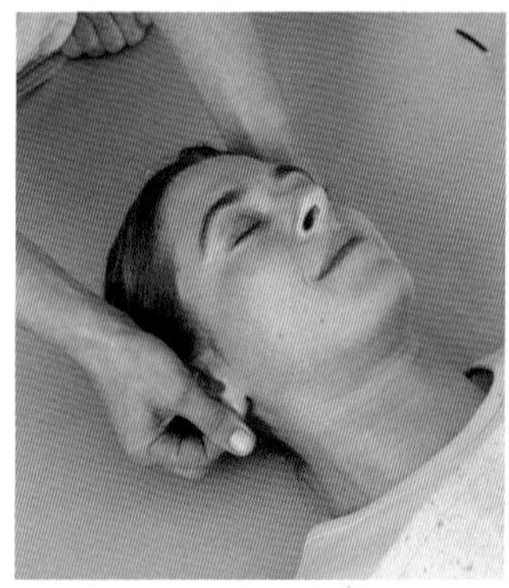
Stroking the earlobes

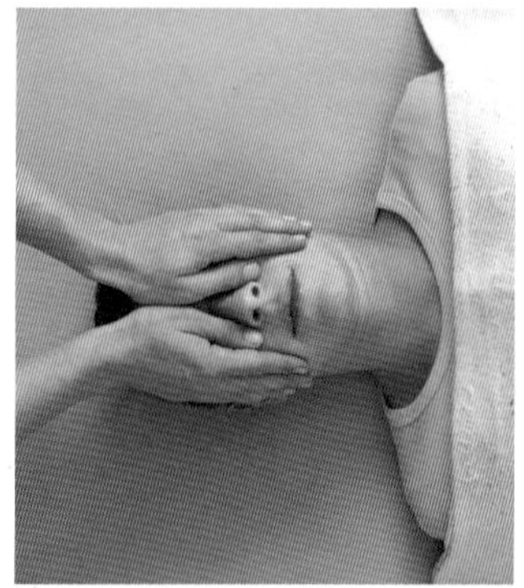
Eye hold

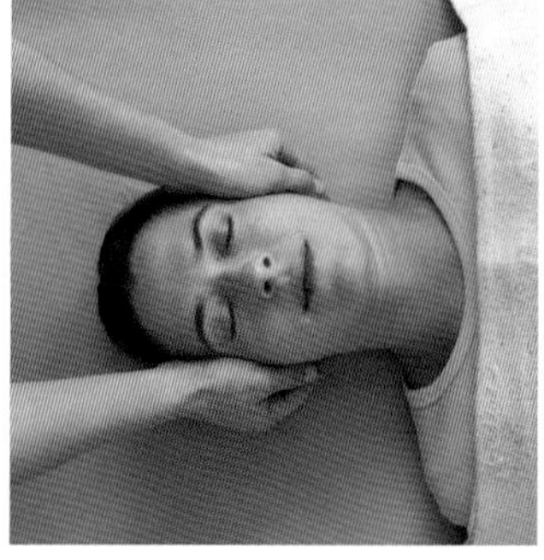
Ear hold

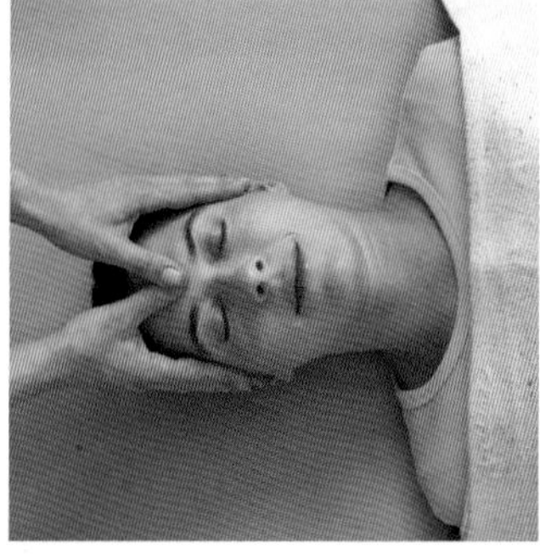
Third eye hold

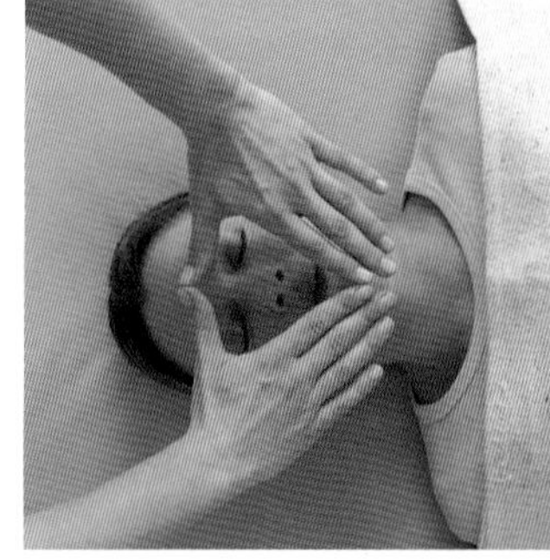
Bodhi mudra

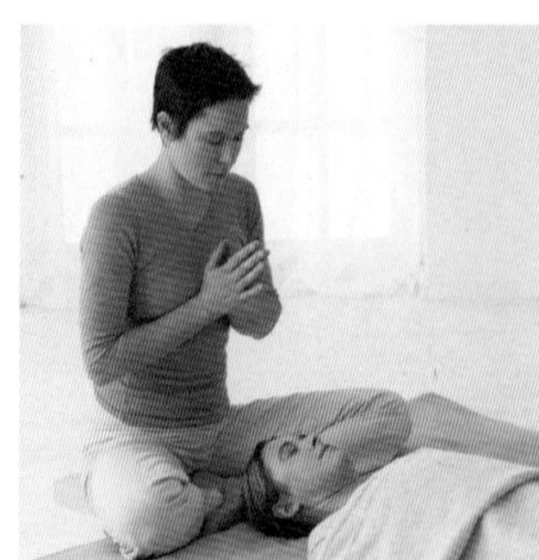
Finishing prayer

Thai Massage for Older People

Receiving massage is even more important later in life, as general wear and tear on the body starts to take effect. Thai massage is particularly supportive for an ageing body – maintaining joint mobility, easing aches and pains and helping you to feel more vibrant and active. The beauty of Thai massage is that even if your strength and physical stamina are not what they used to be, you can still benefit from its gentle motion and passive stretching without any effort or discomfort.

Massage is a lovely way of giving and sharing with parents or grandparents. Thai massage is suitable for any age or fitness level, as you can adapt treatments to suit your partner's needs. If they are very fragile or stiff, do more energy line work and use the gentle, easing stretches rather than the more demanding ones. There is no need to feel timid or over-cautious – just keep communicating with your partner and work with what feels good for their body. However, be sensible and don't choose an older body for your initial practice. Wait until you are more confident with the main routine before applying the adapted versions suggested below.

Getting it right

✗ Do not work on inflamed arthritic joints. With arthritis caused by wear and tear, gently ease through the joints when they are not inflamed.

✗ Never apply pressure on bone or try physically demanding stretches if your partner suffers from osteoporosis or softening of the bones.

✗ Avoid all inverted poses and over-stimulating exercises if your partner suffers from high blood pressure.

✗ Never press directly on any varicose vein.

✓ Check for heart conditions and work appropriately under the guidance of a medical professional.

✓ Have a good supply of cushions on hand for support.

Relaxing Routine

This sequence provides a selective but balanced massage routine. Make sure that your partner has all the padding support they need and is totally comfortable.

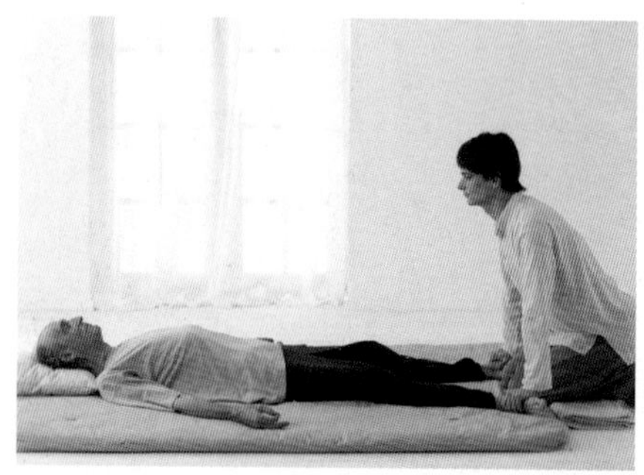

1 Feet – palming the instep Flexibility in all joints is affected by age. Any work that maintains an openness and flexibility in the feet and ankles will have a positive impact throughout the skeletal system. Work through as much of the foot sequence as your partner enjoys.

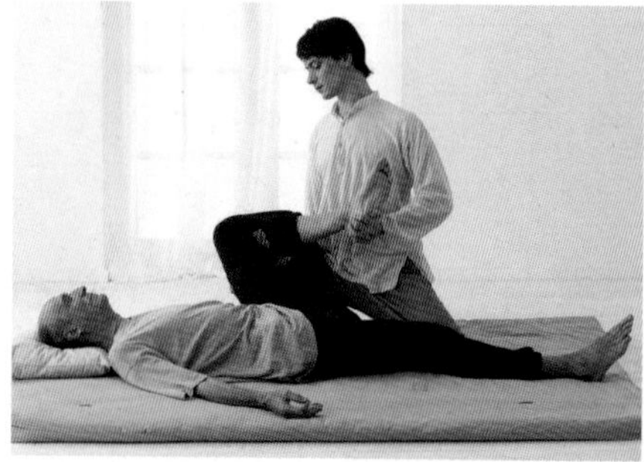

2 Leg circles Working all around the joints helps keep the hips well oiled and mobile, and can also help to relieve stiffness across the lower back. Make sure that you support your own body as you lift and circle the leg in both directions.

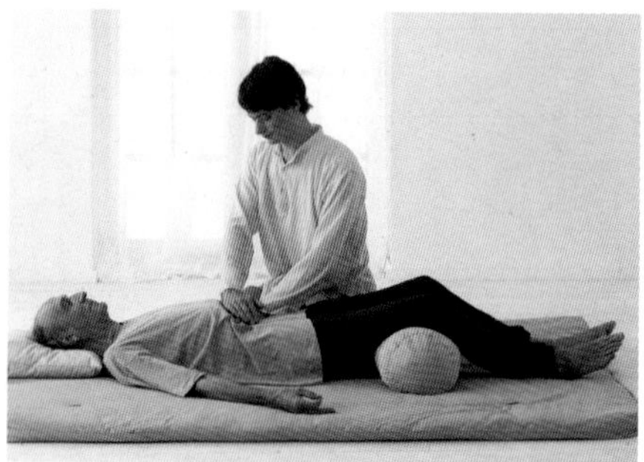

3 Relaxing the abdomen As the body ages, its natural rhythm slows, which can affect internal processes such as the digestion. Maintaining a healthy digestion means nutrients are better absorbed and ensures that the immune system is given adequate support. Start with general circling clockwise around the abdomen; proceed to the deeper work of palming and finger pressing if your partner feels comfortable.

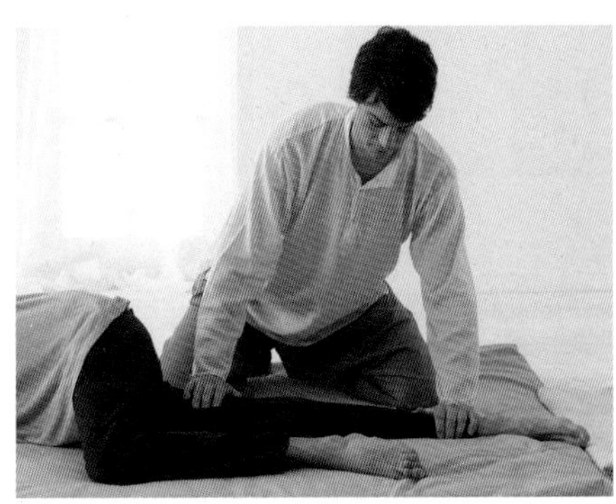

4 Leg lines in side position Your partner may not feel comfortable lying completely flat for very long so you can explore palming the leg lines in the side position.

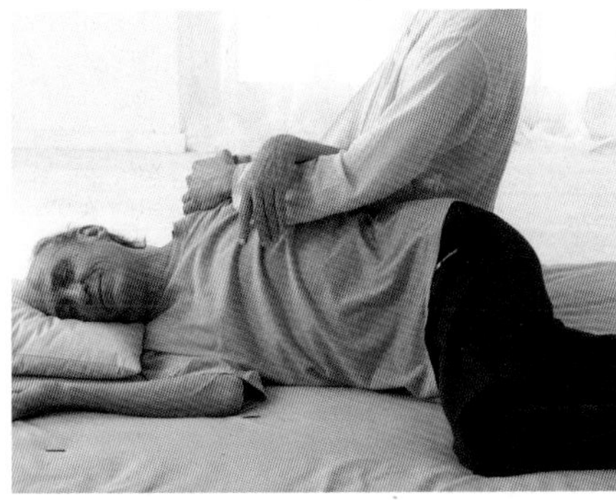

5 Shoulder workout Help to maintain space in the shoulders and neck by spending some time slowly easing through the shoulder joint. Kneel behind your partner and make sure that their neck is well supported by cushions.

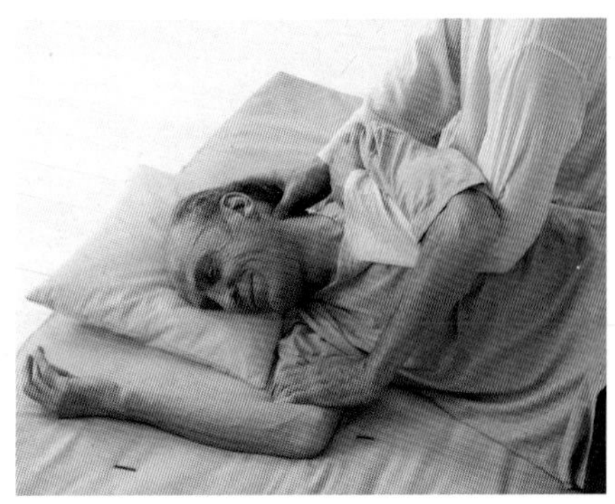

6 Neck release Focused work for the neck can be given in this reclining position, which is more relaxing than sitting. Keep the shoulder well supported from the front and use the hand at the back to work up into and around the occipital ridge at the base of the skull.

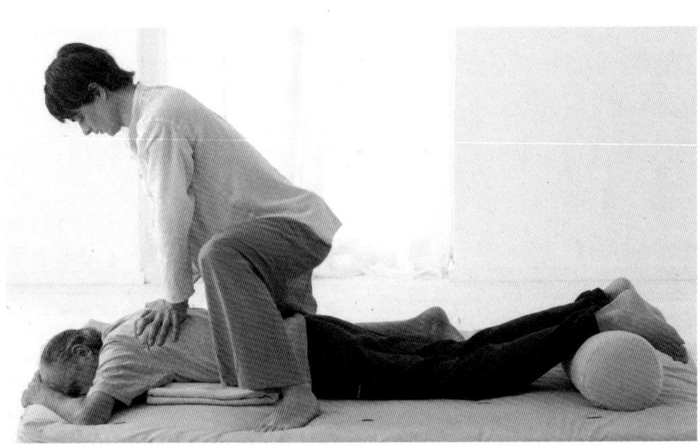

7 Working the back lines (left) Provide plenty of support for your partner's body when they lie on their front. You may need to put more padding under the fronts of their ankles to support their lower back and protect their knees.

Simple Seated Exercises

The versatility of the seated position comes into its own here. Not everyone is able to sit on the floor, so a low chair or stool can be used instead. The important thing is for your partner to feel comfortable so that they can relax more fully into the massage.

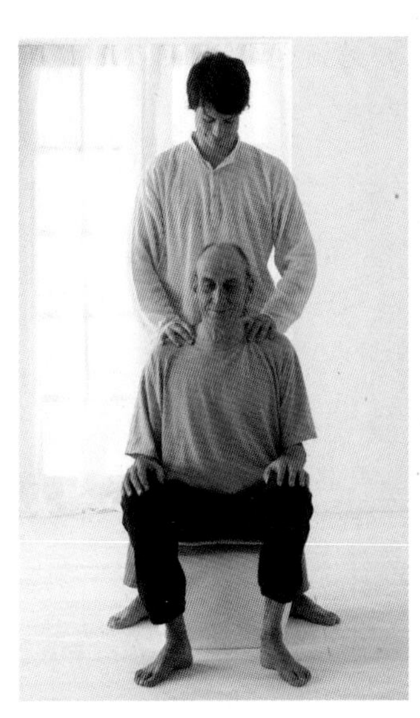

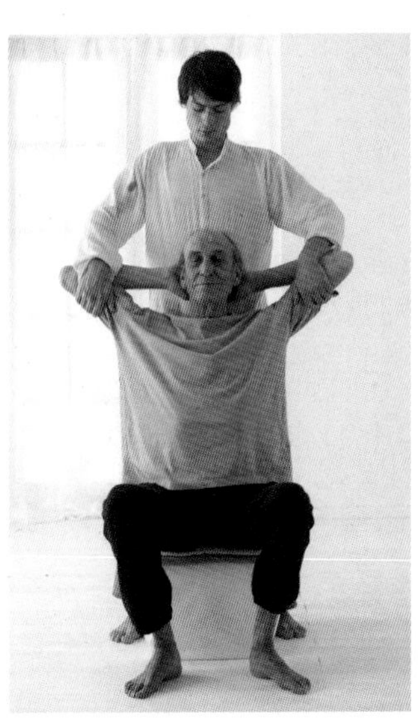

1 Relaxing the shoulders (far left) Work with gentle squeezing and milking techniques to release tension across the top of your partner's shoulders.

2 Hello world (left) (see section in complete body routine on expanding the upper body). Stand with a wide base directly behind your partner and come close in so that they can use your body as support. Ask them to interlace their hands behind their head and clasp around their upper arms. Work into the stretch on both the inhalation and the exhalation, exploring which feels most beneficial for your partner. Whichever way they breathe, encourage their opening to come from the solar plexus up through the centre of the chest and out through the armpits.

Easing Common Conditions

Thai massage is a whole-body treatment that works to rebalance the physical, energetic and emotional bodies. However, if your partner has a headache, back pain or stomach ache, for example, you may want to try easing them by using these short sequences as a guide.

There is no diagnostic tradition as such in Thai Massage, instead we work with the intention to support the body's natural healing ability, by applying the techniques skilfully, appropriately, with awareness and understanding. There is no substitute for the complete rebalancing of energy experienced after receiving a full-body Thai massage. If you wish to use massage to alleviate a long-term condition, such as migraine or back pain, the specific treatment should be incorporated within the full-body massage, by placing an emphasis on particular exercises or on energy line work. If you decide to work in this way you can refer to the energy line and points artwork so that you can start to integrate some basic theory into your practice.

The sequences given below are not fixed plans but guides to help you ease some common conditions. They are shown in the order in which they would occur in a regular full-body massage, working from the feet towards the head. For more detailed technique descriptions, refer to the individual sections of the main routine.

Lower Back Pain

The main relevant treatment lines here are sen sumana, sen ittha and sen pingkhala. The lower back is supported in particular by work on the abdomen, the legs and the hips.

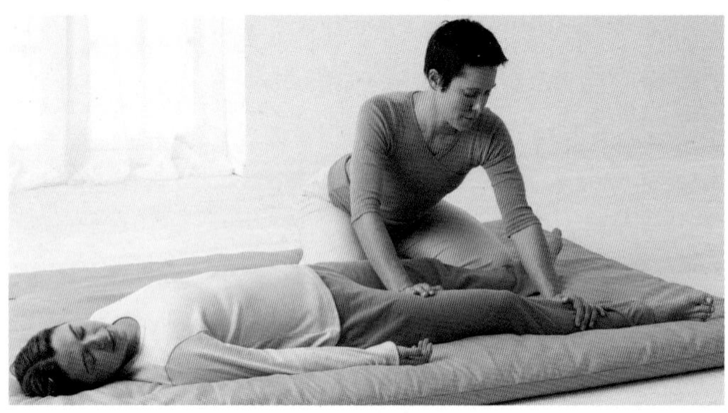

1 Work all the lines on the legs, focusing specifically on the third inside line of the legs (sen sumana).

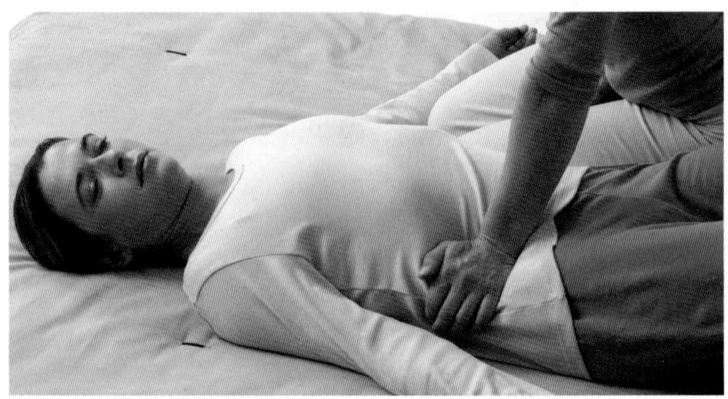

2 Focus on giving repeated abdominal massage. Pain felt in the lower back can often be caused by excess tension in the abdomen and may be relieved by a deep abdominal workout.

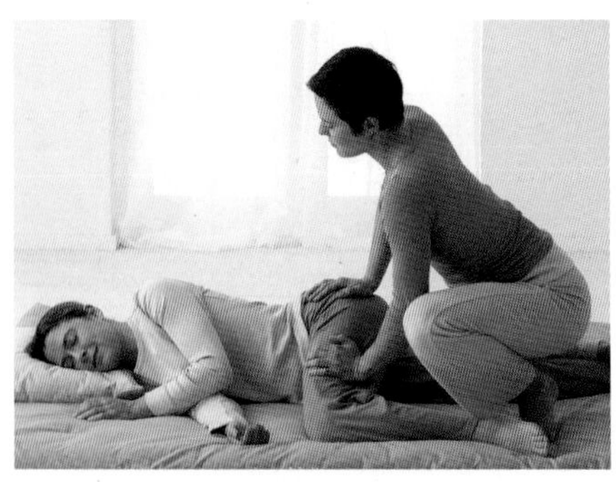

3 Work the third outside line of the leg (sen ittha and sen pingkhala), spending time around the hip area.

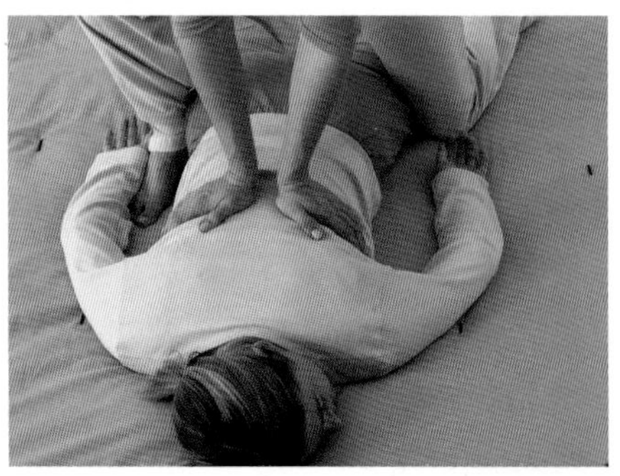

4 Palm and thumb both sets of back lines, especially the first back line (sen ittha and sen pingkhala). Focus on the lower back, rubbing around the buttocks and sacrum.

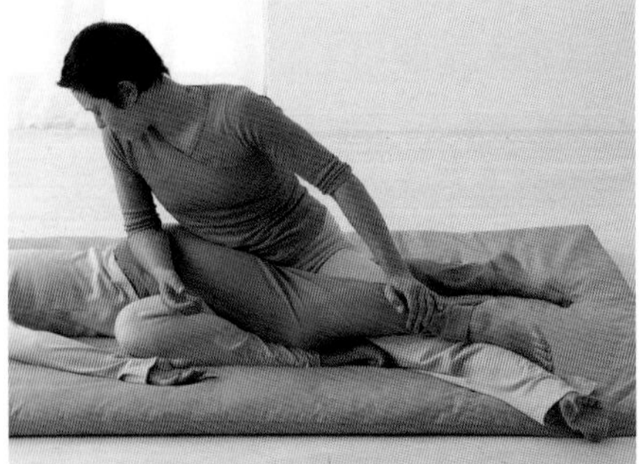

5 Use the forearm to work around the hips and buttocks in the take a break pose (in the sequence for the back of the body).

Knee Pain

Palming and thumbing the leg lines can help to ease knee pain caused by strain or overwork, but do not proceed if serious damage is indicated – if the kneecap is painful when you press directly down on it or move it alternately up and down.

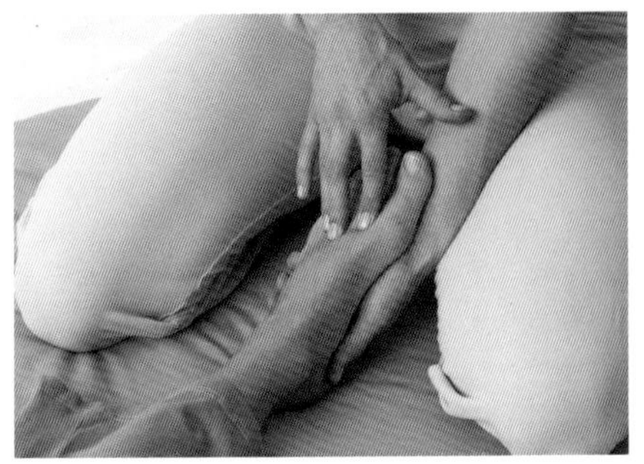

1 Work between the tendons of your partner's feet with your fingers. Use firm pressure but do not press too hard.

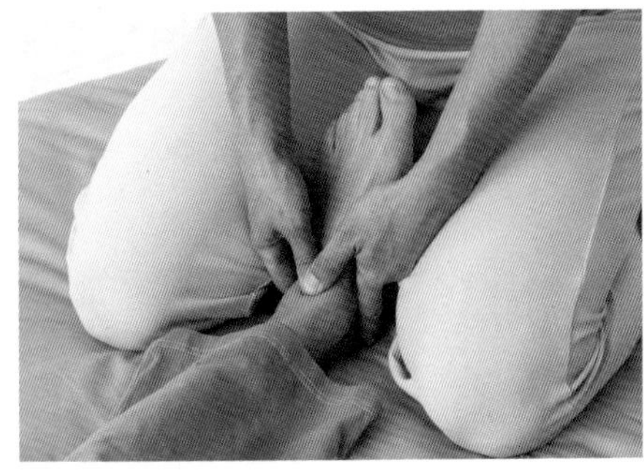

2 Work the knee pain point at the front of the foot. Use repeated pressure, but only hold it for as long as your partner can bear.

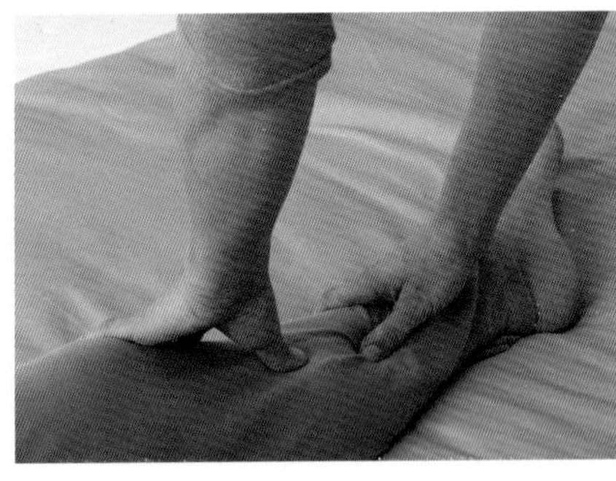

3 Palm and thumb all six leg lines, with particular emphasis on the first outside line (sen sahatsarangsi and sen thawari).

Sciatica

Tension in the lower back and hip can trap the sciatic nerve. This is often experienced as a sharp pain in the hip and down the leg. As well as performing the sequence below, you can also focus your work on sen kalathari.

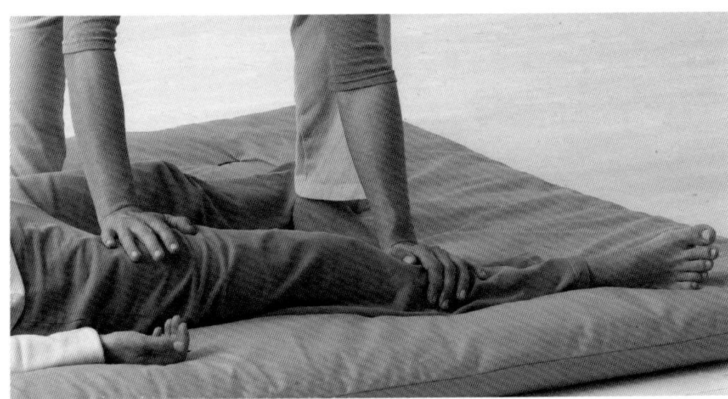

1 When palming and thumbing the leg lines, give particular focus to the second inside line (sen kalathari).

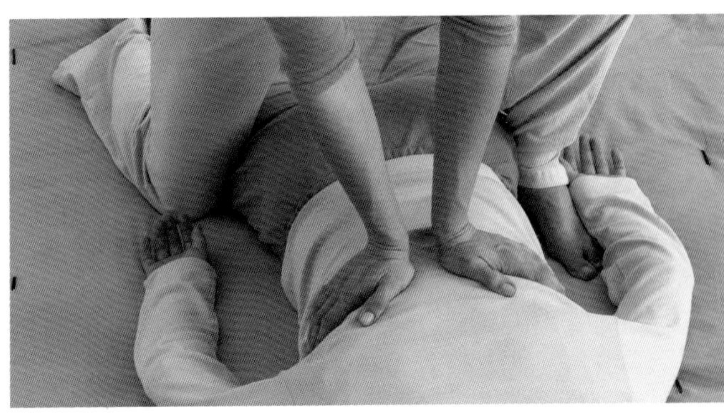

2 Work all around the sacrum, pressing hand over hand on to the bone with firm, gentle pressure, and also work the length of the first line of the back, including the area over the sacral bone, giving pressure in the small dips on either side of the bone.

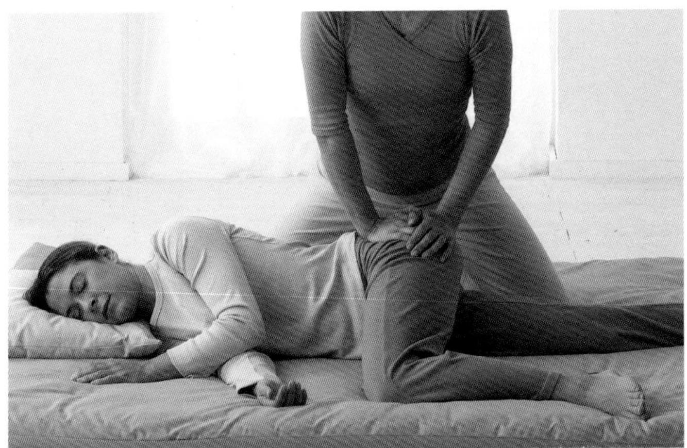

3 Spend time massaging around the hip joint and buttock area to help soften the tissue and release the trapped nerve. Work the third outside line of the leg up into the C-shape around the hip joint.

Sciatica: thumbing the foot points

Work the energy lines on the feet and focus on the point shown, where the fan-shaped massage featured in the foot sequence starts.

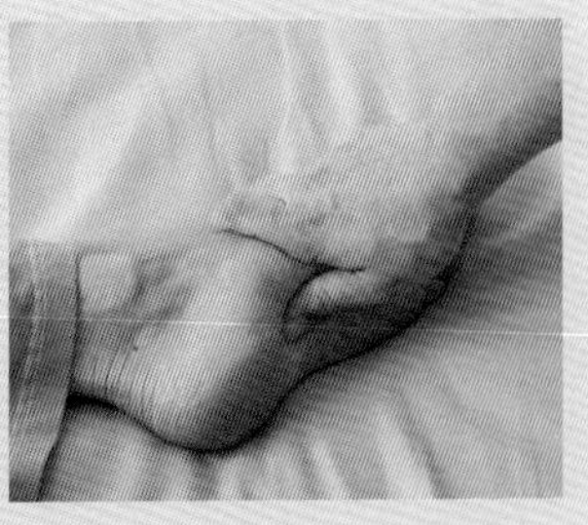

Headaches

These exercises can help a broad range of headaches. It may be best to use them when your partner is not in pain, as prevention rather than cure, as you can work more deeply. It is possible to work deeply if your partner has a headache, but check with them first.

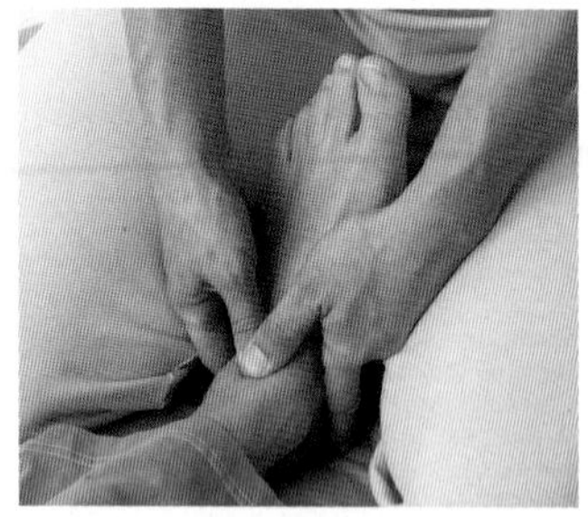

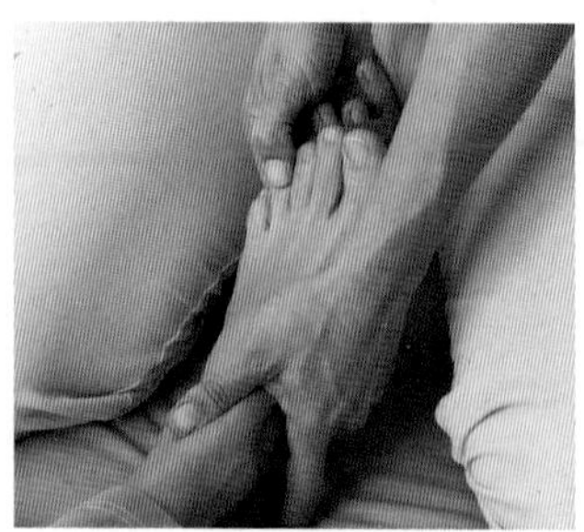

1 (above left) Foot massage can be very soothing, bringing your partner's energy away from their head back down to their roots. Work repeatedly into the knee pain and headache point (page 41).

2 (above right) Squeeze up to the sinus points at the tips of the toes.

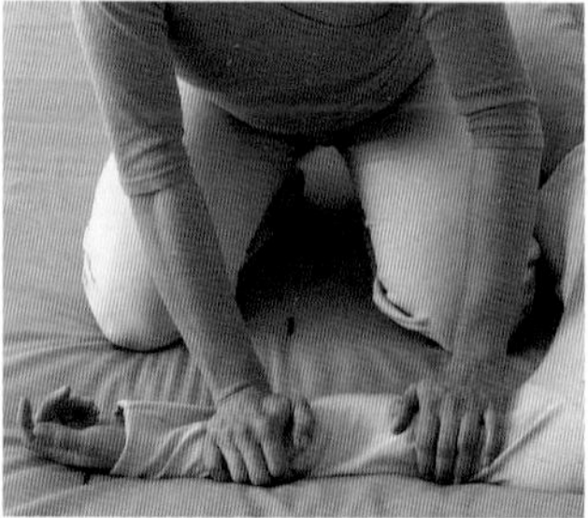

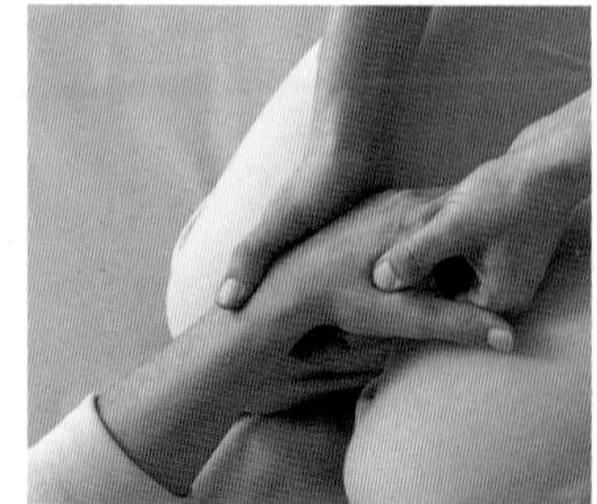

3 (above left) Palm and thumb sen kalathari, to free shoulder tension – tension here and in the back are common causes of headaches.

4 (above right) Work the hands. Focus on the headache points and especially the hegu point (see the hands part of the total routine).

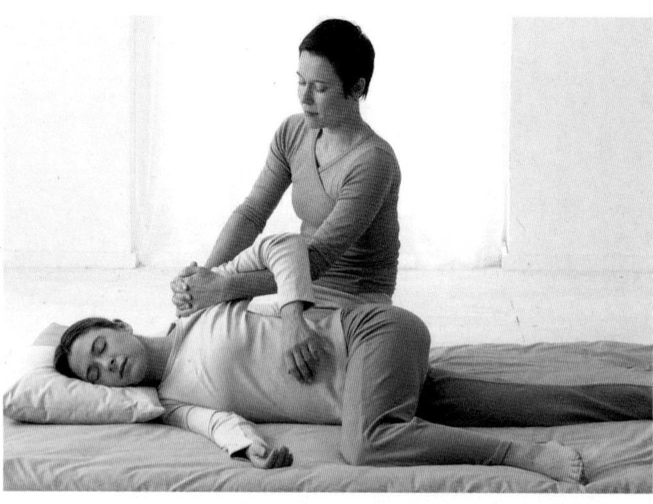

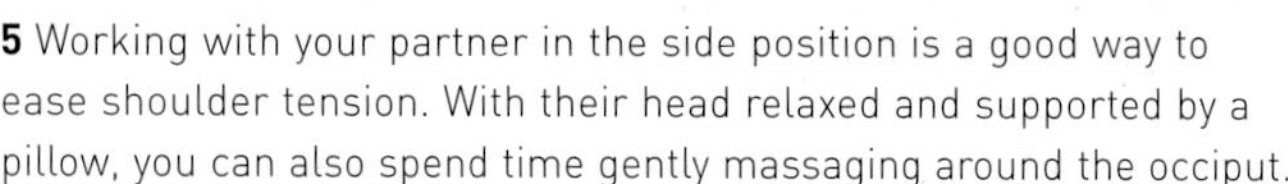

5 Working with your partner in the side position is a good way to ease shoulder tension. With their head relaxed and supported by a pillow, you can also spend time gently massaging around the occiput.

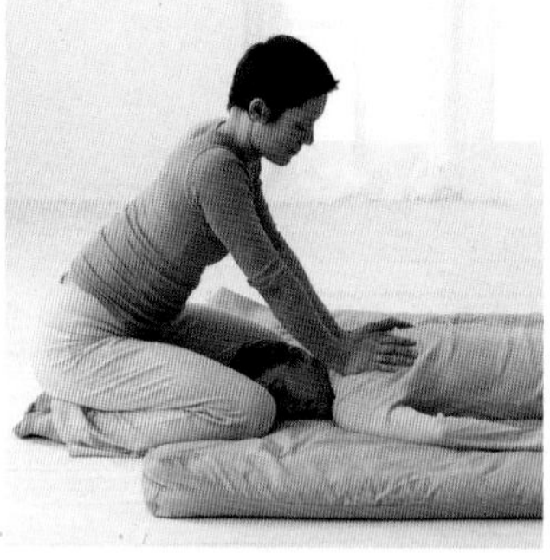

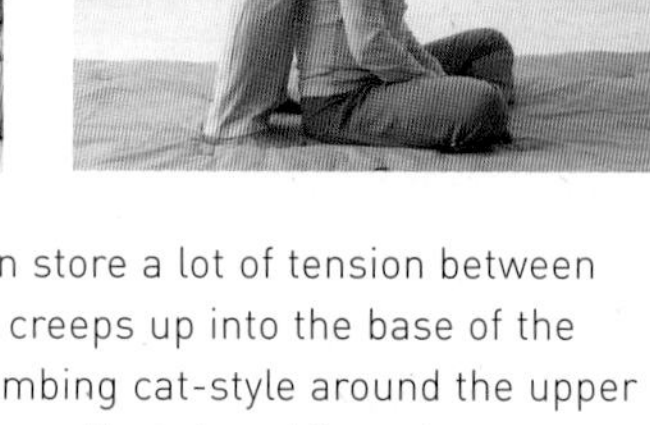

6 (above left) The upper back can store a lot of tension between the shoulder blades, which then creeps up into the base of the neck and head. Palming and thumbing cat-style around the upper spine and between the shoulders on lines 1 and 2 can be very effective for releasing tension.

7 (above right) Work the shoulder acupressure points in the sitting position with palming and thumbing techniques.

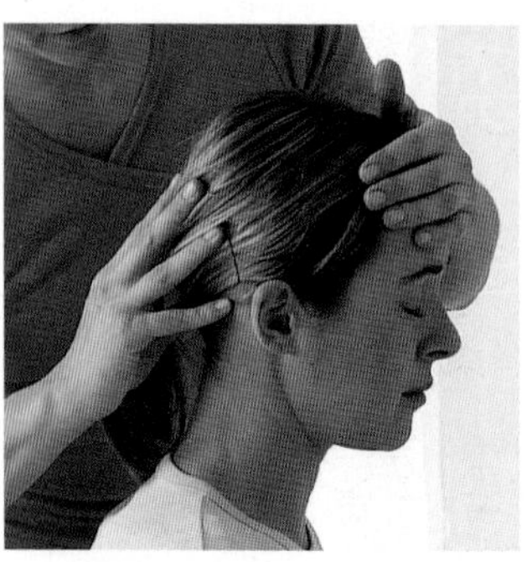

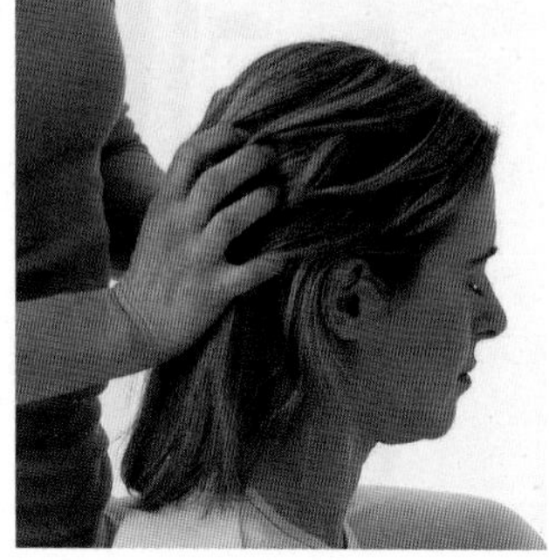

8 (above left) Work around the occipital ridge (see head routine) as this is where tension can become locked right into the neck, restricting vital blood and energy flow to the head area.

9 (above right) Nothing is more relieving for all kinds of headaches than a thorough head massage.

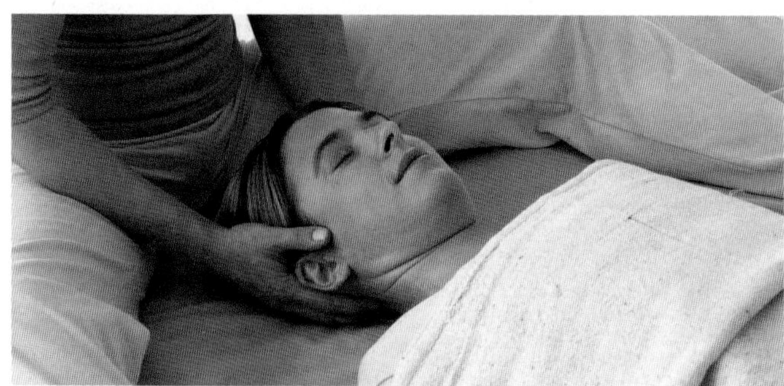

10 Finish off the sequence with a deep relaxing face massage. Start off with the cranial hold and focus on the temples and forehead. Let the eyes rest with the eye hold. Any essential oil that you use for the face massage could also be one chosen to help alleviate the headache. Try a blend of lavender, chamomile and geranium – a few drops of each in a tablespoon or so of carrier oil.

Coughs and Colds

If your partner is suffering from a cold or flu you would not want to give them a full-body Thai massage as it could overload an already compromised immune system. You may, however, find this short sequence useful for alleviating some of their symptoms.

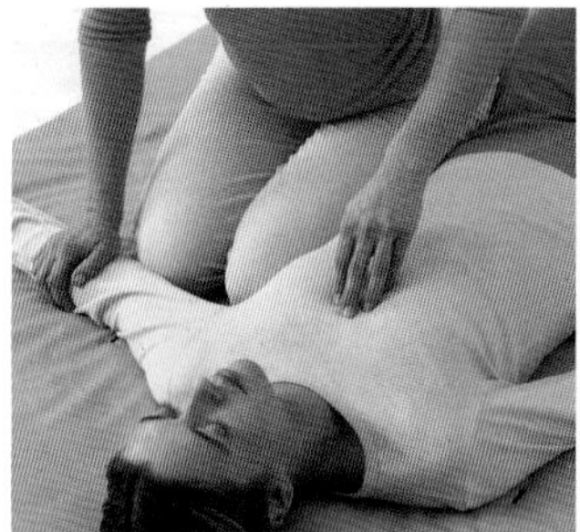

1 Circling the breastbone (sternum) will help boost and support the immune system and get the energy moving through the chest. General rubbing in this area may help to stimulate your partner's breathing if they feel congested and tight across the ribs.

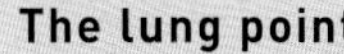

The lung point

There is a reflex point for the lungs on the sole of the foot (right). Pressing and rubbing around this area can help to ease breathing and clear congestion.

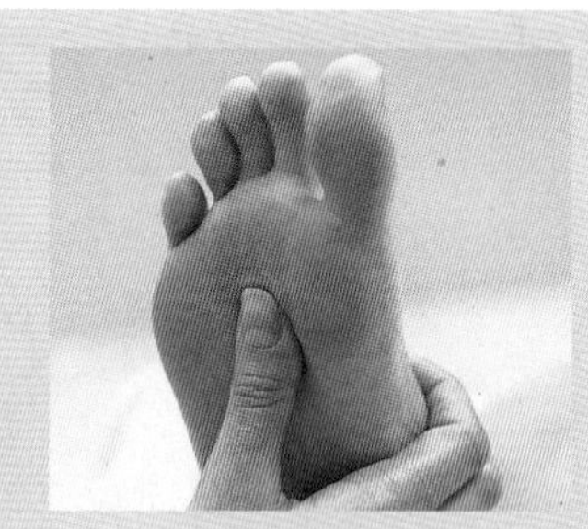

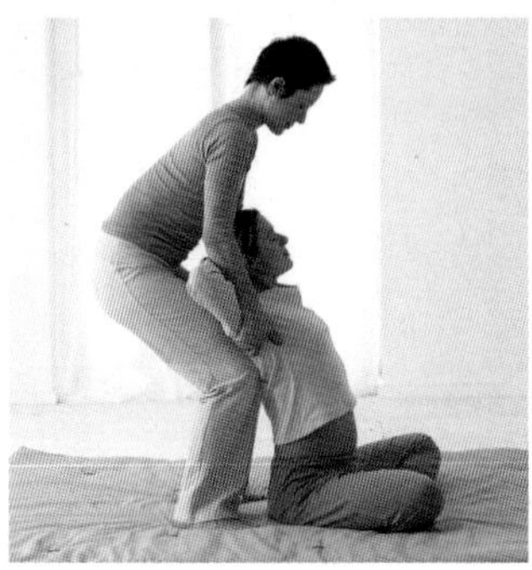

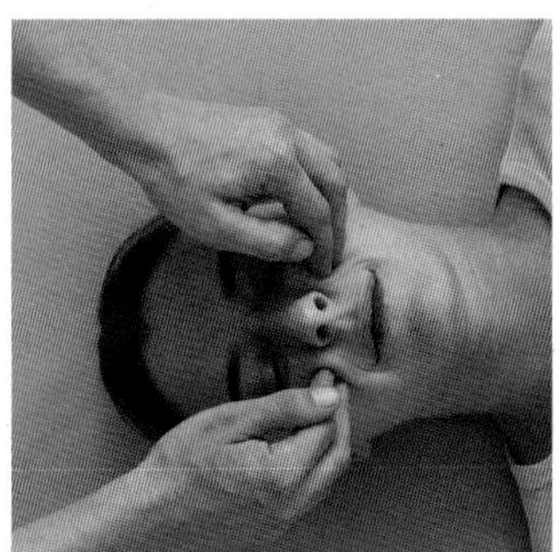

2 (far left) The "hello world" pose (see the Expanding the Upper Body section of the complete body massage routine) opens the lung cavity and encourages deeper breathing in cases of coughs or tightness across the chest.

3 (left) Pressing around the sinuses can feel incredibly releasing for congested head colds.

Constipation and Bloating

In cases of constipation or excess gas the main aim is to stimulate the digestion and release the trapped gases, which often cause a great deal of discomfort.

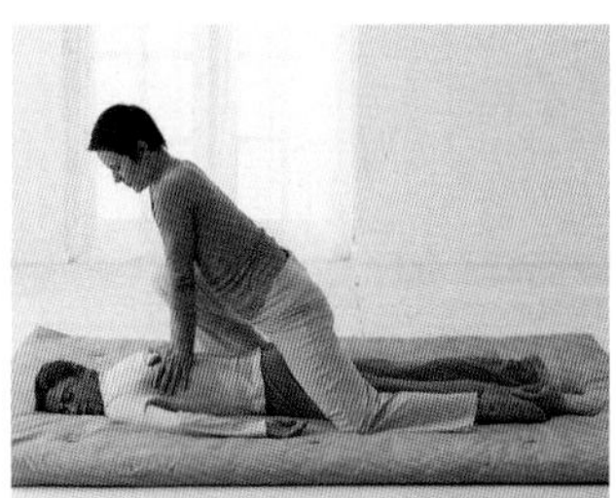

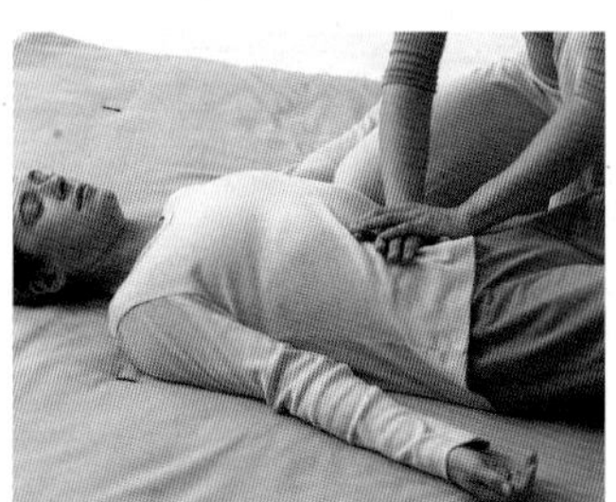

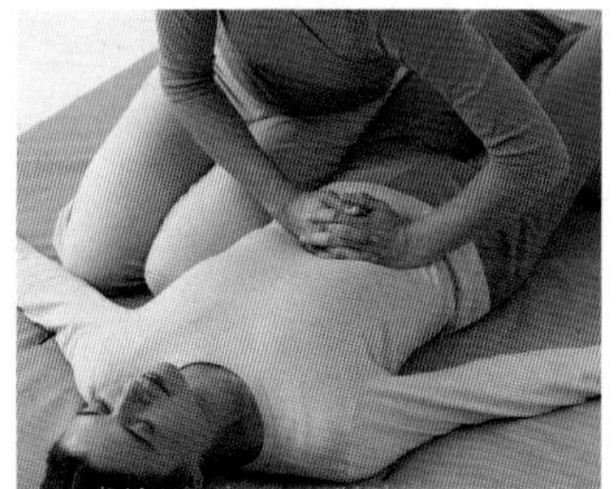

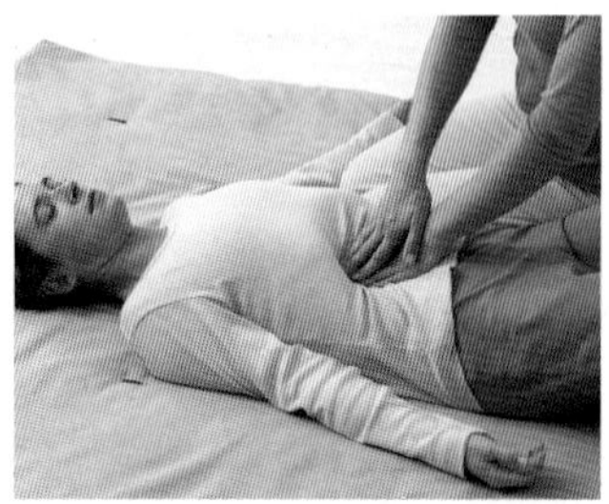

1 (above left) Initially, give your partner a repeated workout on the back lines, placing specific emphasis on line 1 (sen ittha and sen pingkhala) around the area of the lower back.

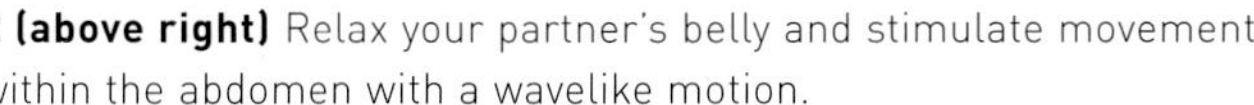

2 (above right) Relax your partner's belly and stimulate movement within the abdomen with a wavelike motion.

3 (above left) The wind-releasing exercise (page 63) is very relieving.

4 (above right) Work clockwise, following the natural direction of your partner's digestion, when palming and finger-pressing. If using oil, try three drops each of marjoram, lemongrass and rosemary in carrier oil, massaged into the belly and lower back.

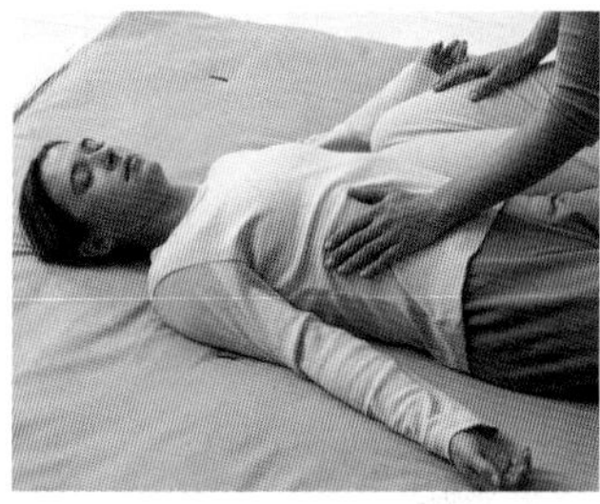

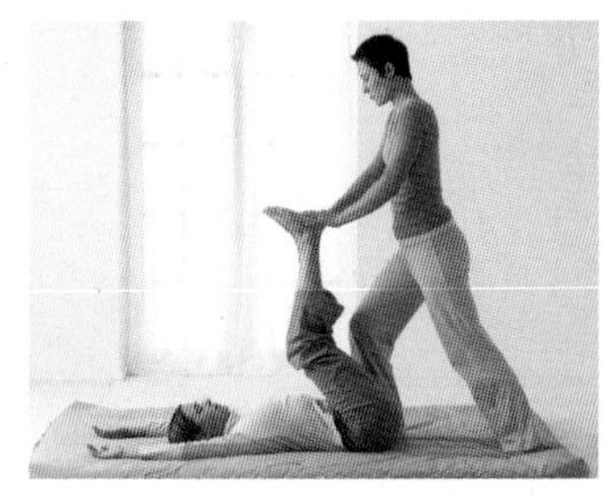

5 (far left) Smooth and soothe an aggravated abdomen with some broad circling movements.

6 (left) The gentle plough (page 55) is a stimulating exercise that can help release wind trapped in the intestines. For a sluggish digestion the whole of the double leg sequence is recommended in order to help stimulate the digestive "fire".

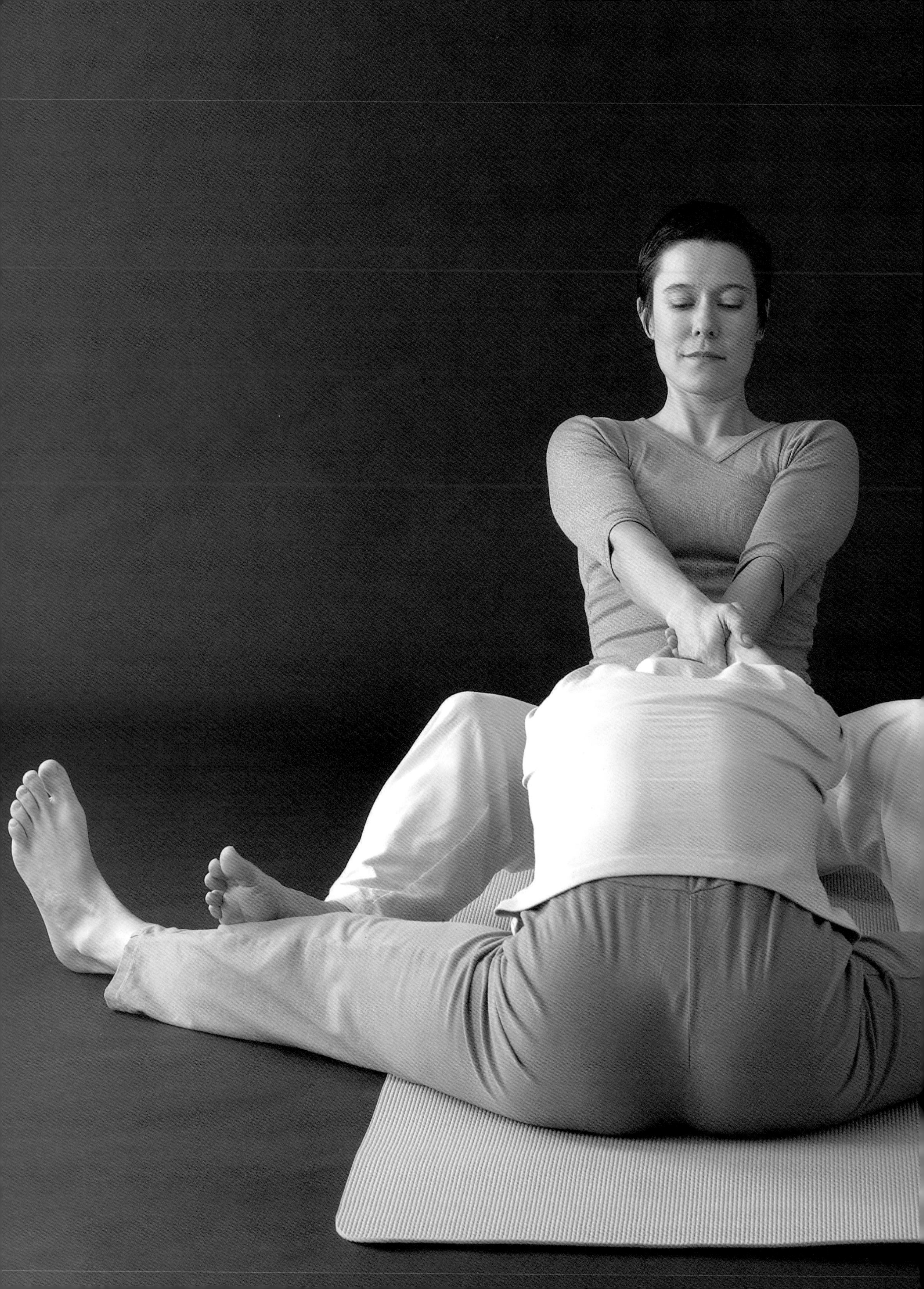

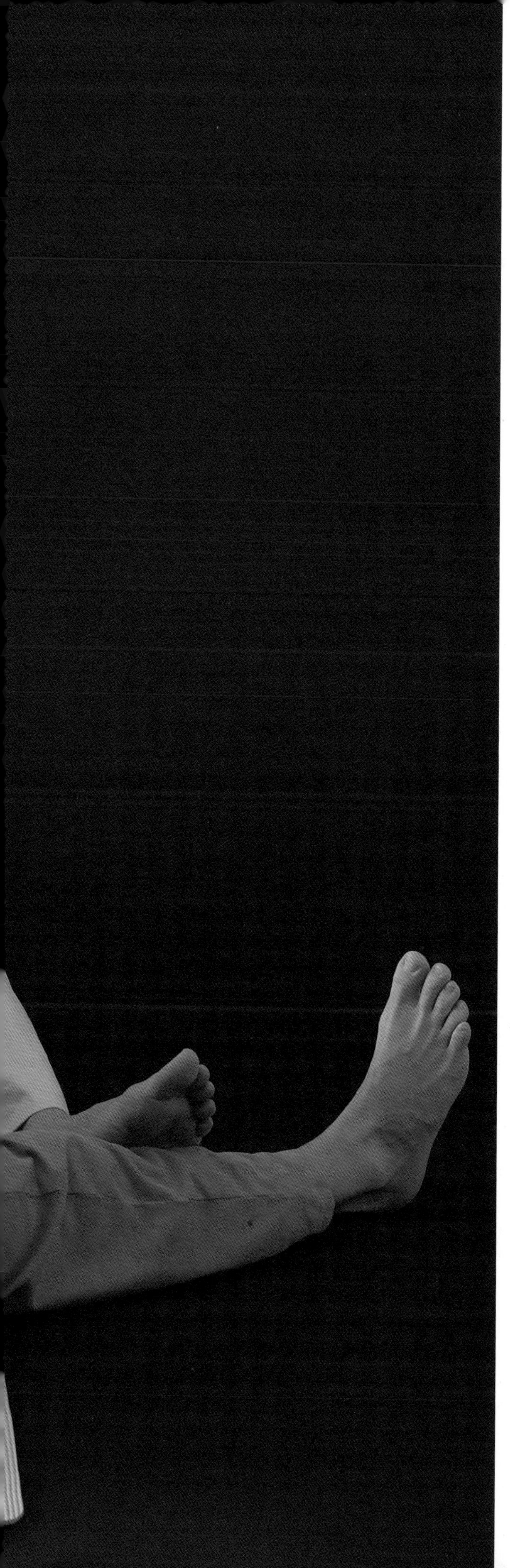

After a Massage

Well done! You have finished the sequence. When you have practised all the aspects of the body separately and feel comfortable with them, you can put the whole sequence together to give a full-body Thai massage. This intense level of working with another person's energy body can leave you in a heightened state of awareness and sensitivity. While this is to be encouraged in your massage practice, it is important that you have the tools to ground, consolidate and contain this sensitivity after a session. Some simple guidelines will help you to integrate and ground this energy after giving a massage, ensuring that you remain in balance yourself.

Post-massage Routines

You can make use of these "post-massage" suggestions after any practice session – no matter how short – to give a sense of completion and containment. Remember to give yourself time for a longer relaxation after giving a full-body massage.

Thai massage is a dynamic and physical form of bodywork. It feels physical to receive and to give. While this aspect is obvious, you should keep in mind that you are also giving your partner an energy workout, and this can in turn stimulate your own energy flow. After a session you may experience heat or a buzzing feeling in your hands and forearms. This is the flow of prana or life energy that is stimulated when you set out with the intention to heal with touch, but it can also be an imprint or absorption of your partner's energy that you have picked up.

It is important to break this energetic connection with your partner, otherwise you can become very unclear about what you are experiencing – whether it is your energy, feelings and emotions or the residual energy pattern of your partner's feelings and emotions.

Below After the massage you need to return to a calm, quiet place – comparable, say, to still serene waters – to centre yourself.

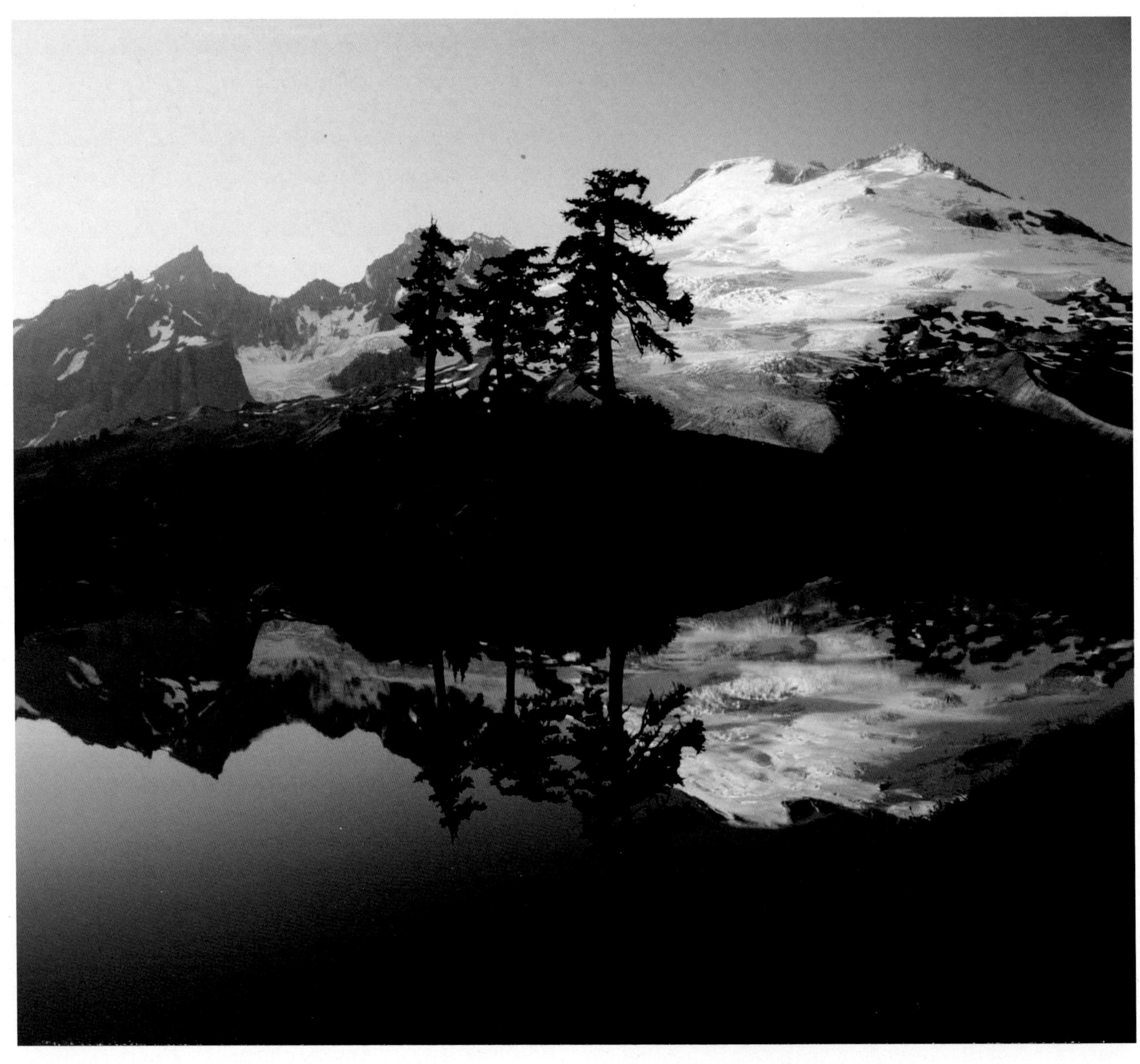

Clearing and Cleansing

Here are some easy techniques that you can employ immediately after massage, while your partner is relaxing. Completing a session in this way helps to establish an energetic boundary that separates the connection made during the treatment.

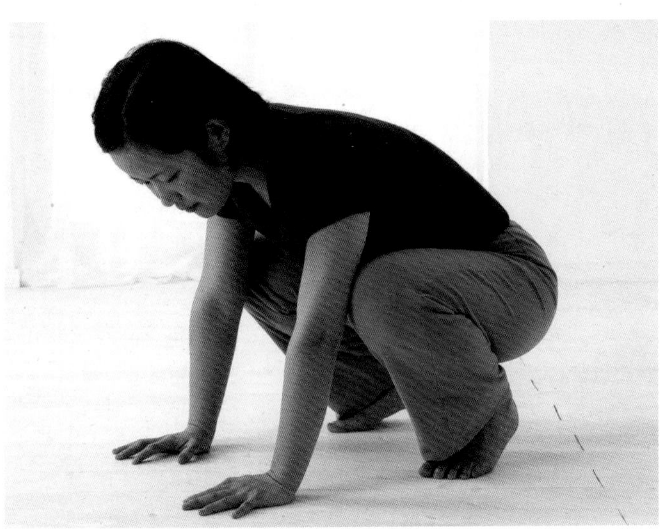

1 Grounding energy This exercise is very simple but highly effective. Just place your hands on the floor and mentally ask that any energy that is not yours, or that is no longer useful for you, be absorbed back into the earth. Stay with this feeling for as long as feels necessary for you. A few moments are usually enough.

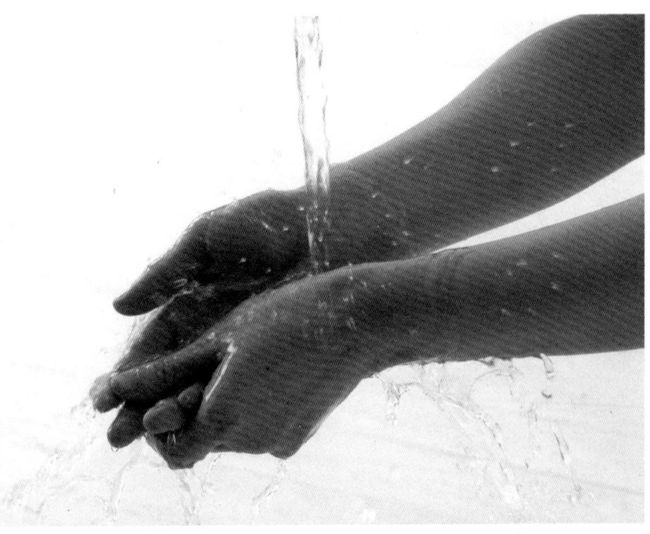

2 Washing the hands This is a practical and hygienic thing to do after giving a massage, but it also has another purpose: flowing water is excellent for cleansing and clearing any residual energy felt in the hands and forearms.

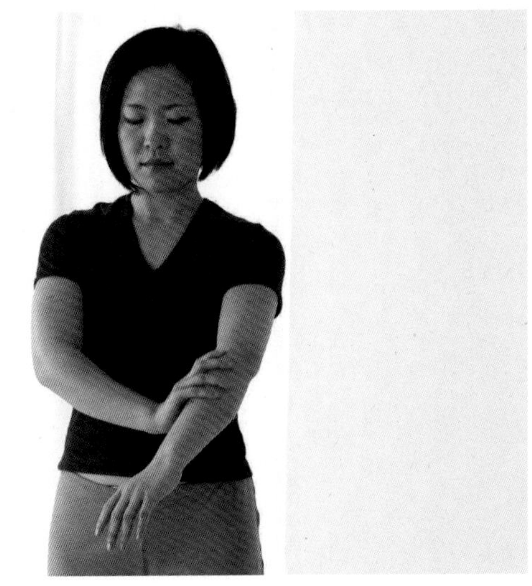

3 Sweeping the hands Sometimes it is not possible to wash your hands immediately after giving a massage. Another technique that is just as effective is to sweep excess energy from your forearms and hands.

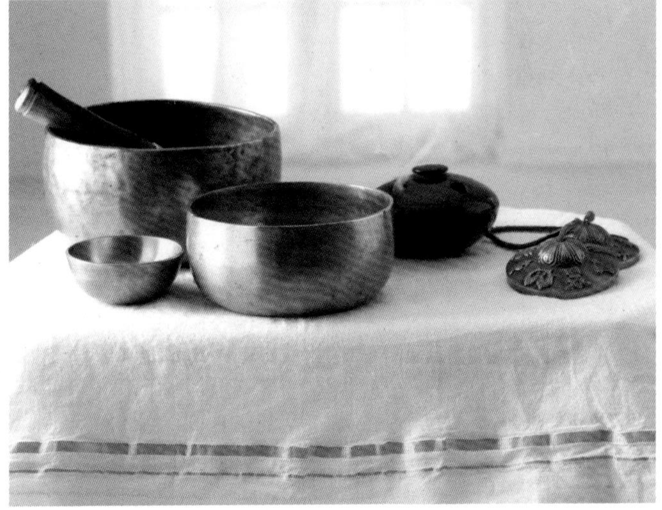

4 Clearing with sound Sound is vibration, and vibration is energy that can be both heard and felt. Using chimes and singing bowls after a session not only produces beautiful sounds but can also be experienced as a soothing resonance in the body. You can use them to clear the energy in a room after a massage or to clear the aura around a person. Traditionally used in Tibet for ceremonial and healing purposes, singing bowls are made of several different metals, corresponding with the chakras, the seven energy centres of the body.

Relaxation Techniques

Just as you would take time for relaxation after any kind of yoga practice, it's a very good idea to take time for relaxation after giving your partner a Thai massage. Below are some suggestions for specific deeper relaxation techniques that allow for physical, mental and emotional release. To feel the full benefit of these techniques, make sure that you find a warm, quiet and comfortable place where you are certain you will not be disturbed. Don't be tempted to skip this stage – it is vital for your personal well-being.

Resting the Body

These gentle poses will alleviate any discomfort or strain in the hips and shoulders and are very relaxing counter-stretches for the half-kneeling and wide-kneeling working postures.

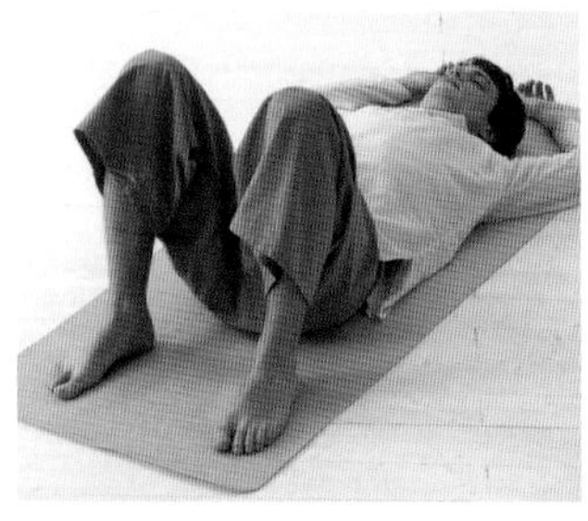

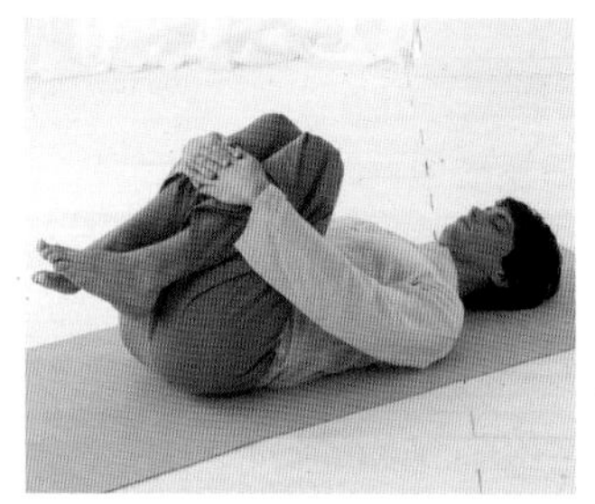

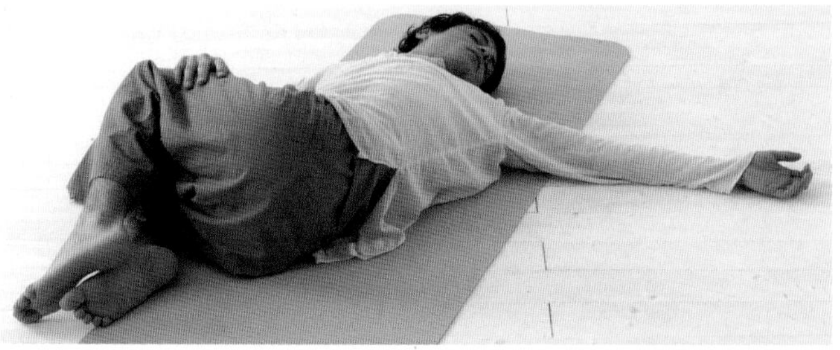

1 (above left) In this pose, your body is completely at rest, fully supported by the floor. Focus on letting your weight drop down through the back of your skull and pelvis.

2 (above right) Here, enjoy the feeling of your lower back and hips broadening and melting into the floor. Breathe, be playful, circle your knees or rock slightly from side to side.

3 With your knees still bent in towards your chest, take your arms out to the sides, palms up. As you breathe out, take your knees to one side and your head to the other; you might want to rest one hand on your leg, as shown. Keep the knees tucked up to protect your lower back. Relax the lower hip and ribs into the floor. Feel a release through the ribs and chest as you end your out-breath. Repeat on the other side.

Deeper Relaxation Techniques

For these two exercises, lie in savasana (corpse pose) with your legs and arms slightly apart, palms facing upwards. Remember to focus on your breathing as much as your movements. Let the breath pass smoothly in and out through your nostrils.

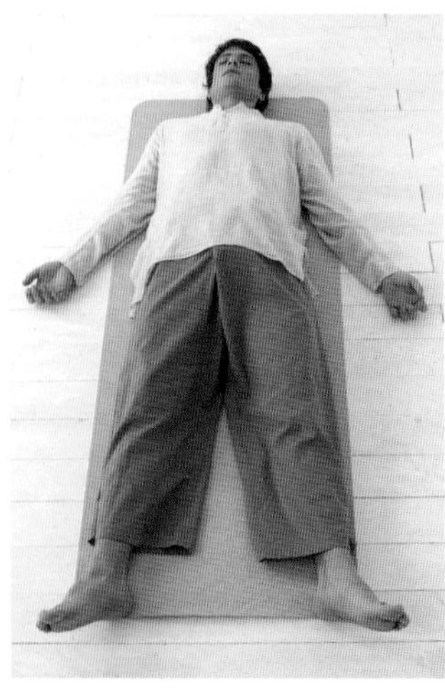

1 Tension and release (left) This quick and simple exercise is perfect if you have only five minutes for relaxation. The idea is to gather tension consciously in your body so that you are aware of when you have let it go. Begin at your feet and work through each part of the body until you reach the head and face.

Inhale and slowly tense your muscles in each body part for as long as you can hold your breath; don't strain. When you need to exhale, release the breath and all the tension at the same time. After working through the whole body, relax for a few moments.

2 Sun and moon (not shown) This visualization exercise helps to bring your right and left sides into balance and can be very rejuvenating. Be comfortable in savasana, close your eyes and focus on the rhythm of your breathing. As you inhale, imagine warm golden sunlight entering the toes of your right foot and then passing through the right side of your body and out through your head. As you exhale, imagine cool, silvery moonlight entering the top of your head and passing down through the left side of the body and back out through your toes. Repeat at least eight times.

Kaya Kriya

Kriyas are yogic cleansing exercises. Kaya kriya means body movement and this particular kriya is a very powerful cleansing technique in which you move the body simultaneously with your breath. Try to keep the in-breath and out-breath of equal length.

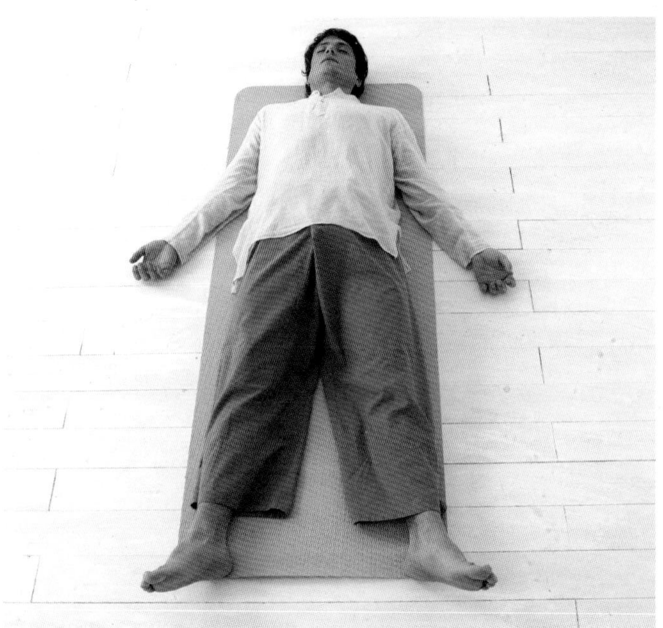

1 Start in neutral position. You will need to adapt savasana slightly, by taking your arms and legs a little further apart.

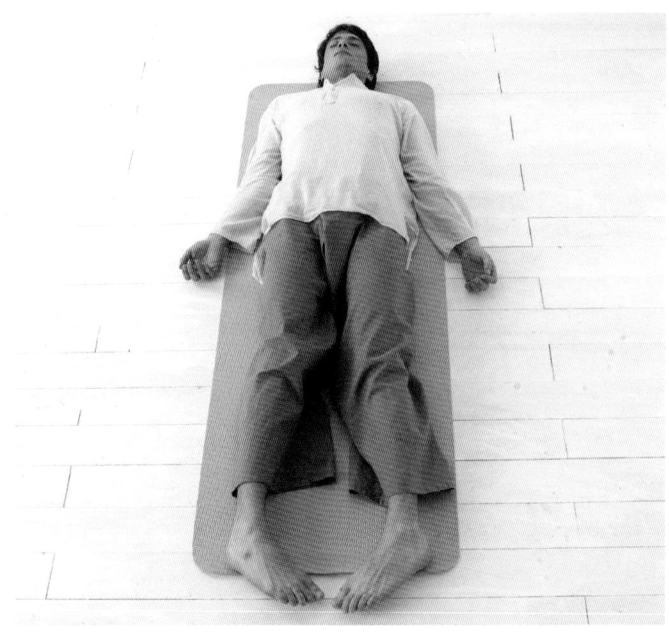

2 As you inhale, roll your feet inwards so that you feel the whole of each leg rotate right up into the hips. As you exhale, roll your feet outwards again and relax.

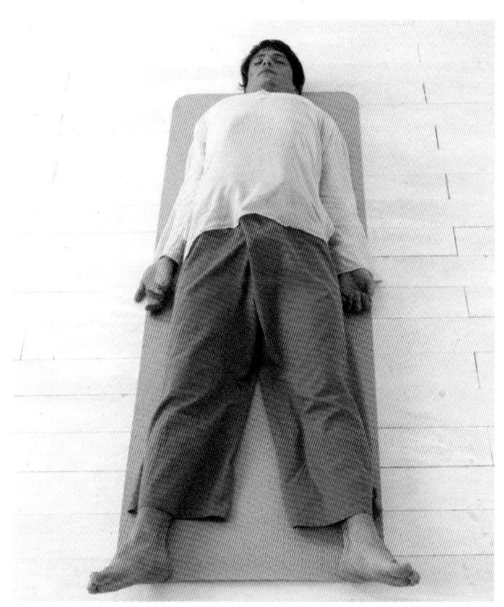

3 Turn your palms face down with your thumbs against your thighs. As you inhale, roll your arms out so that your hands rotate and your little fingers are now against the thighs. As your arms move, your chest will open and lift slightly, drawing your shoulder blades together. As you exhale, roll your arms back so that your chest drops and your palms come to rest face down.

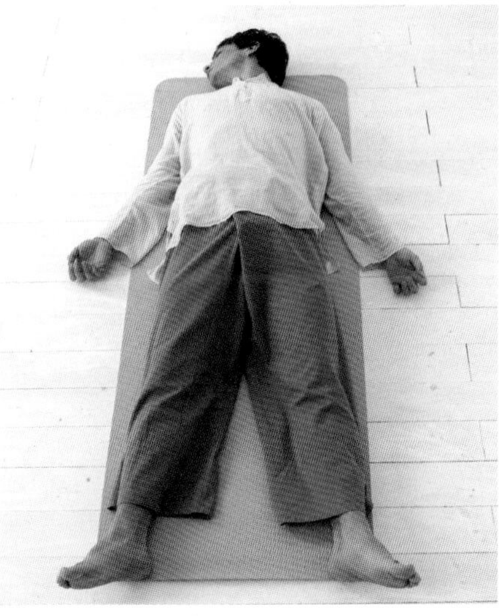

4 As you inhale, slowly roll your head to the right and, as you exhale, roll your head to the left.

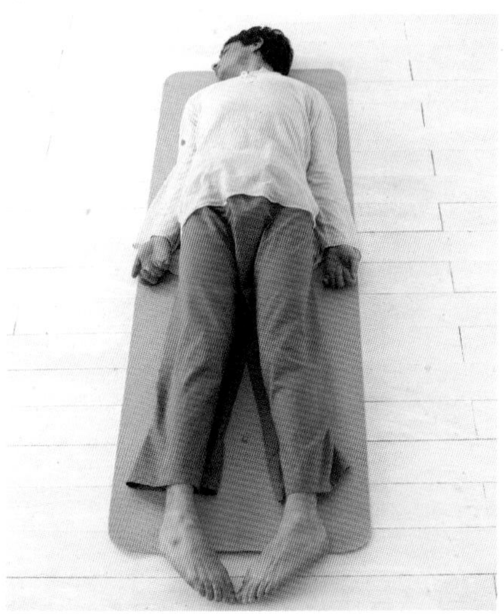

5 Practise each of the previous parts 8–12 times, and then practise all the elements simultaneously for a final 8–12 rounds. Allow the body to relax fully and your breath to flow naturally.

Energy Rebalancing Through Yoga

As practitioners of a profound healing art we have a responsibility to maintain our own physical health and build an awareness of our own bodies and minds that will make us more sensitive to the needs of massage partners. Maintaining a regular physical, energetic and meditative practice will help you to achieve this, and yogic practices such as this version of the classic *Surya Namaskar* routine may be the ideal route for you to try.

In ancient Indian culture, the sun symbolized spiritual awareness and was worshipped daily. Surya namaskar (*surya* means "sun" and *namaskar* means "salutation") is an effective way of loosening, toning, stretching and massaging joints, muscles and organs, harmonizing movement with breathing and rebalancing energy flow within the body. Like Thai massage practice, the routine has its own form, works with energy rebalancing and is underpinned by a smooth and uninterrupted rhythm.

Ideal times to practise this sequence are at sunrise or sunset, but it can be performed at any time, as long as it is on an empty stomach. The full round works both sides of the body. Breathe in and out through your nostrils and let your breath guide you through each movement.

Surya Namaskar – Sun Salutation

Begin this exercise with your right foot, which will be the active foot through one half of the sequence. When you have completed all the postures on one side, repeat with the left foot as the active foot. Finish standing, with your hands in prayer position.

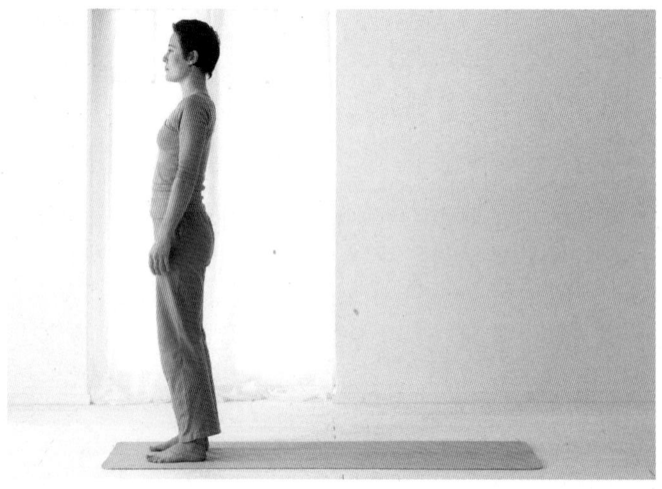

1 Begin with your feet hip-width apart, your body relaxed and your breathing easy. Take time to feel the contact with the earth beneath the soles of your feet. Feel yourself being rooted to the ground, with all the tension in your body flowing out through your feet.

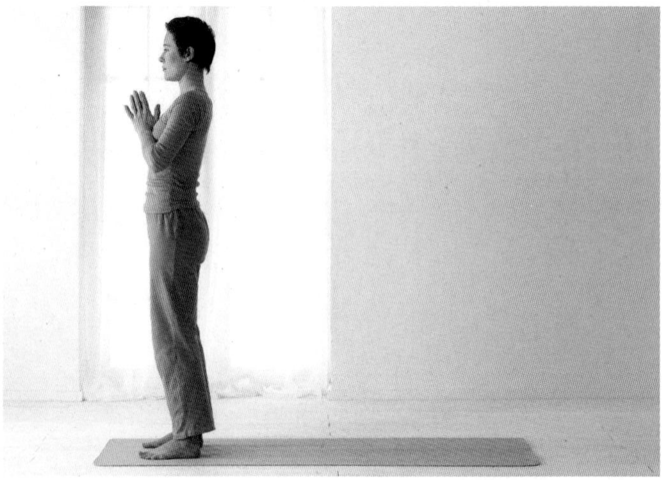

2 Inhale and, as you exhale, bring your hands together in prayer position level with your breastbone, with elbows and shoulders relaxed.

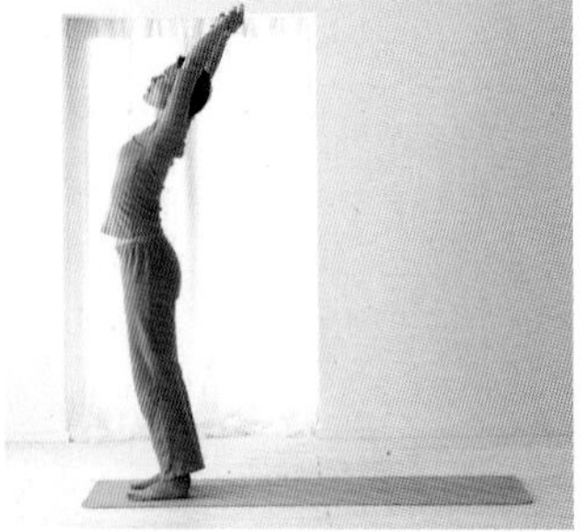

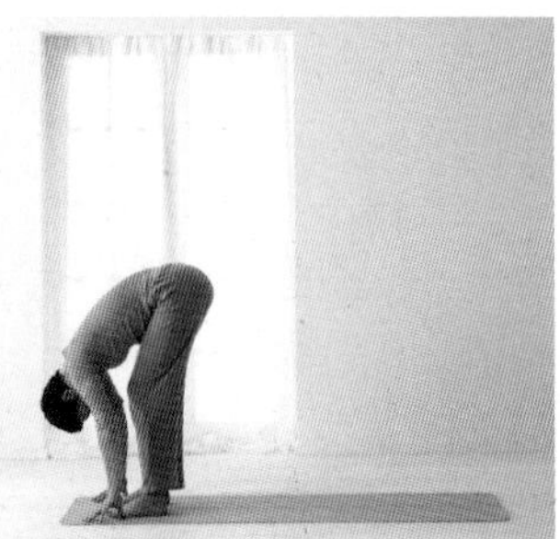

3 (far left) Inhale. Extend your hands straight up, feeling the opening come through the whole of the front of your body.

4 (left) Exhale. Release into a soft forward bend, making sure you fold from your hips, not your waist. Allow your knees to bend if they need to.

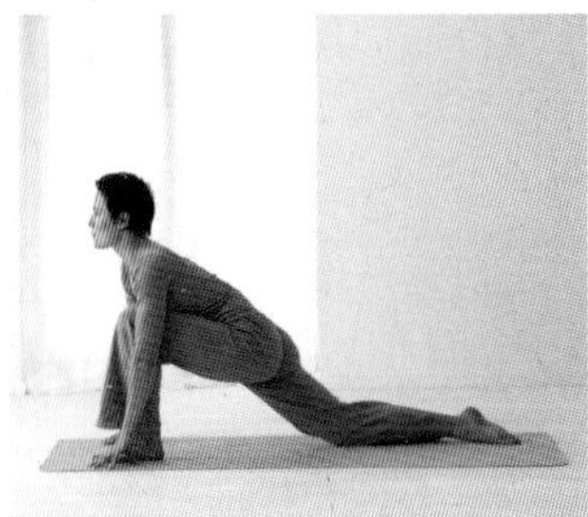

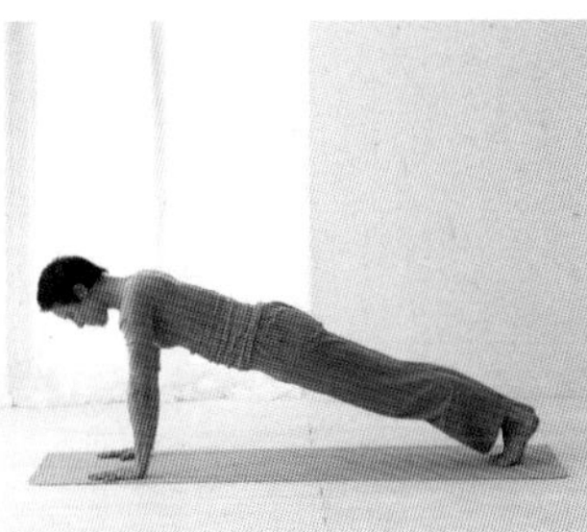

5 (above left) Inhale. Place your fingertips or palms on the floor and take your right foot back. Let your tailbone drop towards the ground. Keep your left foot flat on the ground. Feel the length come from the front of your pubic bone all the way up into the chest.

6 (above right) Hold your breath without straining. Take your left foot back, tuck the toes under and extend into your heels. Check your hips – your body should form a straight line.

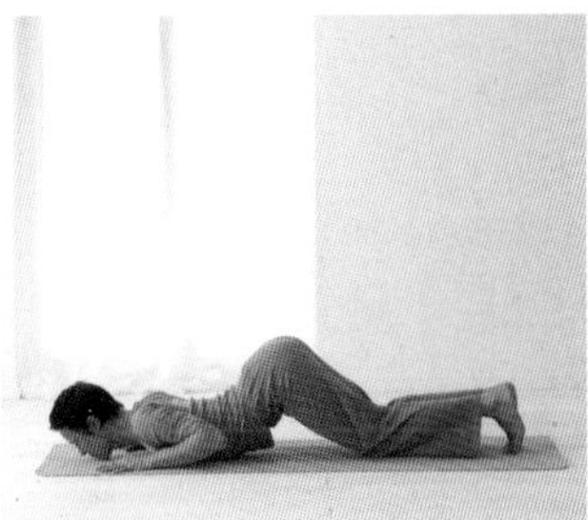

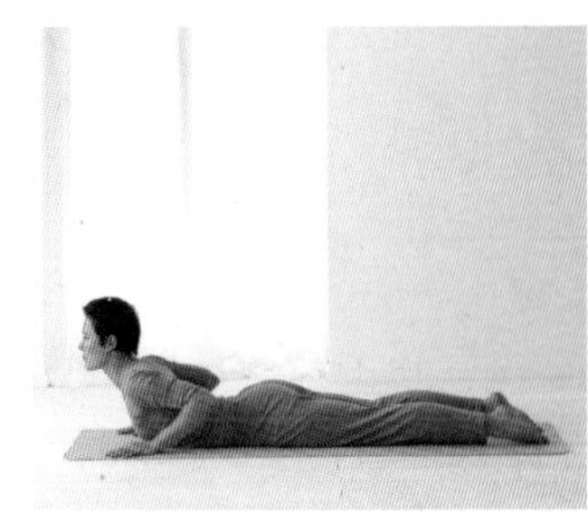

7 (above left) Exhale. Drop your knees, chest, elbows and chin to the ground. Keep your hips up.

8 (above right) Inhale. Slide your hips down and away. Flatten your feet against the mat. Sink your pubic bone into the mat and lift up through the front of your body. Check that your lower back feels comfortable – if not, you have come up too far. Keep your elbows tucked into the sides of your body and your shoulders relaxed away from your ears.

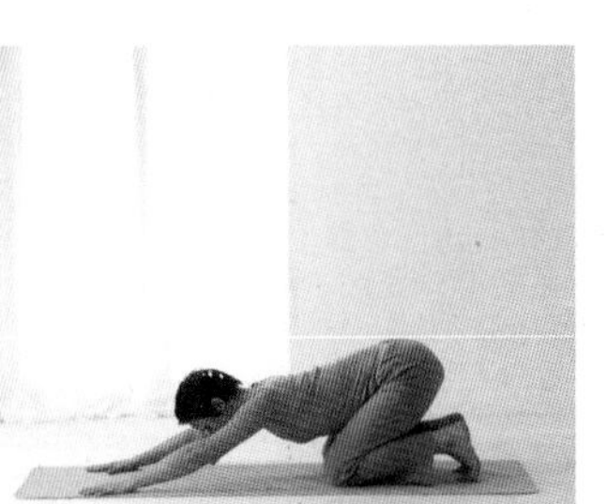

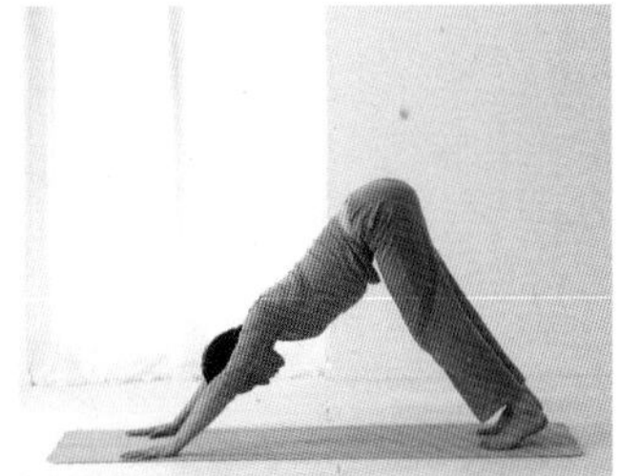

9 (above left) Tuck your toes under and, keeping your hands planted in front of you, drop your hips back towards your heels. Let your hips sink and feel your tailbone lengthen away from your head.

10 (above right) Exhale. With your feet and hands sinking into the mat, let your hips fly up and away towards the sky. If necessary, allow your heels to stay slightly off the mat in order to keep freedom of movement in your hips.

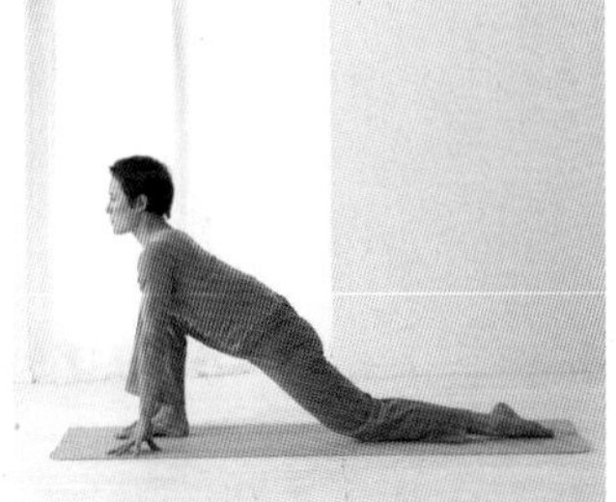

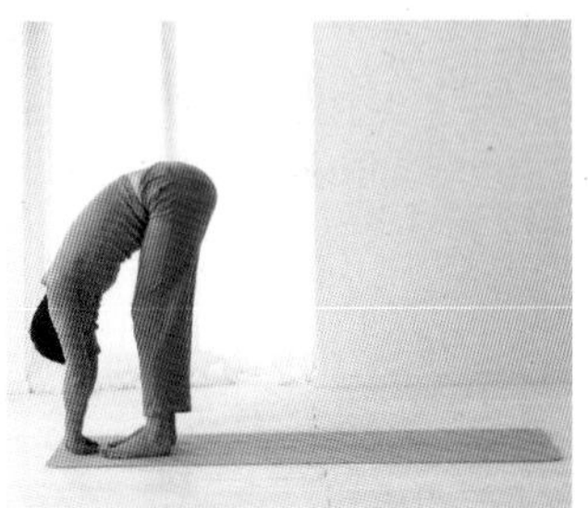

11 (above left) Inhale. Bring your right foot forward in between your hands. Let your tail drop down and the front of your body open.

12 (above right) Exhale. Bring both your feet together and come into a soft forward bend.

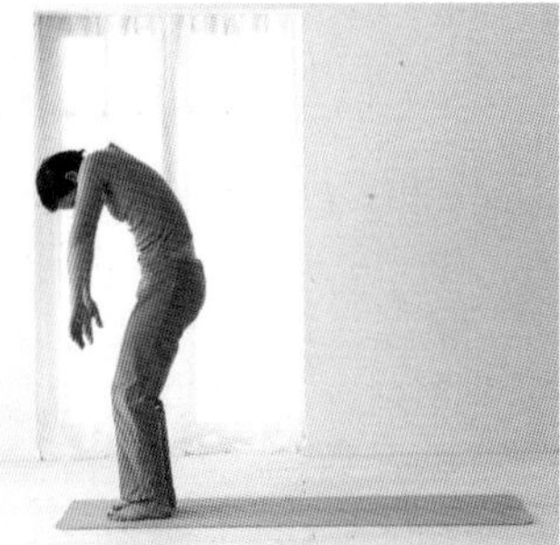

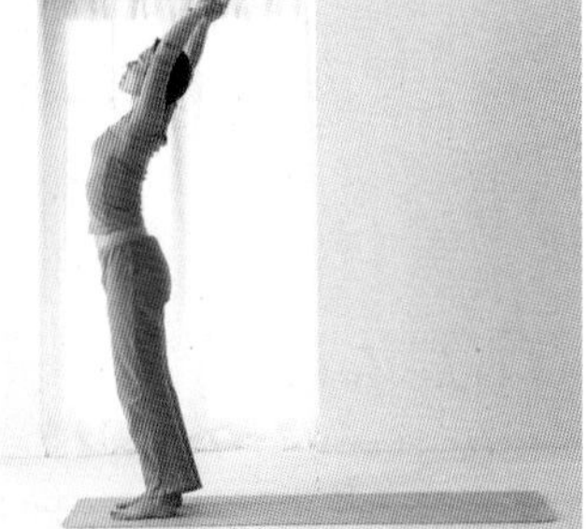

13 (above left) Inhale. Gently roll back up to standing.

14 (above right) Continuing the inhalation, unfold fully, extending your hands up towards the sky.

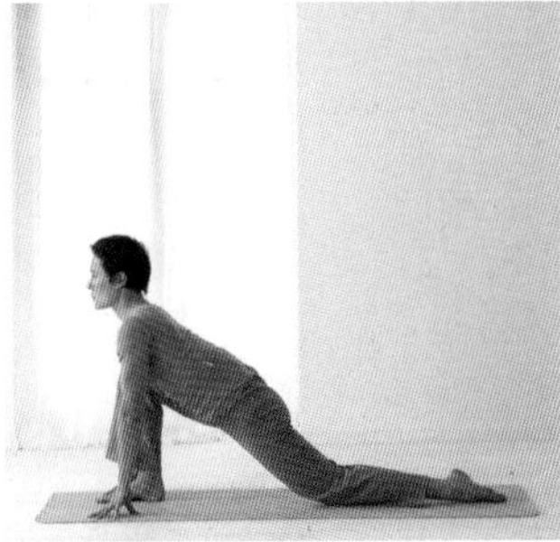

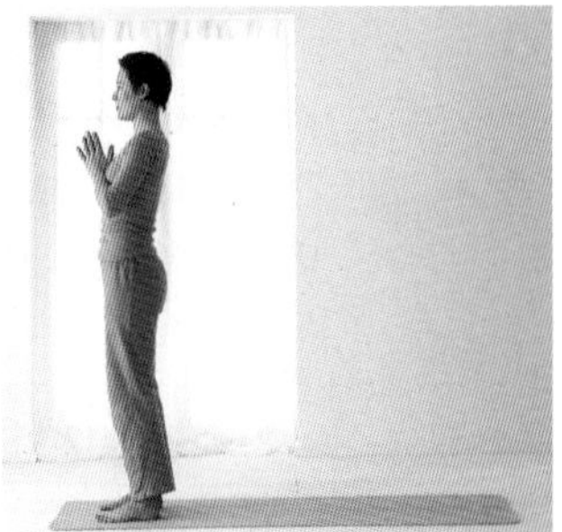

15 (above left) Repeat the sequence, exhaling into forward fold again. This time take your left foot back to continue the movements on the other side.

16 (above right) Complete one whole round, working both right and left feet. Finish in prayer position. Repeat at least six times and then relax in savasana.

Meditation in Motion – Qi Gong

It is very important for the Thai masseur to maintain a sense of balance within their body, and there is a wide variety of energy practices that you can use to achieve this. A particularly beautiful way to experience the subtle flow of energy around the body is by practising the Chinese tradition of *qi gong* – meditation in motion – on which the exercises shown below are based. Qi (or chi) is life energy and gong refers to work or exercise that requires both study and practice.

You can perform these movements after a massage, as a way of calming and grounding the energy stimulated during the session, or even beforehand, as preparation for giving massage.

BUILDING MOVEMENT AWARENESS

These exercises help to cultivate a soft, flowing quality of movement in the body. They can build greater awareness of how the flow of breath is linked with the flow of life energy and how it can permeate through the body to re-energize us. This type of internal exercise is more subtle than the Sun Salutation featured earlier, which is a more dynamic way of balancing internal energy through exercise. Explore both approaches and see which suits you best. Different forms of energy work may suit you better on different days. Try not to become fixed about which practice you adopt, but be sensitive and attentive to your inner cues.

Warm Up

These general movements are an excellent way to stimulate the movement of energy in all of the joints. This brings greater mobility and freedom throughout the whole of the body.

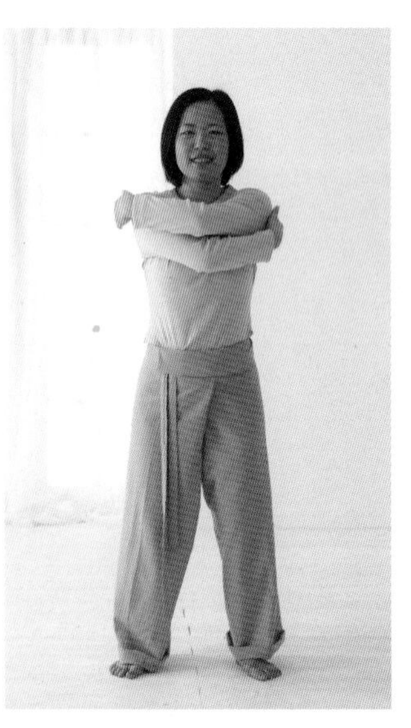

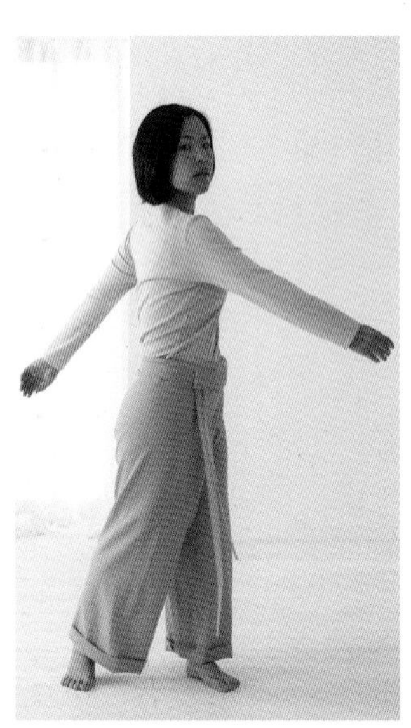

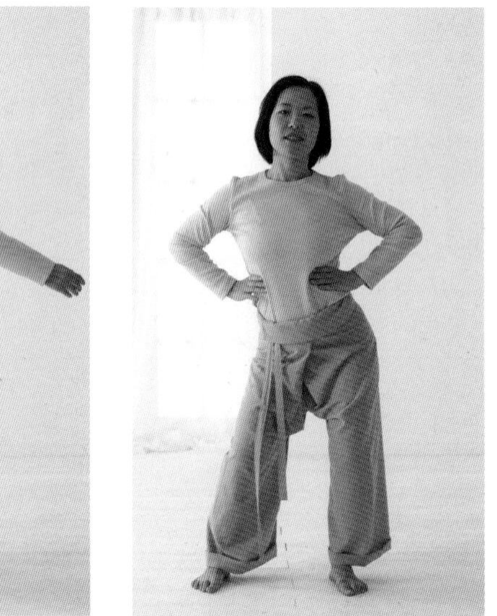

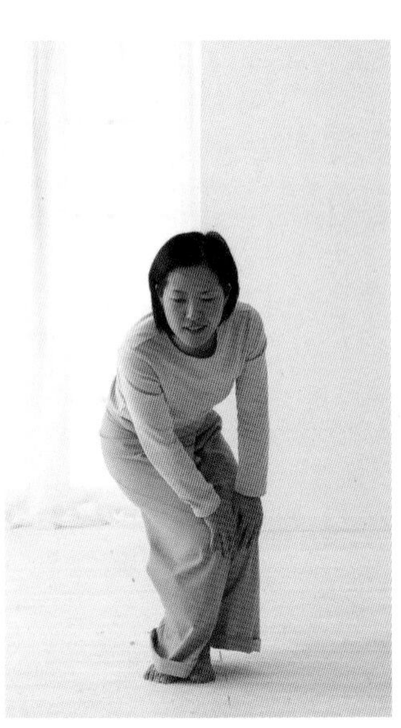

1 (above left) Let your arms swing out and then wrap around your shoulders or ribs in a hugging action. Allow your arms to build their own momentum. Alternate the upper and lower arm.

2 (above right) This is a similar movement to the previous exercise but this time swing both arms to the side, letting them wrap around your body, then swing the other way. To protect your knees, allow your heel to come away from the ground as you swing.

3 (above left) Place your hands on your lower ribs. Looking straight ahead, slowly circle the hips repeatedly in both directions. Try to keep your upper body completely still and move only your hips.

4 (above right) This exercise opens the knee and ankle joints. Bring your feet and knees together. Bend your knees slightly and cup your palms over your kneecaps. Circle your knees in both directions, bringing your heels off the ground if you need to.

Moving Energy

This energizes the hands, arms and chest, bringing lightness to the upper body. Keep your movements quiet, gentle and light as you move between positions. Be attentive to your breath and feel the sensations in your body.

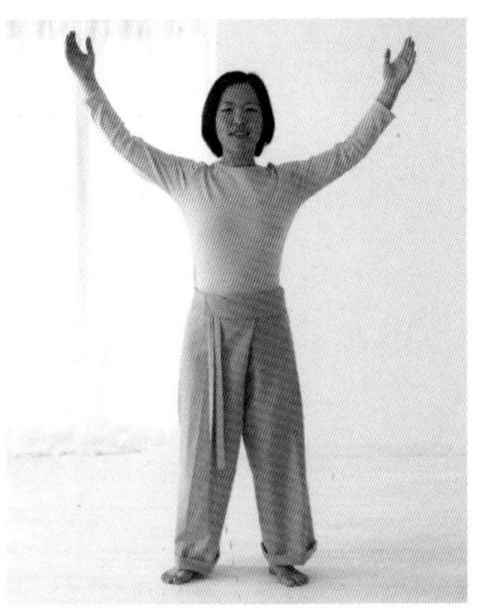

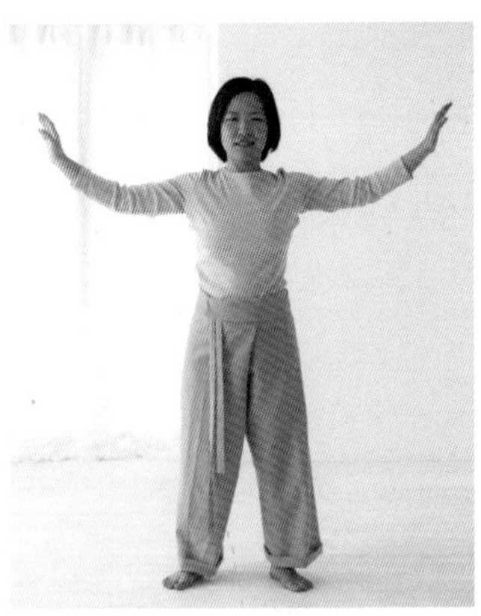

1 (far left) Stand with your feet a comfortable distance apart. Check that your legs are straight without the knees being locked. With your arms hanging by your sides, turn your palms to face the sky. Inhale and slowly raise your arms away from your sides to bring the palms up above your head. Keep your shoulders relaxed and don't overstretch the arms.

2 (left) Exhaling, turn your palms to face downwards and sweep the arms back down to rest either side of your body.

Repeat each movement several times, for as long as feels good to you.

Connecting Heaven and Earth

This re-establishes your link with the earth and the sky. Feel as if you are raising a ball of energy from the ground up the front of your body and releasing it to the sky, then receiving a new ball of energy from the sky and bringing it down the back of your body to the earth.

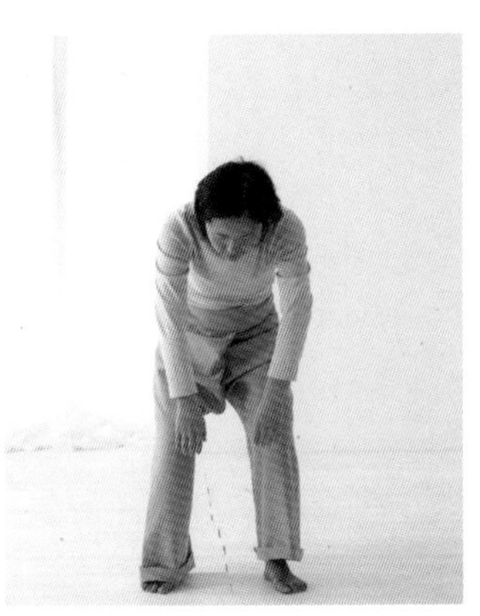

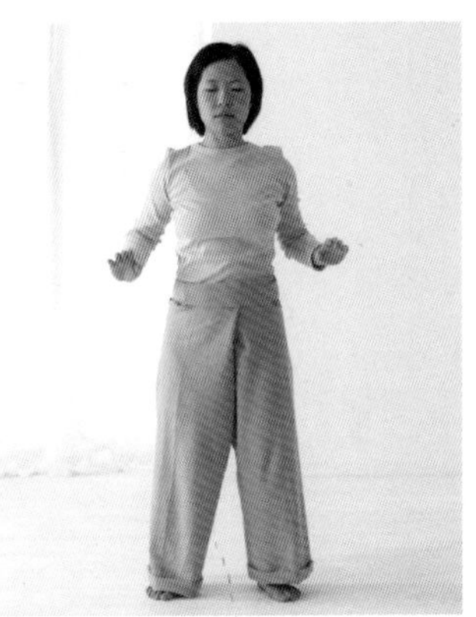

1 (far left) Bend forward, and, as you inhale, draw your hands up from the ground, mirroring the contours of the front of your body without actually touching it. Now continue to extend your arms above your head so that your fingertips are pointing skywards.

2 (left) Exhaling, bring your hands down, mirroring the contours of the back and sides of your body and legs, until you come all the way down to the ground. Continue this cycle of energy from earth to sky and from sky to earth, experiencing your body as a conductor of qi.

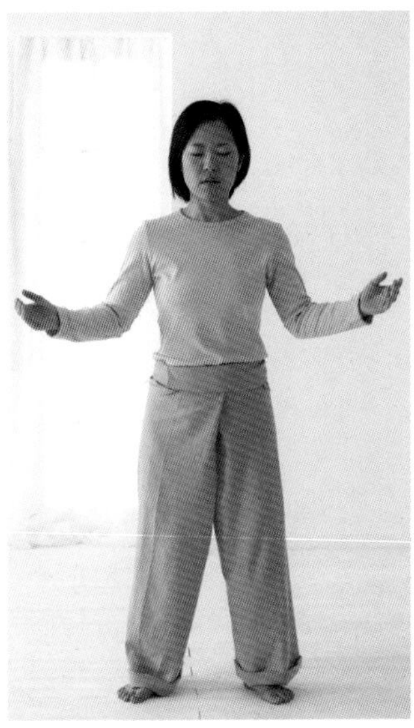

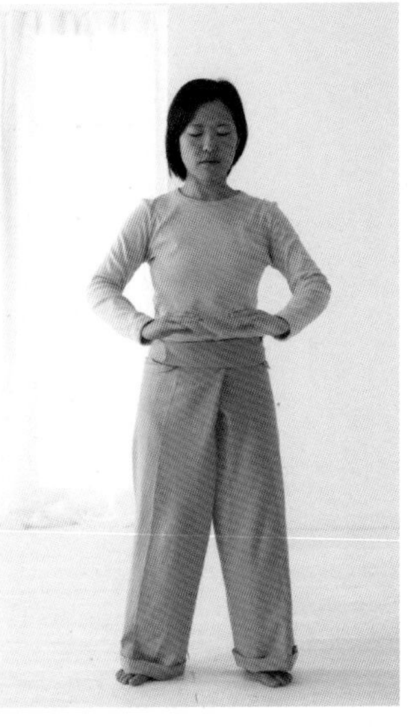

Returning to Your Centre

This grounding exercise works with a small range of circular movement. It focuses on building energy around your abdomen, the body's energetic centre.

1 (far left) As you inhale, turn your palms up to face the sky. Lift your hands up, bringing them no higher than your shoulders. Keep your shoulders completely relaxed and your elbows soft.

2 (left) Exhaling, turn your palms to face downwards and then bring the palms back down until they are level with your abdomen. Repeat this movement several times until you feel that the two halves of the movement have become one continuous flow.

Further Reading

The Art of Traditional Thai Massage by Asokananda. Editions Duang Kamol, Bangkok, 1992.
Thai Traditional Massage for Advanced Practitioners by Asokananda. Editions Duang Kamol, Bangkok, 1997.
Total Body Massage by Nitya Lacroix, Francesca Rinaldi, Sharon Seager and Renée Tanner. Southwater Books, 2004.
Massage for Total Relaxation by Nitya Lacroix. Dorling Kindersley, 1991.
Yoga Mind, Body & Spirit by Donna Fahri. Newleaf, 2000.
The Muscle Book by Paul Blakey. Bibliotek Books, 1992.
Awakening of the Spine by Vanda Scaravelli. Harper Collins, 1991.
The Yoga of Mindfulness by Asokananda. Editions Duang Kamol, Bangkok, 1993.
Qi Gong for Beginners by Stanley D. Wilson. Rudra Press, 1997.
Baby Massage. A Practical Guide to Massage and Movement for Babies and Infants by Peter Walker. Piatkus, 1995.
Thai Massage by Ananda Apfelbaum. Avery Health Guides, 2004.
How to Use Yoga by Mira Mehta. Lorenz Books, 2001.
Emotion and Healing in the Energy Body by Robert Henderson, Healing Arts Press, 2015.
Thai Massage & Thai Healing Arts by Bob Haddad, Findhorn Press, 2013.
Iyengar Yoga by Judy Smith, Lorenz Books, 2023.

Useful Addresses

Europe

Individual Thai massage treatment and information on courses, workshops and retreats in United Kingdom and Denmark:
www.bodywisdom.org.uk

Courses and retreats in Greece:
www.thaimassage.gr

Osteothai courses in France and worldwide:
www.lulyani.com

Abdominal massage and Sen Theory:
www.thaitraditionalyogamassage.co.uk

Thai Energy Bodywork:
www.roberthenderson.info/p/bodywork

Yoga equipment:
The Mad Group (HQ) Ltd
Unit 430 Enterprise Way
Vale Park, Evesham
Worcestershire WR11 1AD
www.mad-hq.com

United States and Canada

Futons and related equipment:
Bodywork Central
4400 Harbord Drive
Oakland
CA 94618
Tel. (510) 540-8200
info@bodyworkcentral.com
www.bodyworkcentral.com

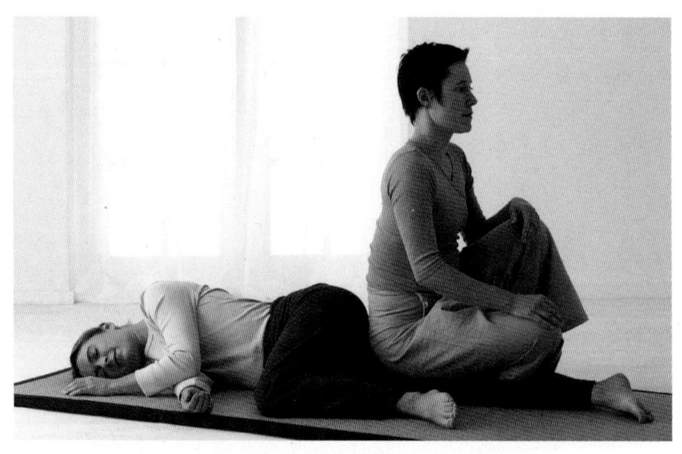

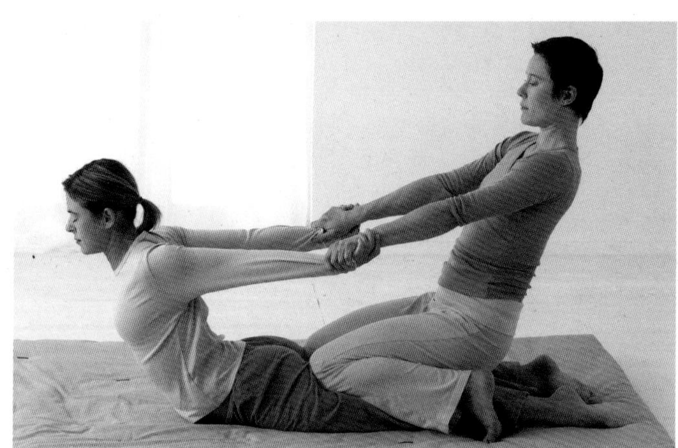

Lotus Palm School of Thai Massage
5244 Saint Urbain
Montreal, Quebec
H2T 2W9, Canada
Tel. (514) 270 5713
info@lotuspalm.com;
www.lotuspalm.com

also Toronto, Ontario
Tel. (647) 352-7256
infotoronto@lotuspalm.com

White Lotus Foundation Retreat Centre
2500 San Marcos Pass
Santa Barbara, CA 93105
Tel. (805) 964-1944
info@whitelotus.org

Naga Center, Portland, Oregon
www.nagacenter.org

Thailand

Thai massage courses:
Sunshine School, Chiang Mai
www.sunshine-massage-school.com

The Foundation of Shivago Komarpa
Old Chiang Mai Medicine Hospital
Near Chiang Mai Cultural Centre
Wualai Road, Chiang Mai

Thai Traditional Medical School, Wat Pho, Bangkok

Worldwide:
www.asokananda.com

Acknowledgements

Author's Acknowledgements

I would like to acknowledge and thank: Asokananda for his guidance, support and dedication to Thai massage; Pitchet Boonthumme, Chaiyuth Priyasith, Claire McAlpine, Sean Doherty, John Stirk, and Silke Ziehl for their gifts of inspiration; my friends and family, for their love and support, especially my sister Fiona for her patience during the photo sessions; the models: Oriol, Spring, Nick and Dagma, and Agoy.com for their beautiful yoga mats.

Publisher's Acknowledgements

The publishers would like to thank the following for permission to reproduce their images:
Page 6 bottom left: Asokananda; Page 12 bottom: © Corbis; Page 13 top left: © Archivo Iconografico, S.A./Corbis; Page 13 bottom right: © Macduff Everton/Corbis; Page 27 bottom right: © Macduff Everton/Corbis. All other photographs are © Anness Publishing Ltd.

Many thanks also to Asokananda, for his helpfulness and for his permission to base the artworks on pages 17–19 on those featured in his book, *The Art of Traditional Thai Massage*.

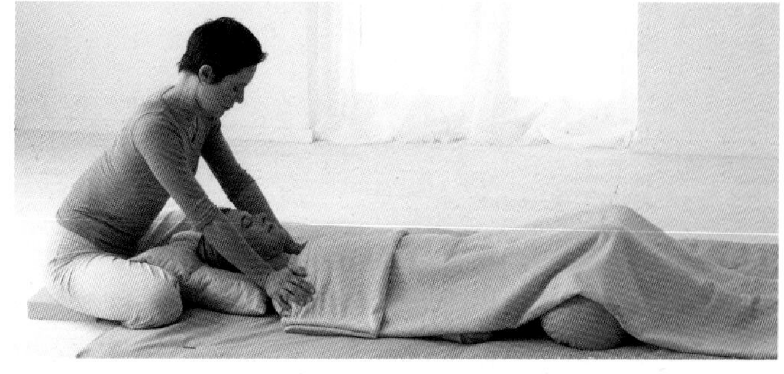

Index

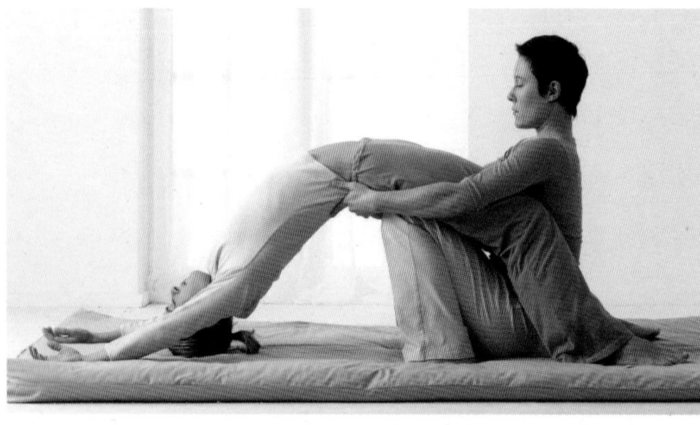

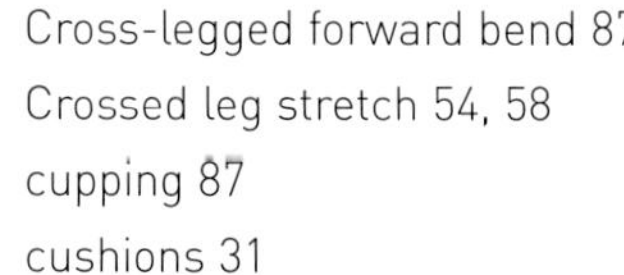

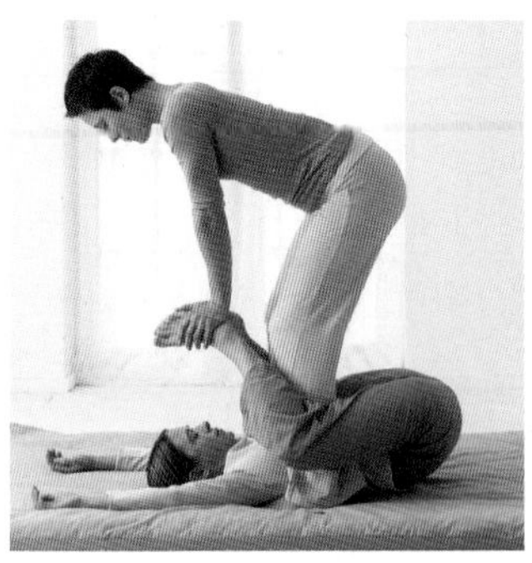

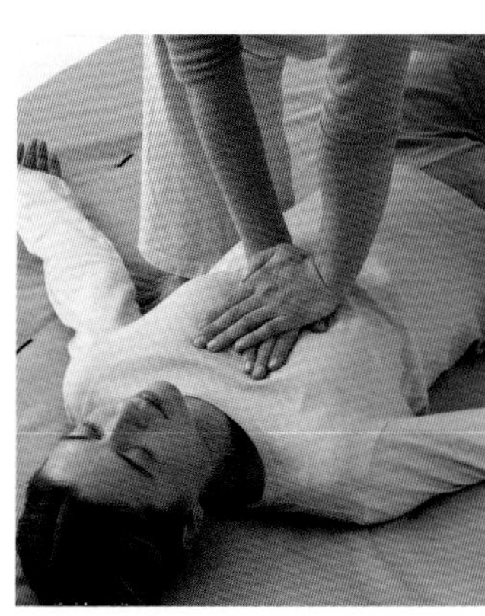

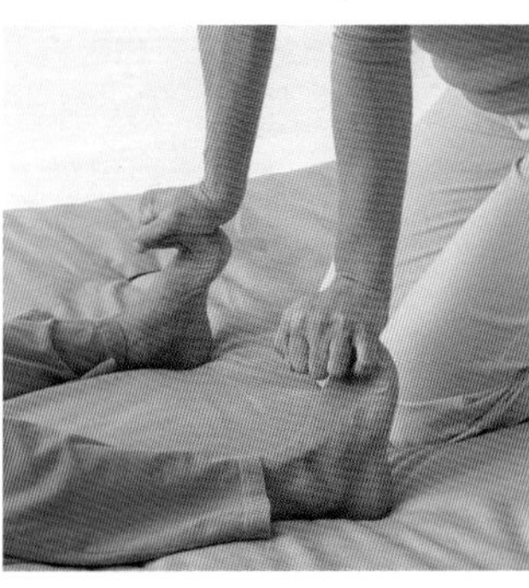

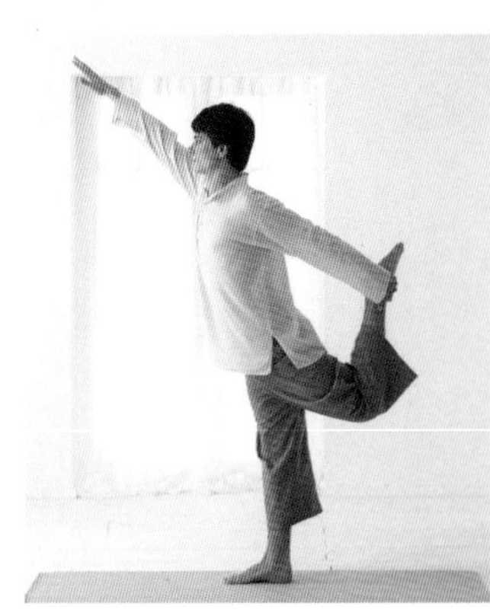

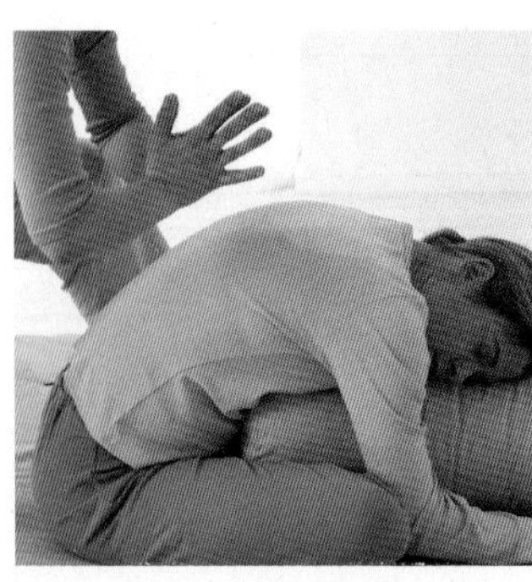

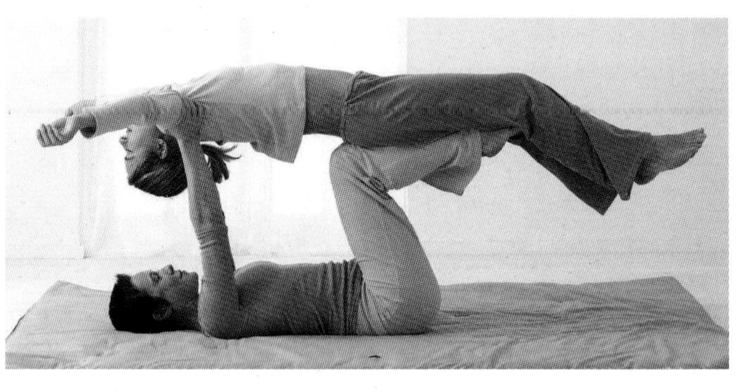